Care of Head and Neck Cancer Patients for
Dental Hygienists and Dental Therapists

Care of Head and Neck Cancer Patients for Dental Hygienists and Dental Therapists

Edited by

Jocelyn J. Harding

Gloucestershire Royal Hospital
Department of Oral and Maxillofacial Surgery
Gloucester
UK

Confident Dental and Implant Clinic
Stroud
UK

WILEY Blackwell

This edition first published 2023

Registered Offices
John Wiley & Sons, Inc., 111 River Street, Hoboken, NJ 07030, USA
John Wiley & Sons Ltd, The Atrium, Southern Gate, Chichester, West Sussex, PO19 8SQ, UK

Editorial Office
9600 Garsington Road, Oxford, OX4 2DQ, UK

For details of our global editorial offices, customer services, and more information about Wiley products visit us at www.wiley.com.

Wiley also publishes its books in a variety of electronic formats and by print-on-demand. Some content that appears in standard print versions of this book may not be available in other formats.

Library of Congress Cataloging-in-Publication Data applied for
Paperback: 9781119795001

Cover Design: Wiley
Cover Images: Courtesy of Jocelyn J. Harding

Set in 9.5/12.5pt STIXTwoText by Straive, Pondicherry, India

Printed in Singapore
M115828_251022

Contents

List of Contributors *ix*
Foreword *xii*
Ewa Rozwadowska
Preface *xiii*

Section 1 Primary Setting *1*

1 The Early Detection of Mouth Cancer: An Initiative for the Whole Dental Team *3*
Philip Lewis

2 Detection and Prevention of Skin Cancer for Dental Hygienists *14*
Greg Knepil

3 Lip Cancer *20*
Alison E. Lowe

4 Smoking and Vaping *23*
Elaine Tilling

5 The Impact of Substance Dependence on Oral Health *29*
Teresa Servas

6 Human Papillomavirus as a Risk Factor for Oropharyngeal Squamous Cell Carcinoma *36*
Elizabeth Marsh

7 Pathologists: The Cornerstone of Head and Neck Cancer Diagnosis and Treatment *44*
Paul Hankinson and Syed Ali Khurram

8 Mental Health and Well-Being Pretreatment *51*
Lauren Barry

9 Flowchart *53*
Stephanie Wright

Section 2 Specialists, Roles, and Departments *55*

10 The Multidisciplinary Team *57*
Lucy Baker

11 History of Oral and Maxillofacial Surgery *60*
Mahesh Kumar

12 **Head and Neck Cancer: Clinical Nurse Specialist Role** *76*
Sonja Hoy and Joanna Rydon

13 **The Role of the Dietitian in the Care of Head and Neck Cancer Patients** *78*
Laura Kent and Hannah Cook

14 **Speech and Language Therapy** *85*
Eve Ferguson and Sarah Hartigan

15 **The Role of the Restorative Dentist in the Management of Head and Neck Cancer Patients** *91*
Michael Fenlon

16 **The Role of the Dental Nurse in an Oral and Maxillofacial Unit** *98*
Laura Holdway

Section 3 Types of Head and Neck Cancer Treatment *101*

17 **Chemotherapy: An Overview** *103*
Helen Davies

18 **Radiotherapy in Head and Neck Cancer** *107*
Muneeb Qureshi, Brindley Hapuarachi, and Bernadette Foran

19 **The Role of Immunotherapy in Head and Neck Cancer Management** *116*
Brindley Hapuarachi, Muneeb Qureshi, and Bernadette Foran

20 **Proton Therapy in the UK** *123*
Karol Sikora and John Pettingell

21 **Transoral Robotic Surgery** *129*
Naseem Ghazali

22 **Photobiomodulation Therapy for Management of Oral Complications Induced by Head and Neck Cancer Treatments** *141*
Reem Hanna

23 **The Hologram, a New Imaging Modality in Head and Neck Cancer** *157*
Mark McGurk

24 **Laryngectomy Care: What Is Required?** *160*
Lauren Smallwood

25 **Mental Health and Well-Being during Treatment** *169*
Lauren Barry

Section 4 Head and Neck Cancer Treatment Complications *171*

26 **Chemotherapy and Risk Assessment in Dental Treatment Planning** *173*
StJohn Crean

27 **Xerostomia, from the Greek (Xero = Dry, Stoma = Mouth) = Dry Mouth** *176*
Leigh Hunter

28 **The Role of Acupuncture in Radiotherapy-Induced Xerostomia** *191*
Andrea N. Beech

29 **Oral Ulceration, Viral Infection, and Candidosis** *194*
Mike Lewis

30 **Halitosis** *197*
Charlotte M. Carling

31 **Oral Mucositis** *205*
Shemifhar Freytes and Alessandro Villa

32 **Nausea and Tooth Erosion** *211*
Lucy Harrison

33 **Osteoradionecrosis** *213*
Imogen Fox

34 **Mucus Secretions and Hypersalivation** *216*
Lucy Baker

35 **Mouth Care and Quality of Life for Patients Living with Head and Neck Cancer** *218*
Jocelyn J. Harding

36 **Obturators** *231*
Rhiannon Jones

37 **Physiotherapy for Head and Neck Cancer Patients: An Overview** *236*
Leah Dalby

38 **Radiotherapy: The Treatment That Keeps on Giving!** *239*
Emma Hallam

39 **Management of Intraoral Hair Growth After Flap Reconstruction** *241*
Susan Smithies

40 **Lifestyle Factors in Oral Cancer** *245*
Mike Nugent

41 **Pain Management for Head and Neck Cancer Patients** *249*
Roddy McMillan

Section 5 Further Considerations, Patient Experiences and Support *253*

42 **Mental Health and Well-Being Post-treatment** *255*
Lauren Barry

43 **Intimacy: Advice for the Patient from a Psychologist** *257*
Jo Hemmings

44 **What Is Palliative Care?** *258*
Emma Husbands

45 **My Cancer, My Journey** *262*
Roy Anthony

46 **Life 2.0: How My Life Has Changed Since My Cancer Diagnosis** *269*
Shrenik Shah

47 **Steve's Story** *272*
Steve Baker

48 **Living with the Legacy** *275*
Debbie Hemington

49 **Look Good Feel Better** *279*
Lisa Curtis

Appendix A: Head and Neck Cancer Charities UK *281*

Index *282*

List of Contributors

Roy Anthony
Retired Dental Hygienist
Stockton on Tees, UK

Lucy Baker
Portsmouth Hospitals University NHS Trust
Portsmouth, UK

Steve Baker
Head and Neck Cancer Survivor
Blackpool, UK

Lauren Barry
York and Scarborough Teaching Hospitals NHS Foundation Trust
York, UK

Andrea N. Beech
Gloucestershire Royal Hospital
Gloucester, UK

Charlotte M. Carling
Dental Hygienist/Therapist
London, UK

Hannah Cook
Gloucestershire NHS Foundation Trust
Gloucester, UK

St John Crean
University of Central Lancashire
Preston, UK

Lisa Curtis
Look Good Feel Better UK
Epsom, UK

Leah Dalby
Leah The Physio
York, UK

Helen Davies
Cardiff and Vale University Health Board
Wales, UK

Michael Fenlon
King's College London
London, UK

Eve Ferguson
Clinical Lead Speech and Language Therapist in Head and Neck
Preston, UK

Bernadette Foran
Weston Park Cancer Centre, Sheffield Teaching Hospitals NHS Foundation Trust
Sheffield, UK

Imogen Fox
Dental Therapist
London, UK

Shemifhar Freytes
Enlivity Corporation
Newton, Massachusetts, USA

Naseem Ghazali
Royal Blackburn Teaching Hospital
Blackburn, UK

Emma Hallam
Nottingham University Hospitals NHS Trust
Nottingham, UK

Paul Hankinson
University of Sheffield
Sheffield, UK

Reem Hanna
Department of Oral Surgery, King's College Hospital NHS Foundation Trust
London, UK
Department of Surgical Sciences and Integrated Diagnostics, University of Genoa
Genoa, Italy

Brindley Hapuarachi
Weston Park Cancer Centre, Sheffield Teaching Hospitals NHS Foundation Trust
Sheffield, UK

Jocelyn J. Harding
Gloucestershire Royal Hospitals
Gloucester, UK
Confident Dental and Implant Clinic
Stroud, UK

Lucy Harrison
Royal London Dental Hospital
London, UK

Sarah Hartigan
Dental Hygienist
Dental Therapist
Manchester, UK

Debbie Hemington
Dental Therapist
London, UK

Jo Hemmings
Behavioural Psychologist
London, UK

Laura Holdway
East Kent Hospitals University Foundation Trust
Ashford, UK

Sonja Hoy
The Royal Marsden NHS Foundation Trust
London, UK

Leigh Hunter
Growing Smiles, UK

Emma Husbands
Gloucestershire Hospitals NHS Foundation Trust
Gloucester, UK

Rhiannon Jones
Cardiff University
Cardiff, UK

Laura Kent
Gloucestershire NHS Foundation Trust
Gloucester, UK

Syed Ali Khurram
Unit of Oral and Maxillofacial Pathology, School of Clinical Dentistry, University of Sheffield
Sheffield, UK

Greg Knepil
Department of Oral and Maxillofacial Surgery, Gloucestershire Hospitals NHS Foundation Trust
Gloucester, UK

Mahesh Kumar
Northwick Park Hospital and the Hillingdon Hospitals NHS Trusts
London, UK

Mike Lewis
Cardiff University
Cardiff, UK

Philip Lewis
Avenue Road Dental Practice
Freshwater, UK

Alison E. Lowe
FitLip, Cardiff, UK

Elizabeth Marsh
University of Derby
Derby, UK

Mark McGurk
Head & Neck Academic Centre, University College London
London, UK

Roddy McMillan
Departments of Oral Medicine and Facial Pain, Royal National ENT and Eastman Dental Hospitals, University College London Hospitals NHS Foundation Trust
London, UK

Mike Nugent
South Tyneside and Sunderland NHS Foundation Trust
Sunderland, UK

John Pettingell
Rutherford Cancer Centres, UK

Muneeb Qureshi
Weston Park Cancer Centre, Sheffield Teaching Hospitals NHS Foundation Trust
Sheffield, UK

Ewa Rozwadowska
Beyond Teeth
Cheltenham, UK

Joanna Rydon
The Royal Marsden NHS Foundation Trust
London, UK

Teresa Servas
Life Over Lemons
Gloucestershire, UK

Shrenik Shah
25-Year Stage IV Vocal Cord Cancer Survivor
Ahmedabad, India

Karol Sikora
Rutherford Cancer Centres, UK

Lauren Smallwood
Highly Specialist Speech and Language Therapist
Newcastle-upon-Tyne, UK

Susan Smithies
University of Liverpool, School of Dental Sciences
Liverpool, UK

Elaine Tilling
Wells, Somerset, UK

Alessandro Villa
University of California San Francisco
San Francisco, California, USA
Miami Cancer Institute, Baptist Health South Florida

Stephanie Wright
Gloucestershire Hospitals NHS Foundation Trust
Gloucester, UK

Foreword

Ewa Rozwadowska

Beyond Teeth, Cheltenham, UK

Many books portray a journey in life as their overriding theme. This book is an accumulation of real-life journeys from the perspective of all those involved in oral cancer – patients, dental professionals in general practice, diagnosticians, surgeons, radiologists, therapists, and those caring for survivors in primary care.

The creation of this book has been a journey in itself. It was born of Joss's passion for educating patients in practical oral care. Hearing the difficult stories of patients, colleagues, and family members with oral cancer inspired her to seek information about how best to help these people. This book is not only the result of Joss's enquiries but also of her ability to engage everyone concerned in dialogue about how to disseminate practical knowledge. It shows how one dental hygienist's inspiration can bring together some of the best minds in the field of oral cancer to collate information relevant to many people.

Patients with advanced oral cancer go on a devastating journey. The chapters recounting personal experiences of people living with cancer serve to remind us of the very human challenges this disease creates. Our professional responsibilities lie not only in using our skills in diagnosis and surgical, therapeutic, and rehabilitation interventions but also in developing professional empathy to support the patients and their psychological and practical needs through all stages of their journey. This book brings together these very personal aspects to improve our understanding of what it is to live with the consequences of oral cancer.

This book also gives us insights into the skills and knowledge of the primary care team and how each of the specialties contribute to the treatment and care of patients – from diagnosis and preparation for surgery, through treatment, and then rehabilitation. Each of these specialists have had their own academic and professional developmental journeys in order to help patients. In these chapters we see how these fields are developing and how we are learning more from each case.

The dental profession has an increasingly vital role to play at both ends of a patient's oral cancer journey. Early diagnosis is essential to trigger the treatment pathways as soon as possible, and soft tissue inspection is now an essential part of each dental examination. Through open collaboration and empowerment, we can use the skills of our dental teams to support oral cancer awareness and preventive initiatives to raise understanding of these conditions in the general population. This book also considers the important role of each dental team member in caring for oral cancer survivors within the setting of our general dental practices.

It has been my great privilege as a general dental practitioner to coach and mentor Joss in her drive to improve the oral care of patients. She has used her passion and her contacts to bring together this version of the oral cancer journey as it stands at present. I know that it is her mission to improve the training of medical students in this topic – may this book inspire policymakers to support her next steps in the journey of preventing these devastating diseases.

Preface

Jocelyn J. Harding

Looking back over my thirty-five year career as a dental nurse and then dental hygienist, qualifying in the Royal Navy in 1992, it is extra-ordinary to see how these roles have evolved and topics expanded. Back then the care of patients with head and neck cancer was not in our curriculum, and the cohort of patients I treated were young and fit. The career path for a dental hygienist on qualifying was non-existent, however, thankfully, with inspirational leaders, the role is now more dynamic and forward-thinking.

My passion for this particular area of care began in the early 1990s with Terry, the first head and neck cancer patient I met. I realised how little I knew about the disease and the long term implications. It was all the more shocking to me as Terry was a dear school friend of my late father, Ian. Terry and his wife, Linda, opened my eyes to the reality of being a patient living with cancer as they shared their experiences of cancer surgery and Terry's long-term complications. This personal connection helped me understand Terry's clinical journey and, more importantly, the emotional rollercoaster this lovely couple had to endure.

A few years later, my clinical skills and knowledge were further tested by Frank, a patient in general practice who needed extensive treatment– surgery, chemotherapy, and radiotherapy for a rapidly progressing squamous cell carcinoma. Frank and his wife helped me realise that we have an ongoing professional responsibility in general practice to help and advise cancer survivors, their close relatives or carers, on managing side effects, for example, limited opening and xerostomia.

I became determined to find and collate practical information for patients and health care professionals to support evidence-based preventive care and treatment pathways for head and neck cancer patients and survivors. This will allow us to improve our monitoring in general practice of the oral health of this group of patients, and consequently, reduce the risk of further dental complications such as rampant caries, extractions, and extensive osteoradionecrosis.

In 2019, as a representative of the British Society of Dental Hygiene and Therapy (BSDHT), I was able to leverage my passion for bringing people and knowledge together. At the updating of Public Health England's Delivering Better Oral Health toolkit (v4) guidelines in the prevention and detection of head and neck cancer, I was honoured to be given this opportunity to press for the inclusion of best practice in the aftercare of head and neck cancer patients at a national level. The door has been opened with a brief statement on this topic; however, I hope to convince the panel to include further information and expand vital aftercare guidance in the future.

One aspect of the care pathway for this cohort of patients rarely considered is the financial burden. Not only does the patient have psychological and physical effects, but there can be an inability to earn an income. Dental care may not be a priority before cancer treatment and the cost of rectifying dental disease and maintaining oral health can be financially prohibitive, resulting in further pain, discomfort, and rampant dental disease, which can often be prevented. I believe it is essential for every dental and health care professional to support the preventive oral care of a head and neck cancer patient before, during, and after treatment by being fully trained in how to manage the day-to-day ravages of this disease and its consequences, thereby reducing the cost to the patient and the NHS.

In 2020, I was accepted for the dental hygienist post with the Oral and Maxillofacial team in Gloucestershire Royal Hospital. This was an opportunity to further expand my knowledge in the range of complicated cases and differing dental needs alongside supporting the patients' physiological and psychological responses to the treatment in a hospital environment. As the department follows the clinical pathways set by the British Association of Head & Neck Oncologists standards 2020, I appreciate the invaluable benefit of improving the patients' outcomes through the collaborative sharing of knowledge by motivated professionals. However, the patient journey is not completed upon discharge from the hospital; the journey is only beginning.

The number of head and neck cancer patients surviving their surgery and attending general practice is increasing. As health care professionals, we must make every contact count and work towards the best patient outcome by giving up to date preventive advice and professional care. Training undergraduate dental professionals in the early stages of their education and encouraging working collaboratively and holistically, regularly updating the latest developments in this field, will support and prepare the clinician for treating and caring for head and neck cancer patients. Science is constantly moving forward and diversifying, significantly improving outcomes in this area of cancer treatment.

As dental professionals, we must aim to support patients and their carers in living with their life-changing conditions and improving their day-to-day well-being, not only with our surgical and technical skills but also with easily understood practical information, explanations, and person-to-person communication. This personal desire to bring together and disseminate expert knowledge about the journey of head and neck cancer patients has led to working in partnership with many health care professionals across the UK and the US in the creation of this book. Reading this book's chapters, I hope you will feel supported and inspired to join us on our journey.

As Elizabeth Lank says in her book, Collaborative Advantage," It goes without saying that a book about collaboration cannot be the product of one person's experience". I want to thank all of the contributors of this book who kindly said 'Yes!' when I approached them to share their knowledge and experience for this project. I am incredibly grateful as these professionals and experts supported this project at the busiest time whilst navigating through a pandemic. A pipe dream of mine would be to see later editions of this book sharing future advancements and developments, which would be wonderful.

I wish to thank Terry, Linda, Frank, Julie, Steve, Shrenik, Roy and Debbie for their honesty in sharing their personal journeys with me. I would like to thank Rob Bate, Mary Anne Freckleton, Rachel S Jackson, Emma Kent and Lisa Kyle for kindly supporting chapters with their wonderful images and figures. Finally, my immediate family, Steve, Mum, James and Emily, deserve a special mention for all the support they have given me and allowances for the time needed to complete a project such as this, along with my dear friends Andrea, Ewa, Nichola, and Sarah. My journey of learning is still ongoing as I am currently studying for my MSc in Advanced and Specialist Healthcare at the University of Kent.

Section 1

Primary Setting

1

The Early Detection of Mouth Cancer: An Initiative for the Whole Dental Team

Philip Lewis

Avenue Road Dental Practice, Freshwater, UK

Early detection of mouth cancer saves lives. It doesn't only save lives, it saves the quality of life both for sufferers and everyone around them. The treatment for mouth cancer discovered early tends to be less aggressive and leads to much better outcomes than when the disease is discovered in its later stages.

The effects on the lives of sufferers, their families, and their friends are profound. Treatment itself can lead to permanent life-changing consequences that might include:

Dry mouth
Difficulty swallowing
Difficulty opening the mouth
Speech impairment
Disfigurement
Loss of teeth and masticatory function
Long-term risk of osteomyelitis following extractions or other surgery after radiotherapy.

During treatment and recovery there may in addition be:

Pain and discomfort at the surgical site
Pain in other areas of the body where tissue has been harvested for repair
Intensely sore mouth (mucositis).

All of these things will have serious emotional impacts and effects on mental health. These will not be confined to the mouth cancer sufferer but also will affect friends, family members, and loved ones. The formerly outgoing individual who now dreads visiting a restaurant because of embarrassment or because of inability to properly taste or enjoy food – and whose reluctance to be seen in public may even extend to family gatherings and other events – will seriously limit the ability of a spouse or partner to take part in these activities themselves.

Sufferer and partner may worry about the outcome of the disease for many years after treatment. There may be financial difficulties. Jobs may be lost as a result of the sickness. Anxiety and distress can lead to despair and depression, which seriously lower quality of life.

Primary care dental teams are uniquely placed to be instrumental in early detection. There are a number of reasons for this:

We see patients regularly. Patients' general practitioners (GPs) may see them more *often*, but crucially we always *look inside their mouths*.
Clinical team members already have a knowledge of the normal appearance of the mouth and will easily spot conditions that look suspicious.
We are familiar with the use of other early detection interventions; for example, we take x-rays, carry out periodontal pocket measurements, and sometimes use techniques such as saliva diagnostics.

Care of Head and Neck Cancer Patients for Dental Hygienists and Dental Therapists, First Edition. Edited by Jocelyn J. Harding.

All team members get to know patients. This may be especially true of non-clinical team members who are often able to immediately recognise changes in facial appearance or in the sound of the voice. It is also often the case that patients will confide in non-clinical team members things they may be reluctant to discuss with clinicians for fear that these things will be considered unimportant.

How often should we carry out examinations? As often as possible! Something that takes so little time does not have to be only reserved for check-up appointments but can easily be included in review and treatment appointments as well. Are you an orthodontic therapist adjusting an appliance? A clinical dental technician providing dentures? A hygienist carrying out a review? There are endless opportunities for a variety of team members to provide this highly important service. Mouth cancer can arise suddenly, so the more often we examine, the better.

Who needs regular exams? Everyone over the age of 16. Mouth cancer is no longer the disease of old men; sadly, we're seeing many more cases among women and the young as well as among people who do not fall into the traditional high-risk groups of tobacco users and spirit drinkers. We know other things are involved: social deprivation, age, gender, infection with some strains of the human papillomavirus, for example, but unfortunately we don't know what we don't know. There are probably other unrecognised risk factors. The bottom line is that the incidence of mouth cancer has increased by about 50% in the last 10 years. That is why everyone (including ourselves) needs regular checks.

Counselling

Dental professionals routinely diagnose conditions such as tooth decay, dental abscesses or periodontal disease. We present our findings to patients who, by and large, will accept this information in a rational way.

A suggestion of suspected mouth cancer is rather different. Prior to the clinical examination, information should be given to the patient about the importance of early detection and the actual procedure. A description of head and neck palpation is especially important for the reasons described later (see Figure 1.1).

"Cancer" is still a very scary word. It is necessary to adopt a sympathetic and supportive approach with patients and especially to advise in advance of the examination the reasons why we may want to carry out further investigations.

Words to use might include:

If we find anything unusual in your mouth, this DOES NOT MEAN you have mouth cancer.

If we're still not sure of a diagnosis, there are many possible reasons for this. That's why we sometimes ask for a second opinion.

The tests help us provide you with the very best service and allow us to identify any problems at a very early stage.

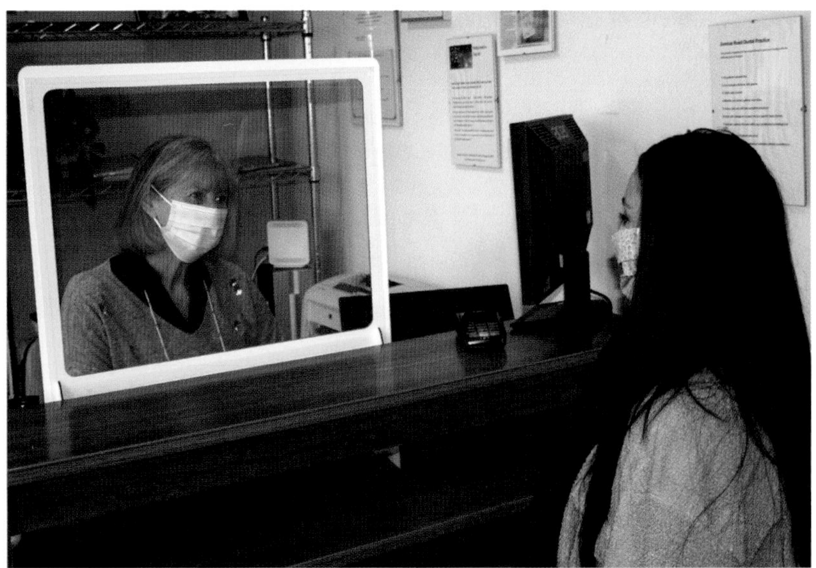

Figure 1.1 Time should be spent with the patient prior to the examination to describe the procedure and provide counselling.

While being gentle in our manner of communication, we must nevertheless stress how important it is for patients to attend follow-up appointments if recommended so that a reliable diagnosis can be reached.

Carrying Out the Examination

The examination is divided into two parts. The first part begins as the patient enters the building and is carried out by whoever meets and greets (see Figure 1.2). This will usually be a non-clinical team member.

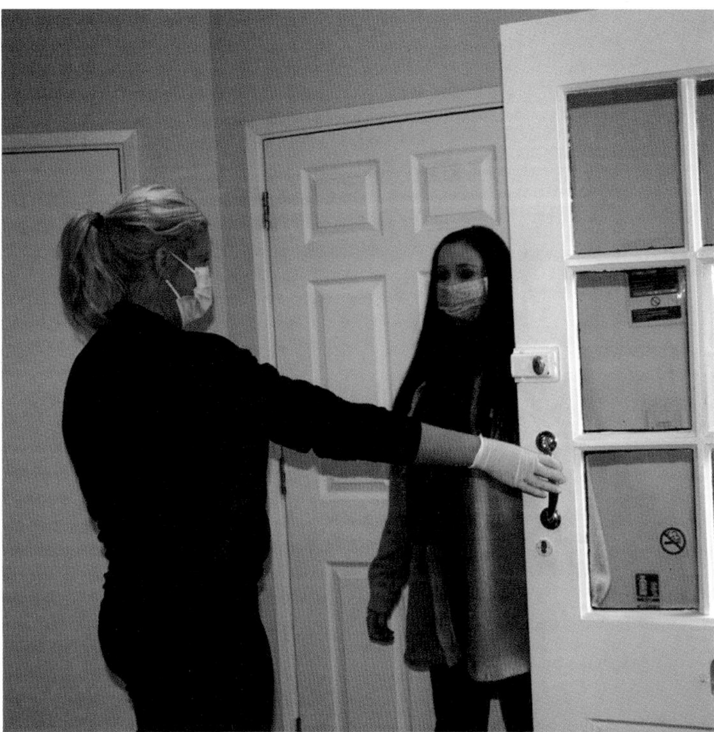

Figure 1.2 The examination begins as the patient enters the building.

We look for obvious asymmetry: listen to their voice – is it hoarse or unusual (if so, for how long?) Are there any unusual blemishes of the skin that we should look at or question the patient about more closely? Do we have any concerns we want to relay to the clinical team?

When the patient enters the treatment room, the clinical team makes these observations again and then seats the patient.

The early detection examination begins with palpation of the head and neck to identify swellings or changes in normal texture. We need to access the tissues right down to the clavicles, so it may be necessary to ask the patient to remove or loosen clothing in this area (see Figure 1.3). It's essential we've told patients in advance that this is planned, or they may be suspicious of the procedure. We stand directly in front to view the head and neck, then, with the patient still sitting upright, we lower the chair back and look again from behind. Observing from a different angle may help to avoid missing swellings. We ask the patient to move the head from side to side. This stretches the skin over the deeper tissues, making subcutaneous enlargements more obvious.

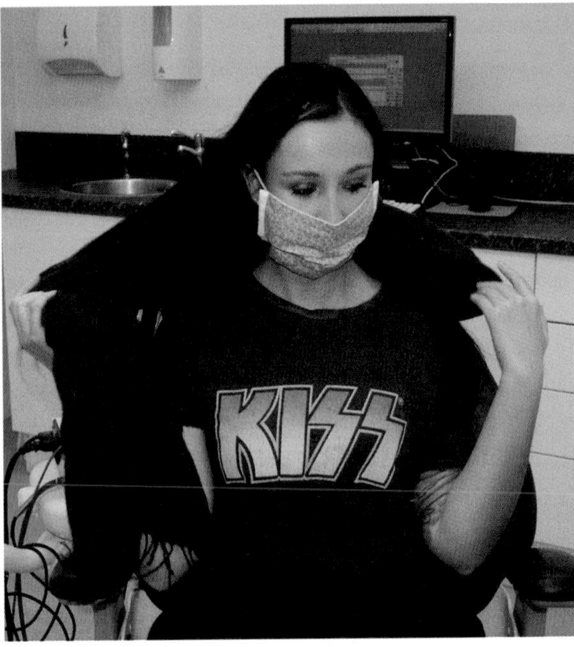

Figure 1.3 The patient should be asked to expose the neck right down to the clavicles.

To palpate we use the pads of the fingers, not the finger tips, which have little tactile sensitivity (see Figures 1.4 and 1.5). The fingers are walked over the tissues with gentle but firm pressure to identify enlarged lymph nodes. Lymph nodes are part of the immune system. They often enlarge when an individual is fighting an infection and are then readily palpable. Infections can either originate from the organs that they drain or primarily within the lymph node itself, referred to as lymphadenitis.

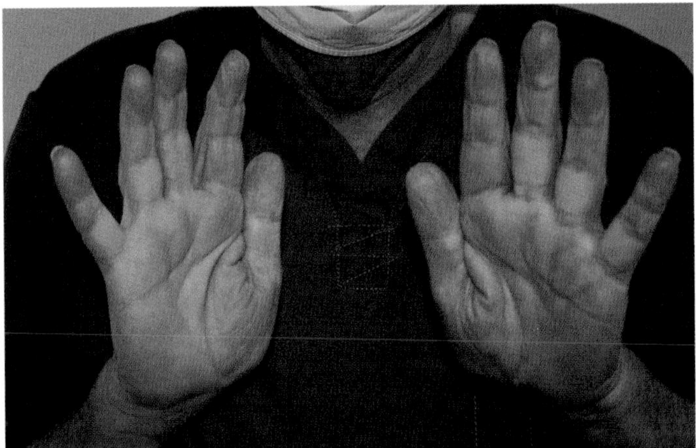

Figure 1.4 Use the soft pads of the fingers to palpate.

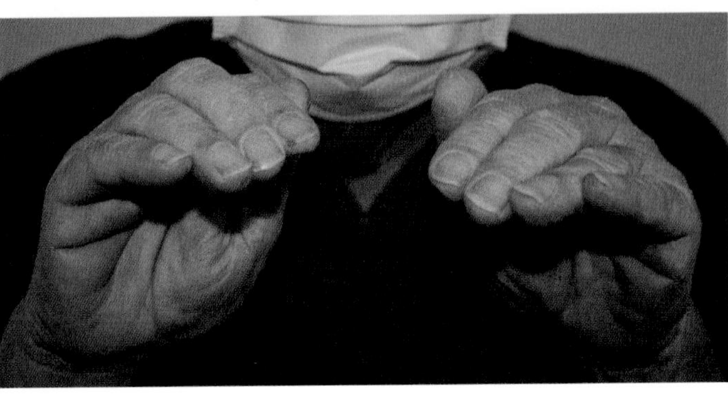

Figure 1.5 The finger tips have little tactile sensitivity.

Lymph nodes that have enlarged because of infection tend to be soft, tender, and warm. The inflammation may spread to the overlying skin, causing it to appear reddened. The nodes return to normal when the infection is over.

Malignancies can also involve the lymph nodes, either primarily, for example, in the case of lymphoma or as a site of metastasis. In either case, these nodes are generally firm, non-tender, matted (i.e. stuck to each other), fixed (i.e. not freely mobile but rather stuck down to underlying tissue), and increase in size over time.

The major lymph node groups are located along the anterior and posterior aspects of the sternocleidomastoid muscle (SCM) and the underside of the jaw. If the nodes are quite big, they may be visible bulging under the skin, particularly if the enlargement is asymmetric (see Figure 1.6).

Examine both sides of the head simultaneously, walking the fingers down the area in question while applying steady, gentle pressure.

The posterior cervical chains extend in a line posterior to the SCMs but in front of the trapezius, from the level of the mastoid bone to the clavicle. Further nodes will be found in front of the muscle.

Additional lymph node chains include:

Tonsillar: located just below the angle of the mandible.
Submandibular: along the underside of the jaw on either side.
Preauricular: and postauricular lymph nodes in front and behind the ear.
Submental: just below the chin.
Supraclavicular: in the hollow above the clavicle, just lateral to where it joins the sternum.

Position of the main groups of lymph nodes

- On either side of the major muscle that turns the head
- Under the jaw and chin
- In the hollow above the collar bones
- In front and behind the ear

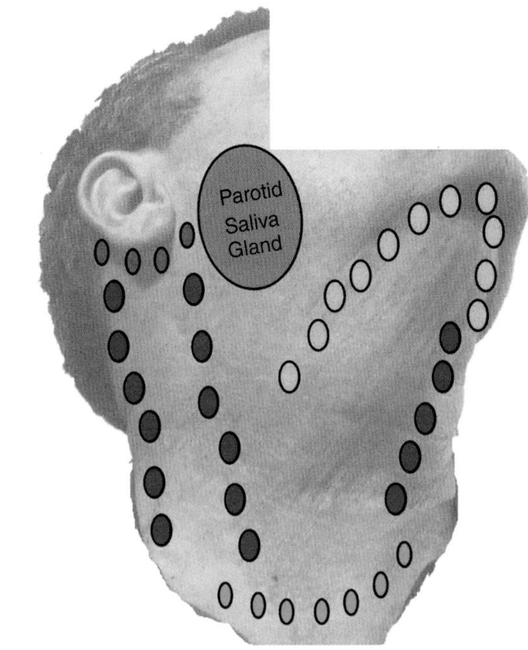

Figure 1.6 Diagrammatic representation of the position of the major lymph node chains.

It is also important to recall that swellings of the salivary glands can be an early indication of tumours, thus it is essential that the examination includes these structures.

Carefully record any unusual findings in the patient records (see Figures 1.7 to 1.14).

Some Areas of Palpation

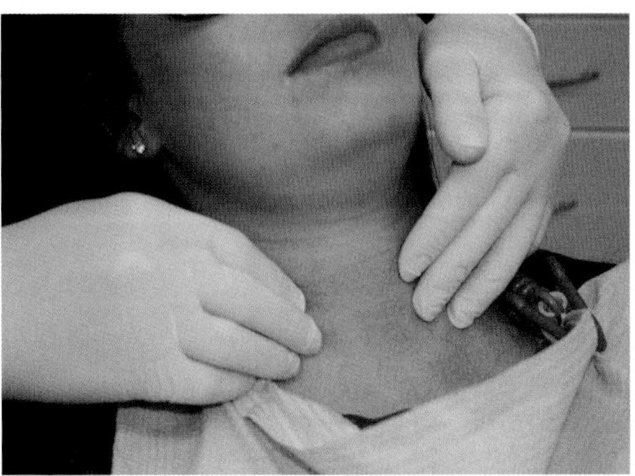

Figure 1.7 Anterior SCM.

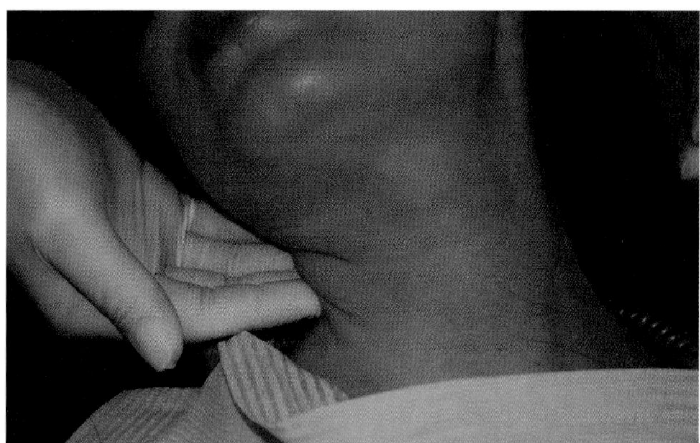

Figure 1.8 Asking the patient to turn the head into your hand allows palpation under the SCM muscle.

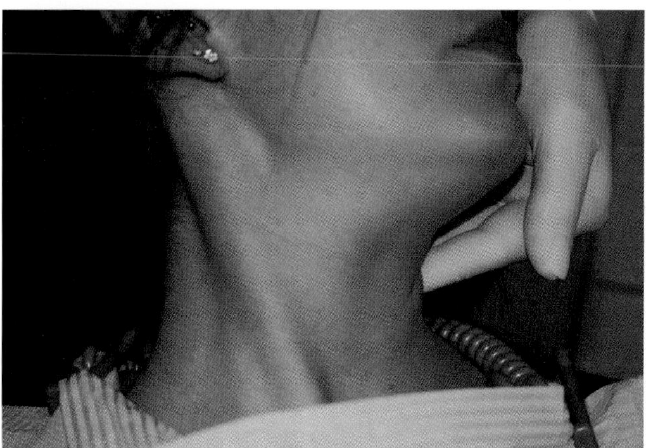

Figure 1.9 Turning the head stretches the skin over the deeper tissues.

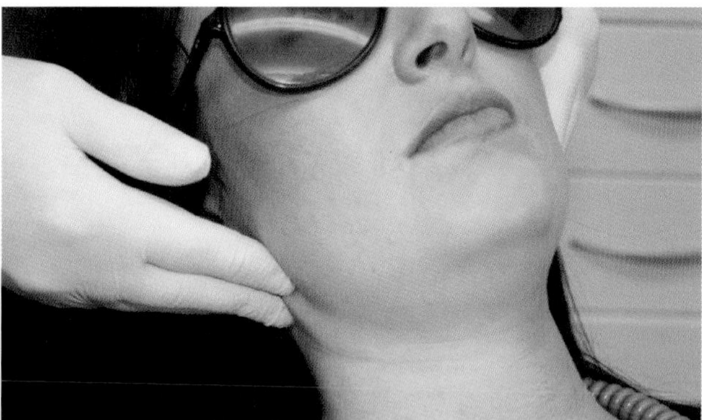

Figure 1.10 Preauricular and postauricular.

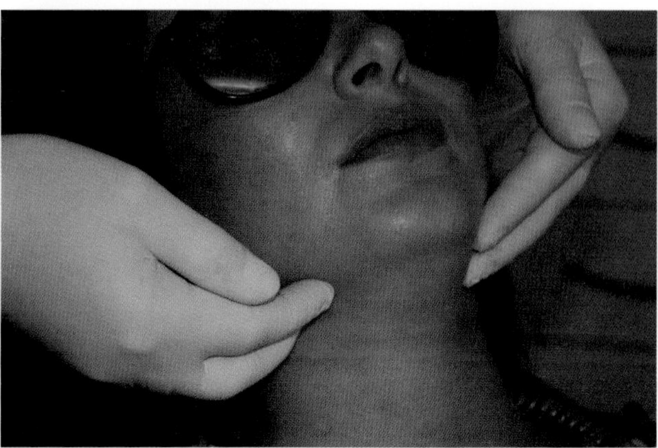

Figure 1.11 Tonsillar.

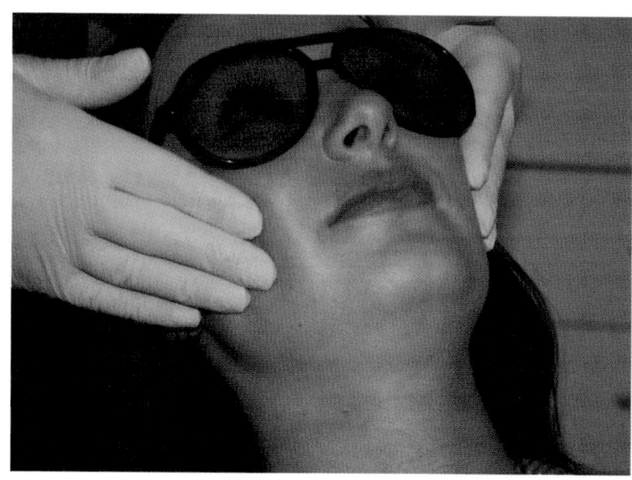

Figure 1.12 Parotids.

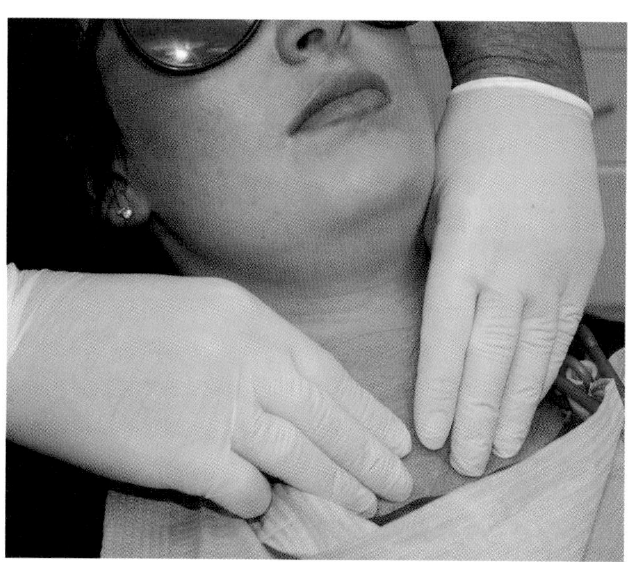

Figure 1.13 Supraclavicular.

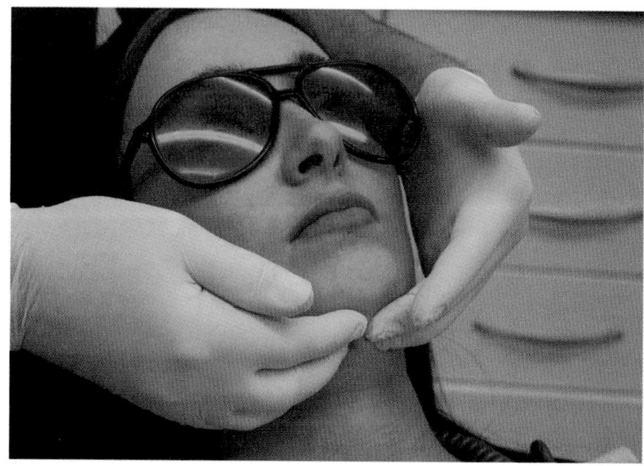

Figure 1.14 Submental and submandibular.

The second part of the examination looks at the intra-oral tissues. We need to assess the lips, labial mucosa and sulcus, commissures, buccal mucosa and sulcus, gingiva and alveolar ridge, tongue, floor of the mouth, and hard and soft palate.

During the intraoral examination, mirrors, spatulas, or even fingers may be used to hold away tissues. It is essential the areas covered by these retractors are also examined as the examination moves on (see Figures 1.15 and 1.16).

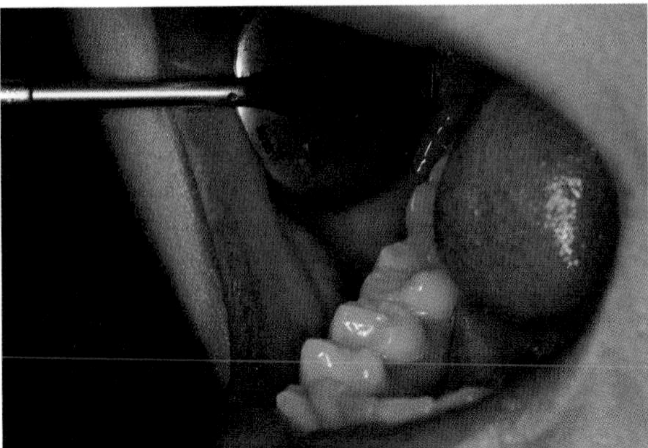

Figure 1.15 Areas of the mouth may be obscured by retraction instruments.

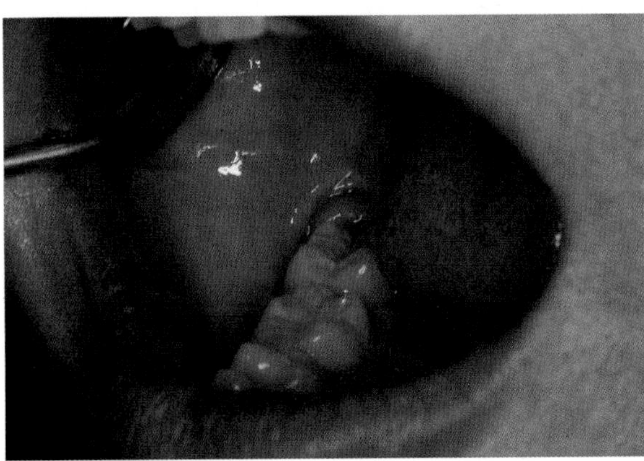

Figure 1.16 Be sure to examine the areas of the mouth that may have been obscured after the instrument has been moved.

With the patient's tongue at rest and mouth partially open, inspect the dorsum of the tongue for any swelling, ulceration, coating, or variation in size, colour, or texture.

The patient should then protrude the tongue. The examiner should note any abnormality of tongue mobility or position. With the aid of mouth mirrors, inspect the right and left lateral margins of the tongue.

Grasping the tip of the tongue with a piece of gauze will assist full protrusion. Palpate the tongue to detect growths. Then examine the ventral surface (see Figure 1.17).

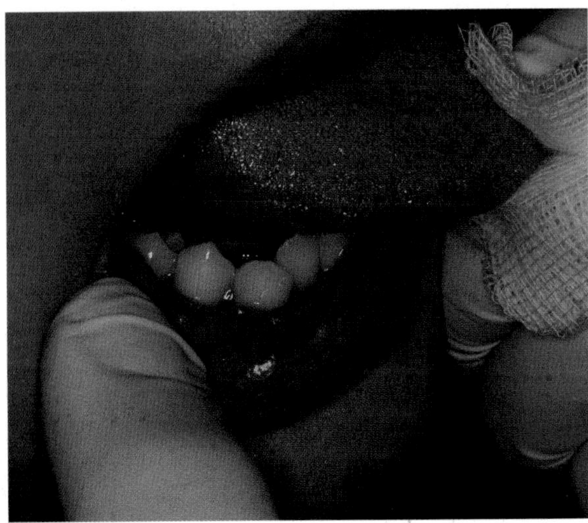

Figure 1.17 Grasping the tip of the tongue with gauze aids manipulation.

With the tongue still elevated, inspect the floor of the mouth for changes in colour, texture, swellings, or other surface abnormalities.

With the mouth wide open and the patient's head tilted back, gently depress the base of the tongue with a mouth mirror. Examine the oropharyngeal tissues, then inspect the hard and soft palate.

Bimanually palpate the floor of the mouth for any abnormalities. Use one hand to support the floor of the mouth while examining with the fingers of the other hand. All mucosal or facial tissues that seem to be abnormal should be palpated.

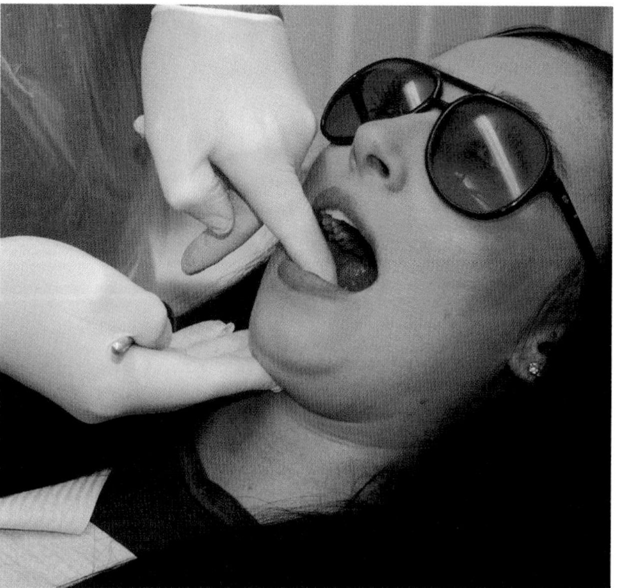

Figure 1.18 Bimanual palpation.

It is important to emphasise the careful examination of the posterior floor of the mouth by placing a mirror on the lateral aspects of the posterior, non-protruded tongue to allow demonstration of this site (See Figures 1.18 to 1.22).

Any unusual findings from the examination should be recorded in the patient's records, as well as a written description recording the shape, texture, colour, and position of lesions. Identifying these on a mouth map is useful. Equally useful is a clinical photograph of the lesion. All of these methods of recording enable clinicians to reliably track the progress of lesions. Arrange to review or refer as appropriate.

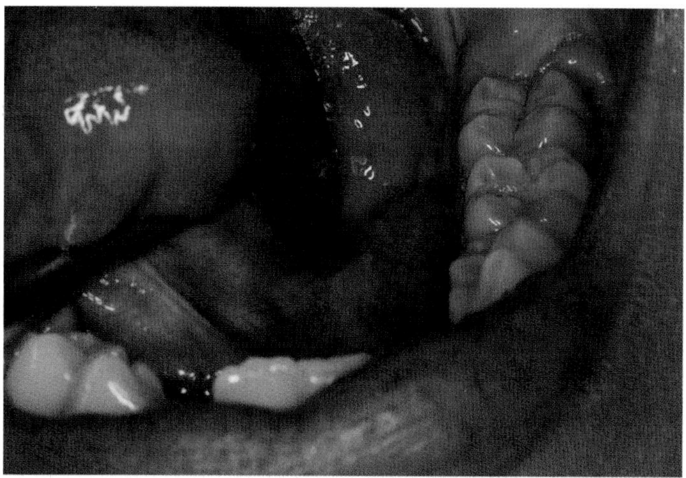

Figure 1.19 Pull the back of the tongue away with a mirror to examine the posterior floor of the mouth.

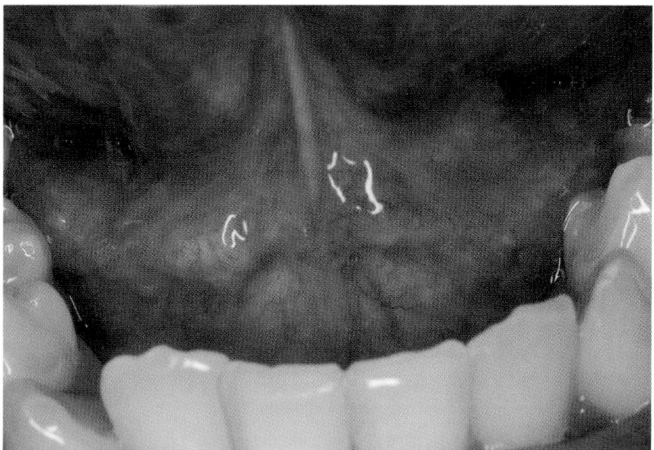

Figure 1.20 The anterior floor of the mouth can be examined by holding the tongue upwards.

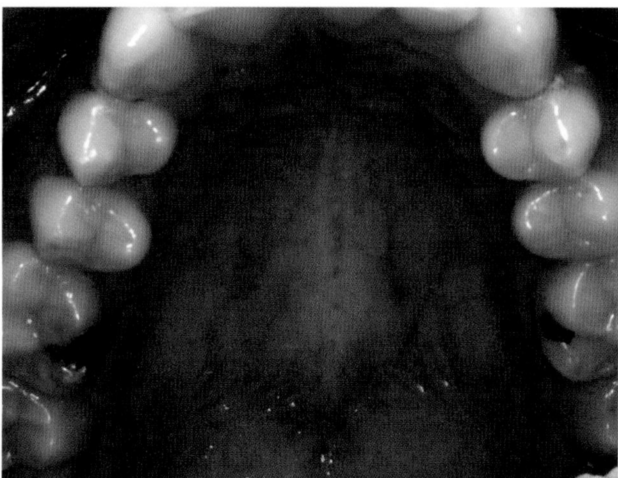

Figure 1.21 Hard and soft palate both need examination.

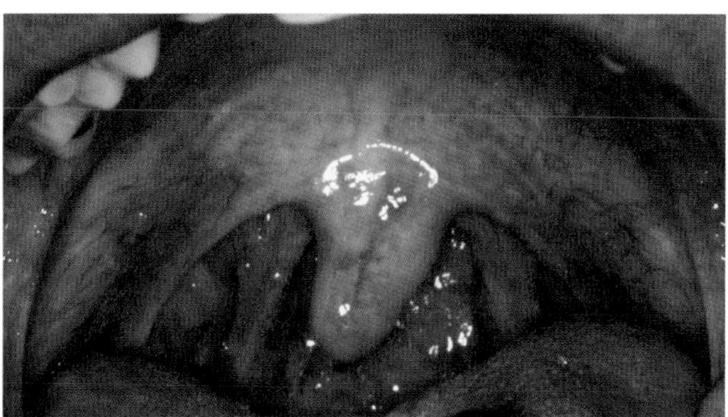

Figure 1.22 Asking the patient to say 'Aah' helps to reveal the anterior pharynx. Pressing down on the tongue with a mirror or spatula at the same time gives a better view.

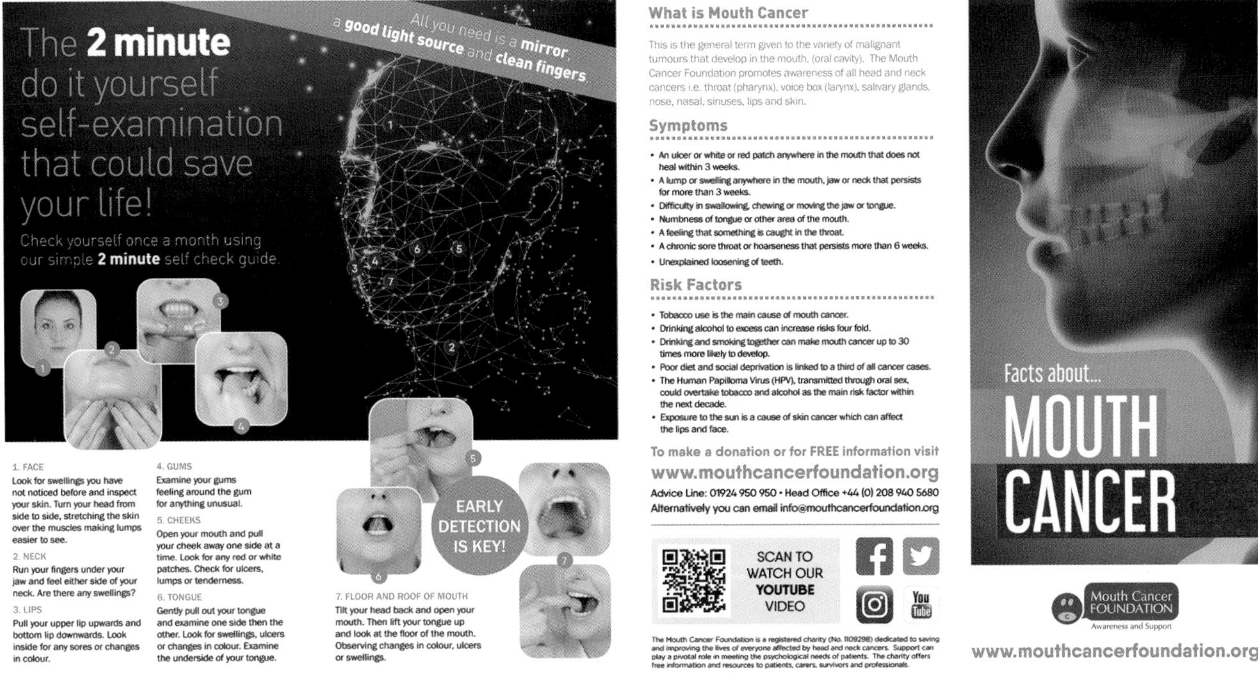

Figure 1.23 Information about self-examination is available from the Mouth Cancer Foundation. *Source:* Mouth Cancer Foundation.

So what are we looking for? Basically, anything we find unusual. Of course there are many innocent things that make the appearance of the inside of the mouth unusual – trauma, for example; however, traumatic injuries will usually heal quickly, and if we suspect that's what we're looking at we can review after a couple of weeks to make sure the problem has resolved.

What we're specifically looking for are:

Red or white patches of no obvious cause
Unexplained lumps
Ulcers that don't heal in a maximum of three weeks
Changes in texture or sensation
Bleeding from the mouth or throat in the apparent absence of gum disease
Teeth that loosen in the apparent absence of gum disease
Hoarseness of the voice
Persistent sore throat
Reports of a feeling of something 'stuck' in the throat.

If anything we find in our examination leads us to believe we may have discovered early mouth cancer, THE PATIENT MUST BE REFERRED IMMEDIATELY FOR A SPECIALIST ASSESSMENT. Rapid referral pathways exist in all health areas but may vary across regions. Find out how to access yours.

Patients should be encouraged to examine themselves regularly at home. Details of how to do this can be found on the Mouth Cancer Foundation website, www.mouthcancerfoundation.org (search for 'Bite Back at Mouth Cancer'; see Figure 1.23).

A full early detection examination including palpation takes less than two minutes.

Factoring that into our routine workflow could save a life and leave us free to continue carrying out all of the other high-quality treatments our patients deserve. Every team member, clinical or non-clinical, has an important role to play. This really is a team effort.

2

Detection and Prevention of Skin Cancer for Dental Hygienists

Greg Knepil

Department of Oral and Maxillofacial Surgery, Gloucestershire Hospitals NHS Foundation Trust, Gloucester, UK

The Role of Hygienists in the Early Recognition and Management of Skin Cancers

Skin cancers are the most common cancer to affect fair-skinned people, and most skin cancers develop on the head and neck. Skin cancers are often slow growing, and frequently patients have visited a dental professional when their skin cancer has been present but before they have visited their GP with a concern. This makes the role of the dental hygienist important in the early detection and raising of concerns about a possible skin cancer, which should prompt a referral to the patient's GP or skin cancer specialist. Health education is also an important preventive measure against the development of skin cancers, and hygienists have an opportunity to educate their patients about risky and healthy behaviours, with particular emphasis on ultraviolet (UV) exposure and protection, self-examination, and vitamin D.

A study of patients undergoing skin cancer surgical removal in Gloucestershire, UK, in 2019 illustrated real-life evidence of the important role hygienists can play in skin cancer management. This study found that two-thirds of the patients were regular dental attenders. Of those regular dental attendees who had visited a dental surgery since the lesion had been identified, one-third had visited a hygienist. Overall, the lesion was only mentioned to 6% of patients by the dentist but was mentioned to the patient by 25% of hygienists. Following a brief educational programme, dental health care professionals felt more confident in raising concerns and discussing health advice regarding skin cancer with their patients (Harte and Knepil 2019).

Skin Anatomy and Physiology

Skin is the largest organ in the body and acts as a waterproof barrier that protects the body from external environmental hazards and prevents loss of water and other bodily substances. The skin is made from three layers called the epidermis, dermis, and subcutis. The epidermis is a thin waterproof layer mostly made of cells called keratinocytes. Keratinocytes change in character as they migrate from the basal layer to the surface, where they are exfoliated. The dermis lies just beneath the epidermis and is a tough fibrous layer, mostly composed of collagen, and contains hair follicles and secretory glands for the skin. The most superficial dermal layer is called the papillary dermis, which interfaces with the basal layer of the epidermis, and the deeper layer of the dermis is called the reticular layer. Deep to the dermis lies the subcutaneous fatty layer, which insulates the body and acts as a protective cushion. As the outermost layer of the body, the skin is subjected to environmental hazards, especially UV radiation, types A and B (see Figure 2.1).

What are Skin Cancers?

Skin cancers arise from the dermal and epidermal layers of the skin, and the most common types are basal cell carcinoma (BCC), squamous cell carcinoma (SCC), and melanoma. Other types of skin cancer exist but are less common (Table 2.1). BCC and SCC are collectively described as nonmelanoma skin cancers (NMSCs) or, more specifically, keratinocyte skin

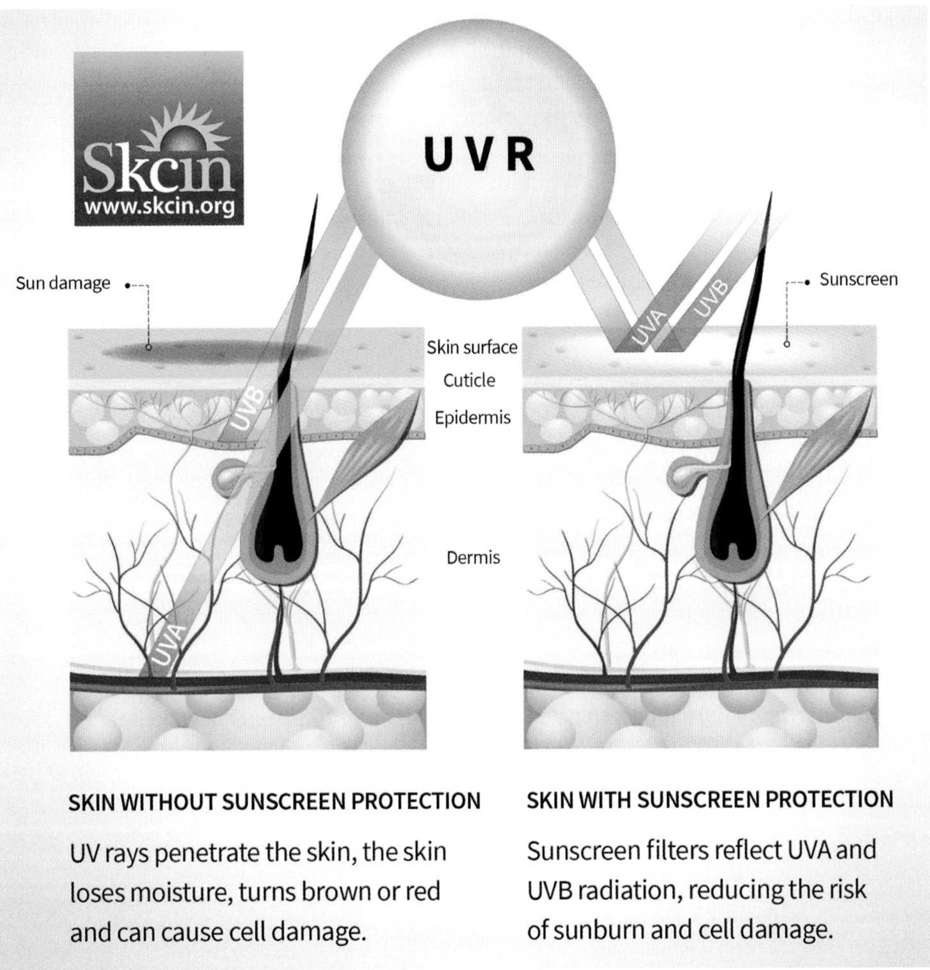

Figure 2.1 Anatomical cross-section of the skin and UVA and UVB penetration. *Source:* www.skcin.org.

Table 2.1 Types of skin cancers.

Name	Derived from	Prognosis	Clinical presentation
Basal cell carcinoma	Basal cells of epidermis	Very rare to metastasise	Variable, pearlescent, arborising telangiectasia, crusting, slow growth
Squamous cell carcinoma	Squamous cells of epidermis	Occasionally metastasises	Crusty, painful nodule, grows quickly
Melanoma	Neuroendocrine cells of dermis	Frequently metastasises	Pigmented patch, superficial spreading, then becomes nodular. Bleeds, itches
Merkel cell carcinoma	Merkel cells in epidermis	Frequently metastasises	Rapid growth, elderly, immunosuppressed patients
Pleomorphic dermal sarcoma	Mesenchymal cells	Occasionally metastasises	Pink nodule, often on scalp. Rapid growth

cancers. They are the most common kind of skin cancers and arise as a result of UV radiation exposure, especially before the age of 20 years, when the skin is immature, but often start to grow later in life. UV exposure may be in the form of multiple severe burns in patients who have a tendency to burn easily, but also with chronic lower levels of exposure, which can also occur in people who tan easily. Two distinct forms of UV radiation exist and have different effects on the skin. Type A (UVA) penetrates deeply into the skin, causes skin ageing rather than burning, and can pass through glass. Type B (UVB) is absorbed in the superficial layer of the skin and causes sunburn, and it is absorbed by glass. Sunscreens have different effectiveness in protecting against UVA and UVB, so it is important to look at the sun factor (numerical) and star rating system (out of five stars), as they may offer different levels of protection. Despite being described with the same collective term, the behaviour of BCC and SCC are quite different, and it is important to understand this behaviour when taking a history and considering how urgently the patient needs to seek specialist advice. Melanomas are also usually caused by exposure to UV radiation, and like NMSC, they are more frequent in older patients; however, they are also an important cause of cancer in younger patients too. Melanomas are one of the most serious skin cancers, as they can metastasise from a very small size and are a frequent cause of death and serious illness from cancer in all ages, making early detection a critical strategy in preventing serious disease.

1) *Basal cell carcinoma (BCC):* BCC is a slow-growing skin cancer most commonly found on the head and neck, and it is extremely rare for it to metastasise to other parts of the body. Due to its erosive effect on surrounding tissues, historically it has been referred to as a 'rodent ulcer', and if left untreated it can cause significant damage to important structures, such as the eyes, ears, and nose. It is thought to arise from UV radiation and usually presents many years after exposure. It is a disease that is common in older-aged people but can occasionally be found in younger patients. Basal cell naevus or Gorlin–Goltz syndrome is a condition where patients develop multiple BCC in addition to odontogenic keratocysts and other diagnostic features. This is an inherited disease, and these skin cancers are often not related to UV radiation damage. Younger patients with multiple BCC especially affecting nonsun-exposed skin should be suspected for this syndrome, and a careful family history is required. Where there is a suspicion of Gorlin–Goltz syndrome, this can be confirmed by genetic blood analysis, and radiology screening for odontogenic keratocysts may be indicated. BCC can have a variety of appearances; however, typically, they will have been present for many months or even years and have a pearlescent raised appearance and diagnostic tree-like branching blood vessels called arborising telangiectasia (Figure 2.2).

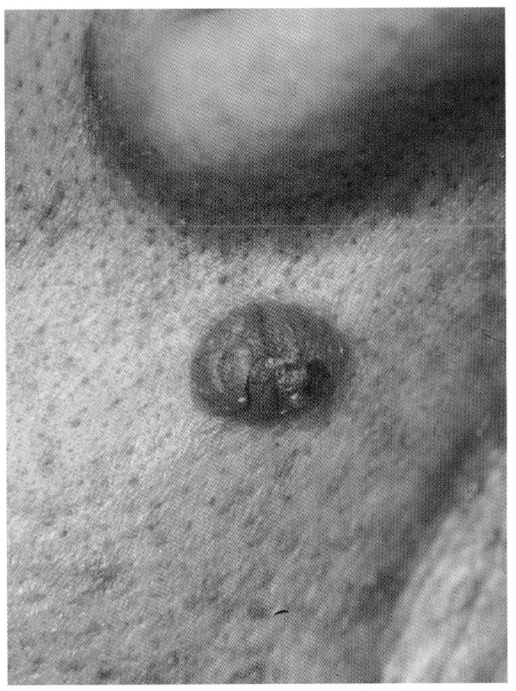

Figure 2.2 Nodular BCC with arborising telangectasia. *Source:* Dr Robert Bates.

2) *Squamous cell carcinoma (SCC):* SCC is a rapidly growing and often painful skin cancer that has a small but important chance of spreading to the lymph nodes and other parts of the body. SCC commonly arises on the head and neck and also other sun-exposed areas such as the hands and the legs. It frequently occurs in older patients and patients who are taking immunosuppressive medications for conditions such as organ transplants or inflammatory conditions such as severe colitis or rheumatoid arthritis. The appearance of SCCs differs from BCCs as they tend to be more crusty (keratotic) and scaly, and they often bleed and are tender, even in places where they are not likely to be traumatised (Figure 2.3).

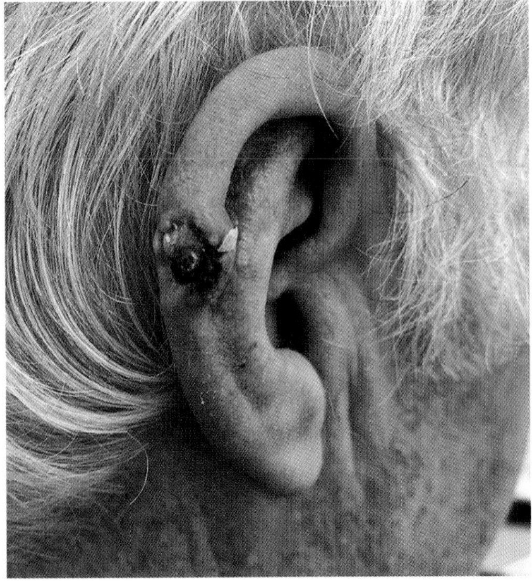

Figure 2.3 Squamous cell carcinoma.

3) *Melanoma:* Melanoma is a rapidly metastasising skin cancer that develops from pigment-producing melanocyte cells. They can arise in pre-existing moles (melanotic naevi) or arise de novo. The prognosis of melanoma is most accurately predicted by measuring the thickness of the lesion below the skin surface by

a specific microscopic measurement called the Breslow thickness. In situ melanoma sits on the skin surface and is considered noninvasive with no potential to spread and, therefore, is not given a Breslow thickness. Invasive melanomas are measured in thicknesses of fractions of a millimetre, and surgical treatment as early as possible provides the best chance of cure. Recently the prognosis for patients with metastatic melanoma who are said to be living with cancer has improved significantly, but not all patients are fit enough to endure the treatment, and some melanomas are not genetically sensitive to some of the new drugs, making early diagnosis important even for patients presenting late (Figure 2.4).

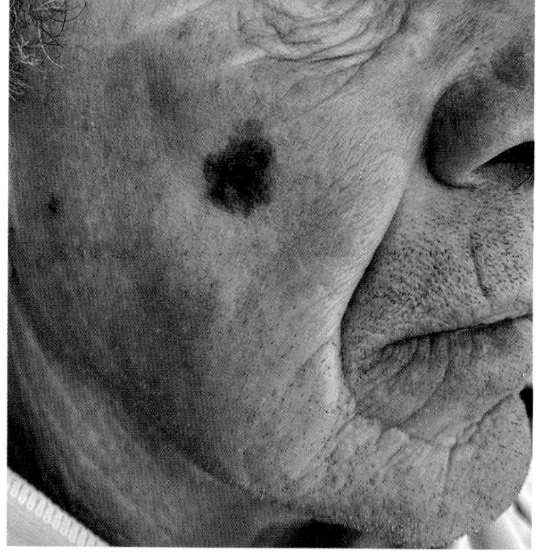

Figure 2.4 Melanoma.

Common Benign Skin Lesions

1) *Actinic/solar keratosis (AK):* AKs are common signs of sun damage in older fair-skinned patients and appear as dry, scaly patches of skin usually less than 1 cm in diameter. They arise in sun-exposed areas of skin and occasionally can go on to develop into skin cancer and are an important index of increased risk of skin cancer over the next five years. They should be differentiated from skin cancers such as SCC. Treatments for these lesions include topical cream chemotherapy agents, cryotherapy, photo dynamic therapy (PDT), and curettage (Figure 2.5).

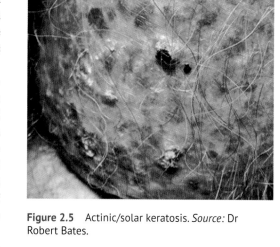

Figure 2.5 Actinic/solar keratosis. *Source:* Dr Robert Bates.

2) *Seborrhoeic keratosis:* Seborrhoeic keratoses are benign pigmented waxy growths with a distinctive appearance that arise later in life and are frequently found on the head and neck and torso. They are not caused by sun damage and should not be a cause for concern; however, they may be confused with melanotic lesions, including melanoma. No treatment is required for seborrhoeic keratoses. However, many patients do not like the appearance, and prominent lesions can be uncomfortable if rubbed by clothing; therefore, surgery, cryotherapy, or curettage can be used to remove them.
3) *Melanotic naevi:* Melanotic naevi are benign growths of melanocytes and are more commonly known as 'moles'. The reason for their development is not fully understood, but they run in families and are associated with UV exposure. They increase in number during childhood and adolescence, especially during puberty, and then much less often after the age of 20 years. The appearance of melanotic naevi varies, and they may be pigmented, skin coloured, flat, or raised; some are hair-bearing. Some patients inherit a condition called atypical mole syndrome, where they have over 100 moles and need to be kept under regular follow-up to detect the early development of melanoma, which is higher in this group of patients.

The Diagnosis of a Skin Cancer

Skin cancers are clinically diagnosed based on the history of the presentation of the lesion, the patient's family history, history of exposure to UV radiation, and appearance of the lesion on clinical examination. Magnified views of the skin can be seen with a special skin microscope called a dermatoscope. Occasionally where there is doubt about the clinical diagnosis, a biopsy may be required. Diagnosis of a skin cancer is a highly skilled procedure that should only be undertaken by a suitably qualified health care professional such as a dermatologist, skin cancer surgeon, specialist skin cancer nurse, or a GP with a specialist interest in dermatology.

How to Manage a Suspected Skin Cancer at a Hygienist Appointment

Skin cancers should only be diagnosed by health care professionals trained and experienced in the diagnosis and management of skin cancer. The role of health care professionals who do not have this higher level of skill and experience is to raise a concern about a suspicious lesion and encourage patients to seek further advice from a suitably trained skin cancer professional. Raising a concern can be as simple as asking patients if they had noticed the lesion of concern before and explaining that it has features that are a cause for concern. Frequently, patients will already be aware of the lesion and need a prompt to visit their GP. Clinical photographs taken with the appropriate consent can also be a useful way to monitor lesions where patients are reluctant to seek further help, and visible changes in appearance may act as a way to persuade a change in patient behaviour. Photos can also be helpful when patients find making a face-to-face appointment with the GP is difficult.

Prevention of Skin Cancer and Promotion of Skin Health

1) *UV protection:* UV radiation is invisible and comes from sunlight. UV light is in three forms: UVA, UVB, and UVC. UVC is screened effectively by the atmosphere, so human exposure to UVC is usually from artificial sources and should not be a concern in normal circumstances. UVA causes ageing of the skin, and UVB causes burning of the skin. Both UVA and UVB have been proven to cause skin cancers through damage to DNA. Children's skin is immature until around 20 years of age and is especially vulnerable to UV damage. Advice on how to reduce exposure to UV is a vital preventive measure against developing skin cancer later in life. Specific measures to be taken include avoiding more than 15 minutes of sun exposure between 11 a.m. and 3 p.m.; using and reapplying adequately strong sunscreen (factor 30 to protect against UVB, and also four- or five-star protection against UVA); wearing protective clothing, including hats that protect the ears and neck and sunglasses; and avoiding using sun beds (Public Health England 2017).
2) *Vitamin D:* Vitamin D is an essential vitamin that grows and maintains bones, muscles, and the immune system. The average person needs 10 μg (or 400 international units [IU]) of vitamin D per day. For most people in the UK, exposure to sunlight is the main source of vitamin D, and therefore patients who avoid UV exposure and rely on diet alone for vitamin D are at risk of vitamin D deficiency, especially during the winter months. Dietary sources of vitamin D include red meat, oily fish, liver, eggs, UV-treated mushrooms, and fortified foods such as breakfast cereal. It is possible to have vitamin D levels checked through a screening blood test; however, taking a daily 10 μg supplement of vitamin D is safe and provides an adequate amount of vitamin D for health (British Association of Dermatologists 2021).

Conclusion

Hygienists spend time in close proximity to their patients' heads and necks, where most skin cancers arise, and can therefore play an important role in the early detection of skin cancers. As health care professionals, hygienists are also trusted advocates for healthy living and can provide valuable education on the prevention of skin cancer and maintaining healthy vitamin D levels. Further training for health care professionals can be provided by the Karen Clifford Melanoma and Skin Cancer Charity (2021).

References

British Association of Dermatologists (2021). Clinical guidelines. www.bad.org.uk/healthcare-professionals/clinical-standards/clinical-guidelines (accessed 12 November 2021).

Harte, M. and Knepil, G. (2019). Skin cancer detection. *Br. Dent. J.* 227: 539. https://doi.org/10.1038/s41415-019-0808-3.

Karen Clifford Melanoma and Skin Cancer Charity (2021). MASCED PRO training for medical & healthcare practitioners. https://pro.masced.uk (accessed 25 November 2021).

Public Health England (2017). Ultraviolet radiation and vitamin D: the effects on health'. https://www.gov.uk/government/publications/ultraviolet-radiation-and-vitamin-d-the-effects-on-health (accessed 14 November 2021).

3

Lip Cancer

Alison E. Lowe

FitLip, Cardiff, UK

Lip cancer can be described as a form of mouth cancer occurring on the outer lip at the intersection between the intra- and extraoral areas of the mouth (National Cancer Institute 2022). It occurs as a result of the abnormal growth of flat cells on the lips (squamous cell carcinoma [SCC]), and although with an annual rate of 12.0 per 100,000 in the UK, it is much less prevalent than other types of mouth cancer (including the inner lip) it can be a preceding factor (Gov.uk 2022). Lip cancer tends to get grouped with either mouth or skin cancer. However, its epidemiology suggests that lip cancer should be considered as a separate entity, rather than being considered as a form of mouth cancer (Scully and Robinson 2017).

To date, it has been difficult to determine the aetiology of the disease, and anecdotal rather than case-controlled epidemiological evidence has often informed its pathogenesis. Indeed, it is still often described as multifactorial and poorly understood, as is the case with many malignant diseases (Stebbins and Hanke 2022).

Nonetheless, sunlight is a recognised aetiological factor. In fact, prolonged and accumulative sun exposure is the most significant carcinogen involved in the development of melanoma and nonmelanoma lip cancers (Moore et al. 2001). Consequently, around a third of lip cancers are found in patients with outdoor occupations, and almost 90% of abnormalities occur on the exposed border of the lower lip, which is at greater risk because it is usually more prominent than the upper lip that is typically angled downwards and protected from the sun by the nose (Karni 2022) (see Figure 3.1).

Dental hygienists and dental therapists frequently talk to their patients about mouth cancer and risk factors such as tobacco, alcohol, and human papillomavirus (HPV), but how often do they mention ultraviolet (UV) damage? In the UK, the incidence of lip cancer is relatively low, but it does exist, and the risk is only going to increase, compounded by climate change, including stratospheric ozone depletion, global warming, and ambient air pollution. Lifestyle habits have also changed following the recent pandemic with people taking up new outdoor hobbies, all leading to greater susceptibility to UV light.

As well as the aforementioned culprits, other risk factors include:

- Being a Caucasian male aged 40+
- Infection with HIV
- Renal transplant due to immunosuppressive antirejection drugs (López-Pintor et al. 2011)
- Blue light (HEV) emitted from digital devices
- Deficiency of the antioxidant vitamins A, C, and E
- Chronic irritation on the lip, for example, by an ill-fitting denture.

Signs and Symptoms

On average, dental hygienists and therapists see their patients every three to six months, and at each visit all patients must have their mouths systematically assessed. This should start with checking the lips, with the mouth both open and closed. It is also important to document the findings, including colour, texture, and any surface abnormalities of the vermilion borders.

Care of Head and Neck Cancer Patients for Dental Hygienists and Dental Therapists, First Edition. Edited by Jocelyn J. Harding.

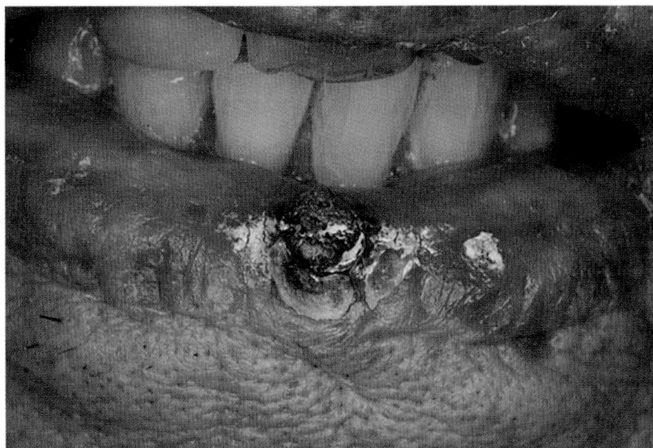

Figure 3.1 Patient with blood-crusted localised swelling. A 75-year-old male complained of a painless 'scab' on his lower lip that had been present for 10 weeks. He had spent long periods of his life outdoors in the sun. Biopsy revealed a squamous cell carcinoma. *Source:* Prof Mike Lewis.

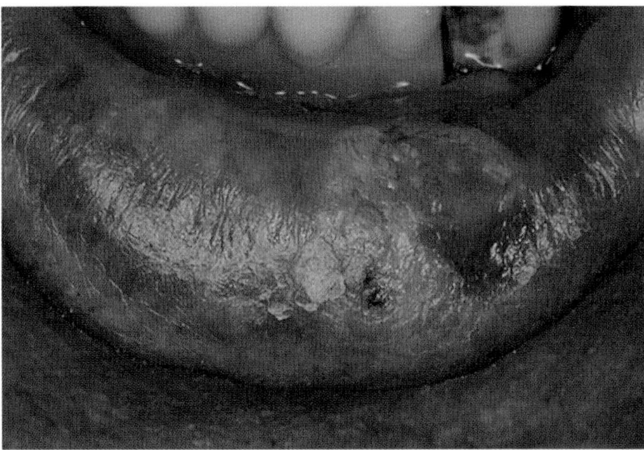

Figure 3.2 Patient with erosive changes on the lip. A 68-year-old male was found to have a symptomless erosion with underlying firm swelling in his lower lip. Unsure how long it had been present. He had smoked roll-up cigarettes for many years. Biopsy revealed a squamous cell carcinoma. *Source:* Prof Mike Lewis.

Lip cancers are usually asymptomatic in the initial progression of the disease, so early detection is crucial (Wilkins 2012). Signs and symptoms to look out for include:

- An area of crusting or discolouration
- A sore on the lip that has not healed
- Leukoplakia and/or erythroplakia
- Bleeding
- Thickening/swelling (see Figure 3.2).
- Tingling, numbness, or pain.

The neck should also be checked for enlarged lymph nodes because lower-lip SCCs often metastasise in this area (Moretti et al. 2011), and remember that lip cancer can occur in conjunction with mouth cancer, so there may be lesions inside the mouth.

Fortunately, because they are in a visible area, cancers of the lip are usually caught early, so treatment is mostly successful. But if not, it can have many functional and cosmetic consequences, including problems with speech, chewing, and swallowing following treatment (Bell et al. 2018). Surgery may also result in disfigurement of the lip and face.

Prevention

As always, prevention is better than cure! The daily use of an SPF lip balm is non negotiable – if you can see daylight, you need SPF! A wide-brimmed hat is recommended when out in the sun, and a healthy diet is always advocated.

Some risks are inescapable, but patients should be encouraged to avoid:

1) Tobacco and alcohol
2) Unsafe sexual practices
3) Sustained exposure to sunlight (especially between 10 a.m. and 3 p.m.).

In many cases, our patients' habits determine their future, so let's advise them what to quit to keep their smoothest muscle fit!!

References

Bell, R., Fernandes, R., and Andersen, P. (2018). *Oral, Head, and Neck Oncology and Reconstructive Surgery*. St. Louis, MO: Elsevier.

Gov.uk (2022). Delivering better oral health: an evidence-based toolkit for prevention. https://www.gov.uk/government/publications/delivering-better-oral-health-an-evidence-based-toolkit-for-prevention> (accessed 29 March 2022).

Karni, R. (2022). Would you recognize lip cancer? Verywell Health. https://www.verywellhealth.com/lip-cancer-symptoms-514436 (accessed 29 March 2022).

López-Pintor, R.M., Hernández, G., de Arriba, L., and de Andrés, A. (2011). Lip cancer in renal transplant patients. *Oral Oncol.* 47 (1): 68–71. https://doi.org/10.1016/j.oraloncology.2010.10.017. Epub 2010 Nov 26. PMID: 21112239.

Moore, S.R., Allister, J., Roder, D. et al. (2001). Lip cancer in South Australia, 1977–1996. *Pathology* 33 (2): 167–171.

Moretti, A., Vitullo, F., Augurio, A. et al. (2011). Surgical management of lip cancer. *Acta Otorhinolaryngol. Ital.* 31 (1): 5–10.

National Cancer Institute. 2022. Head and neck cancers. https://www.cancer.gov/types/head-and-neck/head-neck-fact-sheet> (accessed 29 March 2022).

Scully, C. and Robinson, N.A. (2017). Oral cancer. In: *International Encyclopedia of Public Health*, 2e (ed. S.R. Quah), 348–358. Academic Press.

Stebbins, W. and Hanke, C., 2022. What does skin cancer of the lip look like. https://suupesrasawqw197.blogspot.com/2021/07/what-does-skin-cancer-of-lip-look-like.html> (accessed 29 March 2022).

Wilkins, E.M. (2012). *Clinical Practice of the Dental Hygienist*, 11e. Lippincott Williams & Wilkins.

4

Smoking and Vaping

Elaine Tilling

Wells, Somerset, UK

Smoking

Tobacco smoking remains one of the world's largest health problems. During the twentieth century, it is estimated that around 100 million people died prematurely because of smoking, most of them in rich, developed countries (Jha 2009).

Cigarette smoking causes 30% of all cancer deaths in developed countries (World Health Organization 1997). In addition to lung cancer, cigarette smoking is an important cause of oesophageal, oral, oropharyngeal, hypopharyngeal, and laryngeal cancers as well as pancreatic cancer, bladder cancer, and cancer of the renal pelvis (International Agency for Research on Cancer 1986). Cigarette smoking has also been linked to cancers of the stomach, renal body, liver, colon, nose, and myeloid leukaemia, although the connection to these cancers is weaker (Chao et al. 2000) Carcinogenic compounds in cigarette smoke are thought to be responsible for these cancers (Pfeifer et al. 2002).

Looking more specifically at the effects of smoking on oral health, the evidence for an association between tobacco use and oral diseases has been clearly shown in every surgeon general's report on tobacco since 1964 (US Department of Health and Human Services 2014). The research supports that when smokers are compared with nonsmokers, we see:

- Higher incidence of periodontal disease
- Poorer plaque control
- Poorer wound healing in the mouth
- Higher incidence of tooth loss and implant failure
- Higher incidence of root surface caries
- Higher incidence of mucosal conditions.

Around two-in-three mouth cancers directly caused by smoking, and the risk of being diagnosed with mouth cancer for a smoker is almost double (91%) that of a never-smoker.

The global burden of tobacco-related disease has remained a constant focus of the world's health care authorities for more than 60 years, with a resolution from the World Health Organization (WHO) presenting a Framework Convention on Tobacco Control determined to protect present and future generations from tobacco consumption and exposure to tobacco smoke. This resolution has served to form public policy and legislation around the world in restricting the manufacture, sales and marketing, and taxation of tobacco products that we see today.

Diseases related to smoking in developed countries are important causes of disability and premature death. Health could be improved and life lengthened with the control of cigarette smoking more than with any other single action in preventive medicine.

Care of Head and Neck Cancer Patients for Dental Hygienists and Dental Therapists, First Edition. Edited by Jocelyn J. Harding.

Supporting Patients Who Wish to Give Up Smoking

The need for systemic change towards proactive prevention is recognised in the National Health Service (NHS) 'Making Every Contact Count' toolkit. Health care workers are encouraged to use every opportunity to deliver brief advice to improve health and well-being.

For smoking cessation particularly, we have good evidence that very brief advice (VBA) given by clinicians can often be the trigger to help patients to start the pathway towards stopping smoking. Smokers know that they should give up; what they don't know is how.

The three As used in VBA can be delivered in under one minute of patient consultation time:

- *A*sk: establish and record smoking status
- *A*dvise: let them know that stopping is possible (do not advise them to stop)
- *A*ct: offer help/support – signpost them to smoking cessation services.

The National Centre for Smoking Cessation and Training (NCSCT) is a social enterprise committed to support the delivery of effective evidence-based tobacco control programmes and smoking cessation interventions provided by local stop smoking services. Their online training is excellent and free to health care workers; see https://elearning.ncsct.co.uk/.

The Changing Landscape of Tobacco Use

With market and regulatory pressures to reduce the harms of nicotine delivery by combustion (smoked tobacco), the tobacco product landscape has changed, diversifying into many different products. Nicotine now comes in smokeless tobacco pouches (i.e. snus tobacco), in electric devices that heat nicotine to an inhalable aerosol form from a plug of tobacco (i.e. heated or heat-not-burn tobacco) or from an e-liquid (nicotine vaping device, e.g. e-cigarette, vape, pen, or pod), and in pharmaceutical-grade nicotine replacement therapies (NRTs) (i.e. gum, lozenge, patch, nasal spray, mouth spray, and inhaler).

Despite this diversification, smoked combusted tobacco products remain by far the most common nicotine product used by adults in most places globally. Worldwide, there are approximately one billion smokers, roughly 50% of whom will die from their habit (Drope et al. 2018).

Electronic Cigarettes

The idea of e-cigarettes was first patterned in the US in 1930 but it was not until 2003 that the first commercial device was created, designed by a Chinese chemist who had seen his father die from his lifetime use of tobacco. Hon Lik wanted to find a way of providing smokers with the nicotine that they craved without the known toxins that are present in combustible tobacco.

E-cigarettes, also known as *vapes*, are battery-powered devices that simulate the sensation of smoking (see Figure 4.1). These devices heat a liquid to generate an aerosol, or a 'vapour', which the user then inhales. The liquids typically contain flavourings, additives, and nicotine.

E-cigarettes typically consist of a mouthpiece, battery to heat the contents, and cartridge or tank containing e-liquid solution. In the first generation of devices, the heating element of e-cigarettes was activated automatically when a user inhaled. However, in most recent-generation devices, the user activates heating by pressing a button to vaporise the liquid before inhaling. Refillable e-cigarette devices mean that users are able to choose the strength of nicotine in the liquid they use up to the legal limit of 20 mg/m.

Types of E-Cigarettes

The types of e-cigarettes include the following:

- *'Cig-a-like' products:* The first generation of e-cigarettes were designed to closely resemble tobacco cigarettes. They include nonrechargeable disposable models and reusable models with rechargeable atomisers and replaceable cartridges.
- *'Tank' models or vape pens:* 'Tank' models are an e-cigarette with a rechargeable atomiser and a tank that needs to be filled with an e-liquid (see Figure 4.2).

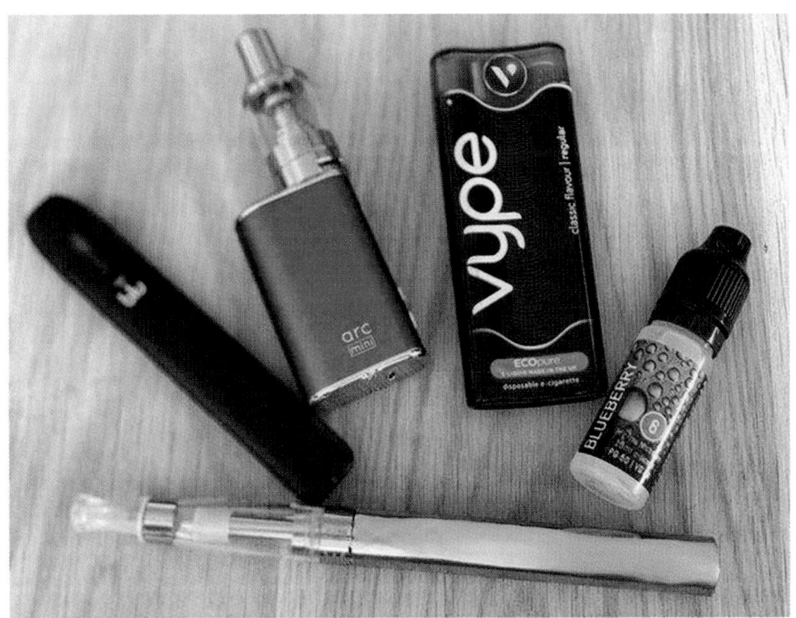

Figure 4.1 Vaping options.

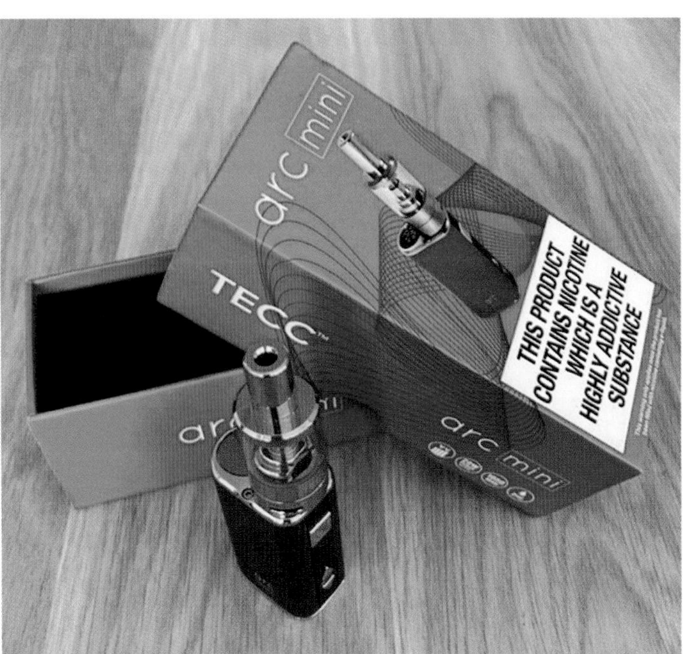

Figure 4.2 A second-generation vaping tank.

- *Pod systems:* These are compact rechargeable devices, often shaped like a USB stick or a pebble and operating with e-liquid capsules. They are simple to use and to maintain (e.g. JUUL).
- *'Mods' or advanced personal vaporisers:* A more complex tank model that can be manually customised, for example, by adjusting the power on the device.

Global e-cigarette use and sales have risen dramatically since records started in 2011, and Euromonitor estimated that there were 55 million vapers in 2021 (Euromonitor International 2021).

The UK is the second largest market in the world for vape products, with an estimated 3.4 million users (Action on Smoking and Health 2019).

The key points regarding e-cigarettes:

- It has been estimated that e-cigarettes are 95% less harmful than ordinary cigarettes (Figure 4.3).
- Almost all e-cigarette users in Britain are either ex-smokers or current smokers.
- There is no evidence that use of e-cigarettes is leading to an increase of smoking in young people in Great Britain.
- The average age range of users in the UK is 35–44 years old.
- The most common reason for vaping in the UK is as an aid to quit smoking.
- There is negligible risk to others from secondhand e-cigarette vapour.
- Seventy-seven percent of vapers use tanks rather than cartridges/JUULs.
- The most popular flavour of vape juice is fruit (in 2015 it was tobacco).

Initially a cottage industry with small independent producers and sellers, the e-cigarette market is now a global industry, with the big global tobacco companies investing heavily in the development and production of e-cigarettes. Compliance with the safety legislation that has been brought in over the last decade has meant that the smaller players in the market have been forced out.

It is clear that e-cigs are an effective tool to help individuals reduce the risks associated with conventional smoking, as the removal of the combustible element of smoking removes the known carcinogens in smoked tobacco. The controversy over the presence of nicotine in e-cigs continues to cause debate. Whilst we know that nicotine is the addictive element of tobacco, new research is emerging that is bringing into question the exact nature of the physiological effects of the nicotine. The research supports that the dependence liability of inhaled nicotine is also influenced by other constituents of tobacco smoke, such as chemicals that inhibit monoamine oxidase (MAO), an enzyme that degrades neurotransmitters released by nicotine. Furthermore, dependence on nicotine from medications (e.g. nicotine patches, gum, and lozenges) that deliver nicotine appears to be low (Prochaska and Benowitz 2019).

Public Health England (PHE) have long supported the use of e-cigs as part of smoking cessation, quoting the 95% less harmful than smoking message and stressing that nicotine is the least harmful element in a cigarette.

E-cigarettes are now tightly regulated in the UK with their marketing, content, and labelling along with mandatory reporting of potential adverse reactions. E-cigs offer smokers a safer option to smoking – harm reduction is a key element of PHE policy on supporting healthier lifestyles. The science on e-cigarettes – although they are not 'harm less' – supports that they are less harmful. The safety for their long-term use is, of course, not yet known.

E-cigarettes are regulated as consumer products under the UK legislation Tobacco and Related Products Regulations 2016 and are currently not used as a licenced medicine for smoking cessation. As of 2021, the NHS are trialling the issue of e-cigarettes for smoking cessation in several hospital pilot sites.

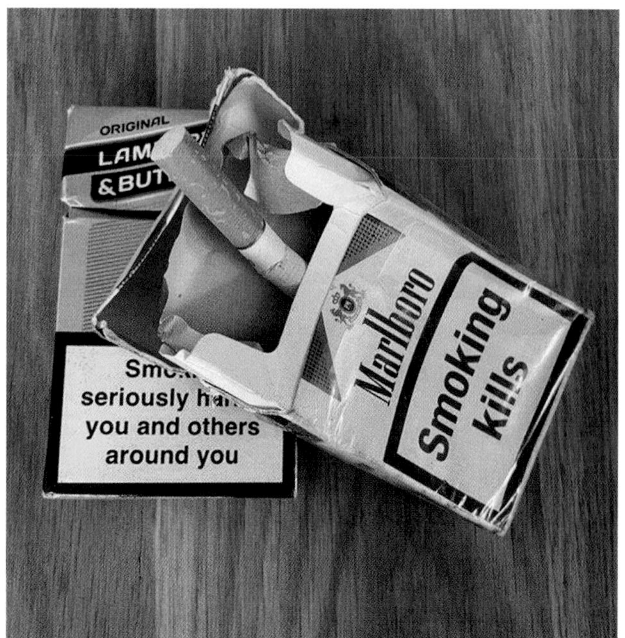

Figure 4.3 Smoking kills – a traditional cigarette.

Nicotine is the least damaging component of a cigarette, and whilst complicit in the role of addiction, it is now thought not to be the only component in the cocktail of chemicals that are delivered in combustible tobacco that enhances addiction to smoked tobacco. The concern regarding its potential to damage the brain tissues of young/adolescent users cited as the rationale for the ban of e-cigarettes in some countries and states in the US is questioned in the scientific community here in the UK (Public Health England 2019). People have been using nicotine for decades. The Scandinavian snus, a nicotine pouch used intraorally, delivers high levels of nicotine daily (see Figure 4.4). We would have seen empirical evidence of damage in its predominantly young users, but we simply don't.

More research is needed in this field, as we appear to be moving away from our original understanding that nicotine was solely responsible for the chemical dependence upon smoked tobacco.

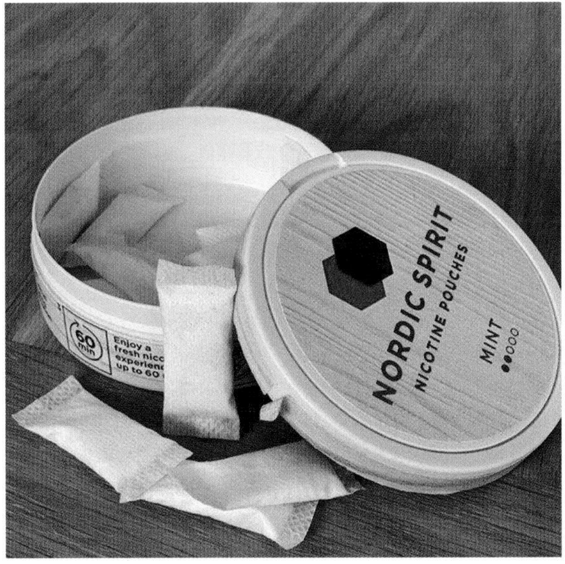

Figure 4.4 Snus – Nordic Spirit.

Cariogenic Potential

Most electronic-cigarette liquids contain propylene glycol, glycerin, nicotine, and a wide variety of flavours, many of which are sweet. Sweet flavours are classified as saccharides, esters, acids, or aldehydes. Various studies investigate changes in cariogenic potential when tooth surfaces are exposed to e-cigarette aerosols generated from well-characterized reference e-liquids with sweet flavours.

A study by Kim et al. (2018) that systematically evaluated e-cigarette aerosols found that the aerosols have similar physiochemical properties as high-sucrose, gelatinous candies and acidic drinks. The data in this research suggested that the combination of the viscosity of e-liquids and some classes of chemicals in sweet flavours may increase the risk of cariogenic potential. However, most studies in this area conclude that clinical investigation is warranted to confirm the data that we see in the laboratory setting.

Respiratory Damage

The respiratory diseases and deaths associated with e-cigarettes in the United States have all been linked to the use of cannabinoids in the e-liquids. Cannabis is widely used legally in the US, and the addition of tetrahydrocannabinol (THC) in e-gigs was originally used with no ill effects. The e-cig market is largely unregulated in the US, and at some point, e-cig manufacturers cut in vitamin E acetate into the liquid to thicken the solution. This was found to be the cause of the incidents related to the condition called 'electronic cigarettes, or vaping, product use-associated lung injury' (EVALI), which have all been discrete to certain areas in the US.

PHE cite that the glycerol used to produce the vapour is the same as that used in stage performances – dry ice. Whilst there is limited evidence for this excipient to cause local irritation and dryness of the respiratory tissue, there is no clear evidence for inflammation of the respiratory cells.

It is clear that legislation and regulation can work to reduce the harm of e-cigs and that their use by smokers to stop smoking or cut down has been a positive step in terms of the reduction in the number of smokers in the UK. In 2019, the proportion of current smokers in the UK was 14.1%, which equates to around 6.9 million. The latest figure represents a significant reduction in the proportion of current smokers since 2018, when 14.7% smoked. This continues the trend in falling smoking prevalence since 2011 (Office for National Statistics 2020).

The role that e-cigarettes can play in a broader public health intervention is yet to be tested. The availability of less harmful noncombusted sources of nicotine such as e-cigs can help smokers transfer their nicotine addiction from combustibles to e-cigs. Many, if not most, people would stop smoking, and the result would be prevention of most tobacco-related disease.

For now, choosing to use e-cigs should be a choice that has the support of health care professionals – reducing the potential for harm and in the hope that nicotine is given up for good. Nicotine for life may be the choice of some, and that too should be supported, as it may be that our understanding of the role of nicotine in the addiction pathway is not as clear as we once thought.

References

Action on Smoking and Health (2019) Use of e-cigarettes (vaporisers) among adults in Great Britain. https://ash.org.uk/wp-content/uploads/2019/09/Use-of e-cigarettes amongst-adults -2019.pdf

Chao, A., Thun, M., Jacobs, E. et al. (2000). Cigarette smoking: cancer risks, carcinogens, and mechanisms. *J. Natl. Cancer Inst.* 92: 1888–1896.

Drope, J., Schuluger, N., Chan, Z. et al. (2018). *The Tobacco Atlas*. American Cancer Society and Vital Strategies.

Euromonitor International (2021) Smokeless tobacco and vapour products https://www.euromonitor.com/smokeless-tobacco-and-vapour-products.

International Agency for Research on Cancer (1986). *IARC Monographs on the Evaluation of the Carcinogenic Risk of Chemicals of Humans*, vol. 38, 37–375. Lyon, France: IARC.

Jha, P. (2009). Avoidable global cancer deaths and total deaths from smoking. *Nat. Rev. Cancer* 9 (9): 655.

Kim, S.A., Smith, S., Beauchamp, C. et al. (2018). Cariogenic potential of sweet flavors in electronic-cigarette liquids. *PLoS One* 13 (9): e0203717. https://doi.org/10.1371/journal.pone.0203717.

Office for National Statistics: 2020; Adult smoking habits in the UK: 2019 https://www.ons.gov.uk/peoplepopulationandcommunity/healthandsocialcare/healthandlifeexpectancies/bulletins/adultsmokinghabitsingreatbritain/2019

Pfeifer, G., Denissenko, M., Olivier, M. et al. (2002). Tobacco smoke carcinogens, DNA damage and p53 mutations in smoking-associated cancers. *Oncogene* 21: 7435–7451. https://doi.org/10.1038/sj.onc.1205803.

Prochaska, J.J. and Benowitz, N.L. (2019). Current advances in research in treatment and recovery: nicotine addiction. *Sci. Adv.* ***5*** (10): eaay9763. https://doi.org/101126/sciadv.aay9763.

Public Health England (2019) Vaping in England: an evidence update February 2019 Annual update of Public Health England's e-cigarette evidence review by leading independent tobacco experts. https://www.gov.uk/government/publications/vaping-in-england-an-evidence-update-february-2019.

US Department of Health and Human Services (2014). *The Health Consequences of Smoking – 50 Years of Progress: A Report of the Surgeon General*. Atlanta, GA: US Department of Health and Human Services, Centres for Disease Control and Prevention, National Centre for Chronic Disease Prevention and Health Promotion, Office on Smoking and Health.

World Health Organization (1997). *Tobacco or Health: A Global Status Report*, 10–48. Geneva: WHO.

5

The Impact of Substance Dependence on Oral Health

Teresa Servas

Life Over Lemons, Gloucestershire, UK

Introduction: Dependency, Substances, and Prevalence

The International Classification of Diseases (ICD) defines substance dependence as a disorder of regulation, arising from repeated or continuous use of a psychoactive substance and consisting of a strong internal drive to use that substance. This is with a manifestation of two or more of the following features: impaired control over substance use; increasing priority of substance use above other aspects of one's life, such as daily activities, responsibilities, and maintenance of health, such that usage escalates despite harmful consequences; physiological features indicative of neuroadaptation, including tolerance, withdrawal symptoms, and repeated use to prevent or alleviate withdrawal. Substance dependence is usually evident over a period of at least 12 months, but a diagnosis is possible when there is continuous use (daily/almost daily) for at least three months (World Health Organization [WHO] 2022a).

Psychoactive substances affect a person's mental processes, including their perception, consciousness, cognition or mood, and emotions (WHO 2022b). Psychoactive substances may be illicit, including marijuana, cocaine, methamphetamine, and opioids, or more commonplace substances, such as alcohol and nicotine.

The effects of psychoactive substances on the individual, and their often illicit nature, are challenges for population research. The Crime Survey for England and Wales works to ascertain representative figures of substance use. Around 3.2 million people (1 in 11) have taken drugs in the last year (Office for National Statistics [ONS] 2020). Cannabis is the most commonly used substance, its prevalence remaining consistent since 1995 with around 2.6 million (7.8%) users and one-third of those being frequent users. Around 873 000 (2.6%) people used powder cocaine, 796 000 (2.4%) people used nitrous oxide, and 471 000 (1.4%) people used ecstasy. While powder cocaine usage has remained consistent, frequent users of other substances have fallen from 14.4% to 8.7% between March 2019 and March 2020.

Treatment statistics provide insight into the prevalence of substance dependency. The National Drug Treatment Monitoring System measured 275 896 adults in contact with drug and alcohol services in 2020–2021 in England (Office for Health Improvement and Disparities 2021a). This rose by 270 750 compared to a year ago. Of those in contact with treatment services, 130 490 enrolled in treatment, including adults returning to treatment following a 21-day break.

The majority of adults in treatment in 2020–2021 were in treatment for alcohol usage (60%). Other substance dependencies included opiates (29%), crack cocaine (20%), cannabis (21%), and cocaine (15%). The most common substance being used among 30–44 year olds was opiates, whereas the large majority of adults 55 years and over reported alcohol as their only problem substance. Adults under 30 years primarily reported problem usage with nonopiate substances and nonopiate substances and alcohol.

The majority of adults receiving treatment reported a mental health need. Mental health needs were most prevalent within the nonopiate and alcohol group (71%), followed by the alcohol (64%) and nonopiate-only groups (64%), and lastly the opiates group (57%). Of those receiving mental health treatment, 55% received it from a primary care setting, such as a GP surgery; 18% were already engaged with a community mental health team or other service. But for 25% with a mental health need identified, no treatment was being received or treatment was being refused (OHID 2021b).

Care of Head and Neck Cancer Patients for Dental Hygienists and Dental Therapists, First Edition. Edited by Jocelyn J. Harding.

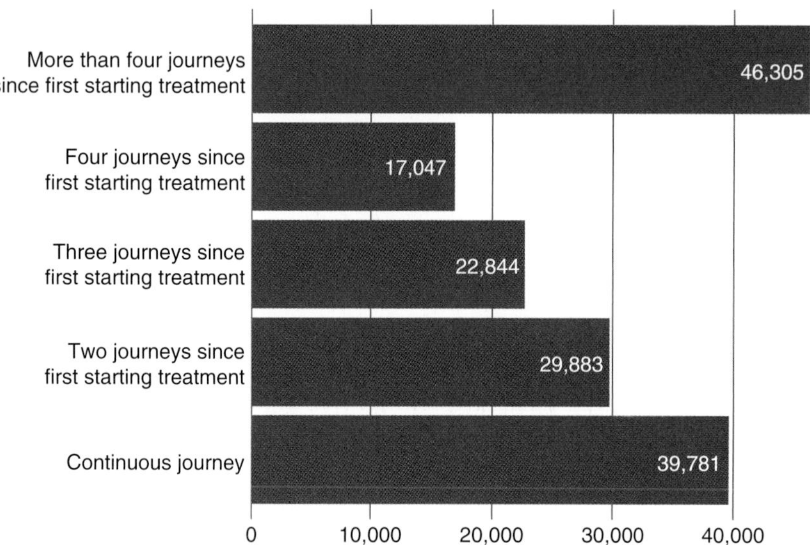

Figure 5.1 Number of previous journeys for people still in treatment at the end of 2020 to 2021 (OHID 2021a).

Substance dependence is a pervasive disease, and long-term treatment journeys are common for people recovering. Figure 5.1 shows the number of people having multiple treatment journeys, and the number of people having a continual treatment journey, across a five-year period. Four or more treatment journeys were had by over one-third of people (41%). Just over a quarter of people (26%) have been in treatment continuously since their treatment started, with 31% of those having been in treatment for five years or more.

Oral Health: Risk Factors and Complications of Substance Use

Substance use negatively impacts oral health, the most common oral health problems being dental caries and periodontal disease (78%), followed by xerostomia (44%), bruxism (17%), and oral mucosal lesions (11%) (Djou and Dewi 2019). A systemic review by Baghaie et al. (2017) found that when compared to the general population, people with substance dependence had greater and more severe caries and periodontal disease, with a mean difference of 5.15 decayed, missing, and filled teeth (DMFT) and a mean difference of 17.83 decayed, missing, and filled surfaces (DMFS). Findings also showed greater tooth loss, noncarious tooth loss, and destructive periodontal disease for patients with substance dependence. The oral conditions (oral hygiene, changes in salivary pH, and cariogenic diets) of patients with substance dependence are what often lead to the progressive caries and maxillofacial infections observed (Cuberos et al. 2020). Poor oral health has recently been linked to a strongly reduced functional diversity of microbiota amongst people with substance dependence. This is such that substance dependence itself decreases the functional potential of the microbiome; people with lower diversity were found to report higher levels of negative reinforcement (i.e. relief usage) with their primary substance (Kosciolek et al. 2021).

Alcohol is easily available and legal to those 18 years and over. It is estimated that 29.2 million adults across the UK will have consumed alcohol in the last week (ONS 2018). UK drinkers favour beer (35%) and wine (32%), followed by spirits (23%), cider (7%), and alcopops (2%) (Drinkaware 2019). While alcohol consumption is commonplace, it does not come without risks; 21% of drinkers are at increasing or high risk due to the number of units they consume (NHS Digital 2017). Increased alcohol consumption (>5 cl per day) is associated with significantly more surface caries and apical lesions but not periodontal disease (Jansson 2008). The significance of alcohol usage in the development of periodontal disease is controversial (Manicone et al. 2017). Research shows that periodontal disease is significantly higher among long-term alcohol users, and people with alcohol dependence specifically, when compared to matched controls, including social drinkers (Hach et al. 2015; Manicone et al. 2017; Priyanka et al. 2017). Alcohol dependence is also associated with more DMFT (Manicone et al. 2017; Priyanka et al. 2017), a lower plaque pH and a lower salivary pH, and a higher prevalence of mucosal lesions (Priyanka et al. 2017). The lifestyle factors and lower oral hygiene among alcohol users and people with alcohol dependence are major contributors of the oral health implications observed (Jansson 2008; Manicone et al. 2017).

Cannabis is drug derived from a plant; it can be smoked, eaten, or vaped (FRANK 2022a). When smoked without a filter, this increases the amount of smoke the user inhales. This usage has been found to cause stomatitis, leukeodema of the buccal mucosa, and hyperkeratosis (Cuberos et al. 2020; Versteeg et al. 2008). In addition, smoked cannabis is a carcinogen and is associated with an increased risk of oral cancer, including dysplastic changes (leukoplakia and erythroplakia) and premalignant lesions of the oral mucosa (Cho et al. 2005). Krogh et al. (1987) found evidence that certain strains of *C. albicans* and of other yeasts may play a part in the development of oral cancers. Further oral health implications of Cannabis include xerostomia, an increased risk of caries, and periodontal disease (Cho et al. 2005; Versteeg et al. 2008). It is thought that the short-term xerostomia, which is caused by delta-9-tetrahydrocannabinol (THC), together with lifestyle factors such as more sweet beverages, less tooth brushing, and fewer dental visits are responsible for a higher prevalence of dental decay (Schulz-Katterbach et al. 2009).

Cocaine is a stimulant drug with a white powdery appearance (FRANK 2022b). It is normally taken intranasally by snorting or orally by rubbing into the gums, though it can also be smoked as crack or freebase, or injected (FRANK 2022c). Pure cocaine has a pH of 4.5 and can disintegrate enamel when ingested, snorted, or taken orally (Krutchkoff et al. 1990). The oral health problems associated with crack/cocaine use include periodontal problems, caries, and lesions in the oral mucosa (Cherobin et al. 2019; Brand et al. 2008). Regular cocaine use can lead to orofacial effects such as perforation of the nasal septum and palate (Brand et al. 2008). Crack cocaine users have 46% more frequent tooth loss and a greater severity of periodontal disease (Antoniazzi et al. 2021). A greater probing depth is observed in substance-dependent crack/cocaine users, but destructive periodontal disease has not been found to be associated with the addiction (Cury et al. 2017b). Cury et al. (2017a) have found a greater proportion of DT but fewer FT/MT. This may be indicative of a dental care need within this population; after all, crack cocaine users are less likely to use dental care services (Antoniazzi et al. 2021). Lesions are observed in patients topically applying cocaine to the oral and/or nasal mucosa, including erythematous lesions, gingival recession, and bone sequestration, the likely cause being vasoconstrictor activity of cocaine (Gandara-Rey et al. 2002). The most prevalent lesions are traumatic ulcer and actinic cheilitis, followed by fistulae associated with retained dental root, the addiction being associated with the oral mucosal lesions observed (Cury et al. 2018).

Methamphetamine is a stimulant drug that is swallowed, snorted, or injected (FRANK 2022d; FRANK 2022e). Methamphetamine users have an average of 2.1–4.58 more MT when compared with controls (Baghaie et al. 2017; Shetty et al. 2010). Interestingly, users who inject are found to have significantly more MT than those that smoke methamphetamine. This is despite the corrosive effects of methamphetamine on the oral tissue and may be down to the severity of the addiction (Shetty et al. 2010). Users are four times as likely to have caries with an average of 2.6 more DT than controls and are twice as likely for their decay to be untreated (Shetty et al. 2016; Baghaie et al. 2017; Shetty et al. 2016). The rampant caries observed may be due to poor oral hygiene, the effects of methamphetamine having a long duration, and the hyperactivity causing dehydration (Hamamoto and Rhodus 2009). The reduction in salivary flow causes xerostomia and results in a reduced buffering ability (Heng et al. 2008). The continued use of methamphetamine makes it difficult for users to increase their salivary flow, hindering oral hygiene (Hamamoto and Rhodus 2009). Methamphetamine users also experience bruxism and excessive tooth wear (Hamamoto and Rhodus 2009; Shetty et al. 2010). Even when compared with users of other substances, methamphetamine users experience significantly more jaw clenching, grinding, frequent chewing, and temporomandibular joint (TMJ) tenderness (McGrath and Chan 2005). It should be noted that the popularly referenced phenomenon of 'meth mouth' is contested within the research literature. Rossow (2021), for example, contrasts the intraoral photos in which almost all teeth are severely affected by decay or are missing crowns with epidemiological studies that find DT scores to be in the magnitude of 2–5 and the average MT scores to range from 3 to 5 (Shetty et al. 2015; Smit and Naidoo 2015; Rommel et al. 2016; Ye et al. 2018). When compared to the use of other illicit drugs, methamphetamine use is not associated with a greater need for oral health care (Robbins et al. 2010). The construction of the 'meth mouth' diagnosis has been interpreted to be part of a drug scare (Murakawa 2011).

Dental Professionals: Support for Patients Who Use Substances

People with substance dependence have lower levels of health and report a more frequent need for physical and oral health care compared to the general population (Robbins et al. 2010; Sheridan et al. 2001; Truong et al. 2015). They present with greater and more severe dental caries but fewer restorations (Baghaie et al. 2017). Rossow (2021) highlights that the irregular lifestyle, poor economy, and mental health problems that are connected with substance use are key facilitators for the dental health problems observed, due to their influence on oral hygiene, sugar intake, and frequency of dental visits (Figure 5.2).

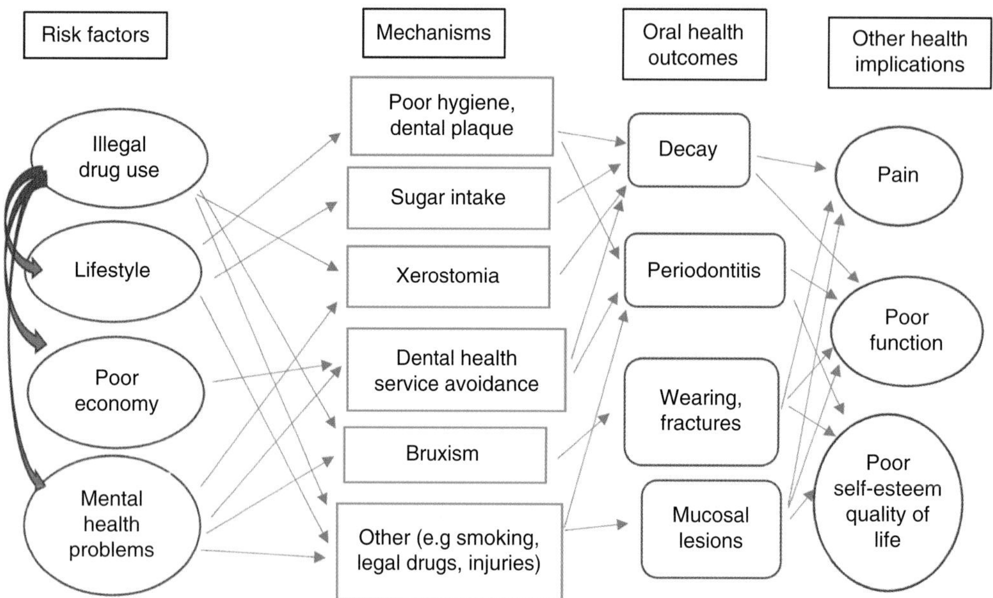

Figure 5.2 An illustration of underlying mechanisms for oral health problems and their sequelae among people with drug use disorders (Rossow 2021).

Despite the need for care, people taking substances are less likely to visit a dentist or seek dental treatment, even when they experience pain, and typically have difficulty accessing dental treatment (Baghaie et al. 2017; Laslett et al. 2008; Rossow 2021; Sheridan et al. 2001). A factor contributing to dental avoidance amoung substance users is heightened dental anxiety (Åstrøm et al. 2011; Dawkes et al. 1995; Scheutz 1986; Titsas and Ferguson 2002). Managing dental pain for substance users is complex, and pain magnifies the anxiety (Titsas and Ferguson 2002). People who are substance dependent may be self-medicating to manage painful medical and dental conditions, or they be unable to tolerate pain and fearful of treatment, anticipating subadequate pain management (Cuberos et al. 2020; Sainsbury 1999). Patients using substances may also experience psychiatric difficulties. For example, cannabis intoxication can cause acute anxiety, dysphoria, and psychotic-like experiences such as paranoid thoughts, and methamphetamine intoxication can cause psychosis and paranoia (Cho et al. 2005; Hamamoto and Rhodus 2009). It is vital that dental professionals assess a patient's substance use history prior to treatment, especially when using anaesthetics. The effect of local anaesthetics can be reduced for patients using opioids, including methadone (Titsas and Ferguson 2002). Local anaesthetics containing epinephrine can prolong tachycardia for patients using cannabis, and those with vasoconstrictors can result in cardiac dysrhythmias, myocardial infraction, and cerebrovascular accidents for patients using methamphetamine (Cho et al. 2005; Hamamoto and Rhodus 2009). Patients using cocaine are also at increased medical risk, including cardiovascular complications, during dental treatment, especially with local anaesthetics containing epinephrine or epinephrine-impregnated retraction cords (Blanksma and Brand 2004; Blanksma and Brand 2005). It is advised that dental treatment is delayed by 6–24 hours after use (Brand et al. 2008; Hamamoto and Rhodus 2009).

Dental anxiety and poor experiences with the perceived attitudes of dental workers are key factors leading to insufficient dental follow-up (Åstrøm et al. 2022). In a recent study of dentists' and dental hygienists' attitudes towards patients with substance use disorders, Åstrøm et al. (2021) found slightly negative attitudes towards medically assisted rehabilitation patients. The beliefs that 'completion of treatment is often unsuccessful', and that 'information on illict drug use and oral health is difficult to understand' were associated with their negative attitudes. Such negative attitudes can actually diminish patients' feelings of empowerment and their treatment outcomes (Van Boekel et al. 2013). Negative attitudes might exist due to a lack adequate education, training, and support structures for engagement and work with patients with substance use disorders (Åstrøm et al. 2021; Van Boekel et al. 2013). While this may be the case, findings from the 1990s suggest that most dentists would actively welcome training focused on substance misuse (Dawkes et al. 1995). Education of patient substance use for dental professionals is growing. Recently, an investigation into the content and stratergies that are used in dental schools' curriculum in the US found that 81% incorporated substance use disorder (Odusola et al. 2021). The substances that were most frequently taught included opioids, alcohol, nicotine, and marijuana.

Clinical examination accompanied with a detailed medical history is essential. A nonconfrontational and judgment-free questioning style is needed for the identification of patients using substances (Cuberos et al. 2020). Interviewing methods applied within clinic can bolster dental care and well-informed treatment plans. Dental professionals should evaluate the extent to which patients can actively participate in their treatment plan; plans should be feasible and simple, with pain management and the prevention of orofacial infections prioritised (Cuberos et al. 2020). Patient-centred interviewing in particular acknowledges and validates a patient's unique life experiences, strengthening the replationship between clinician and patient, and encourages postive communication, overall, helping to overcome barriers to care plan adhereance (Schatman et al. 2020). Another standardised tool is Screening, Brief Intervention, and Referral to Treatment (SBIRT), which can be applied directly when working with patients who use substances. It includes questionnaires that identify a continuum of substance use, protocol-driven brief intervention, and referral options for patients. SBIRT improves attitudes and helps dental professionals to feel more prepared to manage patients with substance dependence (Odusola et al. 2020).

An integration of care for patients who are substance dependent can benefit their oral and general health (Rossow 2021). It is therefore imperative to signpost patients who are using substances to their GP, where the pathway to support can begin. The collaboration of dental professionals with other services, such as community pharmacies, could increase the uptake of dental services among drug users, and drug users should be encouraged to use the free dental treatment available to them through the National Health Service (Sheridan et al. 2001). Cuberos et al. (2020) recommends a multidisciplinary approach for dental management for patients already in contact with treatment services. This includes regular communication with a patient's GP and pharmacist and is important when pain management is needed to prevent poly-pharmacy, drug interactions, and overdosing.

References

Antoniazzi, R.P., Palmeira, R.V., Schöffer, C. et al. (2021). Use of crack cocaine increases tooth loss. *Am. J. Dentist.* 34 (6): 317–321.

Åstrøm, A.N., Skaret, E., and Haugejorden, O. (2011). Dental anxiety and dental attendance among 25-year-olds in Norway: time trends from 1997 to 2007. *BMC Oral Health.* 11 (1): 1–7.

Åstrøm, A.N., Özkaya, F., Virtanen, J., and Fadnes, L.T. (2021). Dental health care workers' attitude towards patients with substance use disorders in medically assisted rehabilitation (MAR). *Acta Odontol. Scand.* 79 (1): 31–36.

Åstrøm, A.N., Virtanen, J., Özkaya, F., and Fadnes, L.T. (2022). Oral health related quality of life and reasons for non-dental attendance among patients with substance use disorders in withdrawal rehabilitation. *Clin. Experiment. Dent. Res.* 8 (1): 68–75.

Baghaie, H., Kisely, S., Forbes, M. et al. (2017). A systematic review and meta-analysis of the association between poor oral health and substance abuse. *Addict.* 112 (5): 765–779.

Blanksma, C.J. and Brand, H.S. (2004). Effects of cocaine use on oral health and implications for dental treatment. *Nederlands. Tijdschrift Voor. Tandheelkunde.* 111 (12): 486–489.

Blanksma, C.J. and Brand, H.S. (2005). Cocaine abuse: orofacial manifestations and implications for dental treatment. *Int. Dent. J.* 55 (6): 365–369.

Brand, H.S., Gonggrijp, S., and Blanksma, C.J. (2008). Cocaine and oral health. *Brit. Dent. J.* 204 (7): 365–369.

Cherobin, T.Z., Stefenon, L., and Wiethölter, P. (2019). Oral lesions in crack and cocaine user patients: literature review. *Oral Heal. Dent. Sci.* 3 (1): 1–5.

Cho, C.M., Hirsch, R., and Johnstone, S. (2005). General and oral health implications of cannabis use. *Aust. Dent. J.* 50 (2): 70–74.

Cuberos, M., Chatah, E.M., Baquerizo, H.Z., and Weinstein, G. (2020). Dental management of patients with substance use disorder. *Clin. Dentist. Review* 4 (1): 1–8.

Cury, P.R., Oliveira, M.G., de Andrade, K.M. et al. (2017a). Dental health status in crack/cocaine-addicted men: a cross-sectional study. *Environ. Sci. Pollut. Res.* 24 (8): 7585–7590.

Cury, P.R., Oliveira, M.G.A., and Dos Santos, J.N. (2017b). Periodontal status in crack and cocaine addicted men: a cross-sectional study. *Environ. Sci. Pollut. Res.* 24 (4): 3423–3429.

Cury, P.R., Araujo, N.S., das Graças Alonso Oliveira, M., and Dos Santos, J.N. (2018). Association between oral mucosal lesions and crack and cocaine addiction in men: a cross-sectional study. *Environ. Sci. Pollut. Res.* 25 (20): 19801–19807.

Dawkes, M., Sparkes, S., and Smith, M. (1995). Dentists' responses to drug misusers. *Health Trend.* 27 (1): 12–14.

Djou, R. and Dewi, T.S. (2019). Oral manifestation related to drug abuse: a systematic review: Manifetasi oral terkait penggunaan obat-obatan terlarang: Sebuah tinjauan sistematis. *Dentika: Dent. J.* 22 (2): 44–51.

Drinkaware (2019). Alcohol consumption UK. www.drinkaware.co.uk/research/research-and-evaluation-reports/alcohol-consumption-uk (accessed 15 June 2022).

FRANK (2022a). Cannabis. https://www.talktofrank.com/drug/cannabis (accessed 15 June 2022).

FRANK (2022b). Cocaine. https://www.talktofrank.com/drug/cocaine (accessed 5 June 2022).

FRANK (2022c). Cocaine: how do people take it? https://www.talktofrank.com/drug/cocaine#how-do-people-take-it (accessed 15 June 2022).

FRANK (2022d). Methamphetamine. https://www.talktofrank.com/drug/methamphetamine (accessed 18 June 2022).

FRANK (2022e) Methamphetamine: how do people take it? https://www.talktofrank.com/drug/methamphetamine#how-do-people-take-it (accessed 18 June 2022).

Gandara-Rey, J.M., Diniz-Freitas, M., Gandara-Vila, P. et al. (2002). Lesions of the oral mucosa in cocaine users who apply the drug topically. *Medicina. Oral.: Organo. Oficial de la Sociedad Espanola de Medicina Oral y de la Academia Iberoamericana de Patologia y Medicina Bucal* 7 (2): 103–107.

Hach, M., Holm-Pedersen, P., Adegboye, A.R.A., and Avlund, K. (2015). The effect of alcohol consumption on periodontitis in older Danes. *Int. J. Dent. Hyg.* 13 (4): 261–267.

Hamamoto, D.T. and Rhodus, N.L. (2009). Methamphetamine abuse and dentistry. *Oral Dis.* 15 (1): 27–37.

Heng, C.K., Badner, V.M., and Schiop, L.A. (2008). Meth mouth. *NY State Dent. J.* 74 (5): 50.

Jansson, L. (2008). Association between alcohol consumption and dental health. *J. Clin. Periodontol.* 35 (5): 379–384.

Kosciolek, T., Victor, T.A., Kuplicki, R. et al. and Tulsa 1000 Investigators(2021). Individuals with substance use disorders have a distinct oral microbiome pattern. *Brain, Behavior, Immun. Health.* 15: 100271.

Krogh, P., Hald, B., and Holmstrup, P. (1987). Possible mycological etiology of oral mucosal cancer: catalytic potential of infecting Candida aibicans and other yeasts in production of N-nitrosobenzylmethylamine. *Carcinogenes.* 8 (10): 1543–1548.

Krutchkoff, D.J., Eisenberg, E., O'Brien, J.E., and Ponzillo, J.J. (1990). Cocaine-induced dental erosions. *N. Engl. J. Med.* 322: 408; Cited in: Teoh, L., Moses, G., McCullough, M.J., 2019. Oral manifestations of illicit drug use. *Aust. Dent. J.* 64(3), pp.213–222.

Laslett, A.M., Dietze, P., and Dwyer, R. (2008). The oral health of street-recruited injecting drug users: prevalence and correlates of problems. *Addict.* 103 (11): 1821–1825.

Manicone, P.F., Tarli, C., Mirijello, A. et al. (2017). Dental health in patients affected by alcohol use disorders: a cross-sectional study. *Eur. Rev. Med. Pharmacol. Sci.* 21 (22): 5021–5027.

McGrath, C. and Chan, B. (2005). Oral health sensations associated with illicit drug abuse. *Brit. Dent. J.* 198 (3): 159–162.

Murakawa, N. (2011). Toothless: the methamphetamine "epidemic,""meth mouth," and the racial construction of drug scares. *Du. Bois. Rev.: Soc. Sci. Res. on Race* 8 (1): 219–228.

NHS Digital (2017). Health Survey for England, 2017: adult health related behaviours – tables (version 2). Table 13: Summary of weekly alcohol consumption, by age and sex. https://digital.nhs.uk/data-and-information/publications/statistical/health-survey-for-england/2017#resources (accessed 16 June 2022).

Odusola, F., Smith, J.L., Bisaga, A. et al. (2020). Innovations in pre-doctoral dental education: influencing attitudes and opinions about patients with substance use disorder. *J. Dent. Educ.* 84 (5): 578–585.

Odusola, F., Kaufman, J., Turrigiano, E. et al. (2021). Predoctoral substance use disorders curricula: a survey analysis and experiential pedagogy. *J. Dent. Educ.* 85 (10): 1664–1673.

Office for Health Improvement and Dispartities (2021a). National statistics: adult substance misuse treatment statistics 2020 to 2021: report. https://www.gov.uk/government/statistics/substance-misuse-treatment-for-adults-statistics-2020-to-2021/adult-substance-misuse-treatment-statistics-2020-to-2021-report (accessed 31 March 2022).

Office for Health Improvement and Dispartities (2021b). Adult substance misuse treatment statistics 2020 to 2021: data tables. https://www.gov.uk/government/statistics/substance-misuse-treatment-for-adults-statistics-2020-to-2021 (accessed 12 April 2022).

Office for National Statistics (2018). Adult drinking habits in Great Britain: 2017. www.ons.gov.uk/peoplepopulationandcommunity/healthandsocialcare/drugusealcoholandsmoking/bulletins/opinionsandlifestylesurveyadultdrinkinghabitsingreatbritain/2017#in-great-britain-an-estimated-292-million-adults-drank-alcohol (accessed 15 June 2022).

Office for National Statistics (2020). Drug misuse in England and Wales: year ending March 2020. www.ons.gov.uk/peoplepopulationandcommunity/crimeandjustice/articles/drugmisuseinenglandandwales/yearendingmarch2020 (accessed 1 June 2022).

Priyanka, K., Sudhir, K.M., Reddy, V.C.S. et al. (2017). Impact of alcohol dependency on oral health – a cross-sectional comparative study. *J. Clin. Diagnost. Res.* 11 (6): ZC43–ZC46.

Robbins, J.L., Wenger, L., Lorvick, J. et al. (2010). Health and oral health care needs and health care-seeking behavior among homeless injection drug users in San Francisco. *J. Urban Health* 87 (6): 920–930.

Rommel, N., Rohleder, N.H., Wagenpfeil, S. et al. (2016). The impact of the new scene drug "crystal meth" on oral health: a case–control study. *Clin. Oral Invest.* 20 (3): 469–475. Cited in: Rossow, I., 2021. Illicit drug use and oral health. Addiction, 116(11), pp.3235-3242.

Rossow, I. (2021). Illicit drug use and oral health. *Addict.* 116 (11): 3235–3242.

Sainsbury, D. (1999). Drug addiction and dental care. *New Zealand Dent. J.* 95 (420): 58–61.

Schatman, M.E., Patterson, E., and Shapiro, H. (2020). Patient interviewing strategies to recognize substance use, misuse, and abuse in the dental setting. *Dent. Clin.* 64 (3): 503–512.

Scheutz, F. (1986). Anxiety and dental fear in a group of parenteral drug addicts. *Europ. J. Oral. Sci.* 94 (3): 241–247.

Schulz-Katterbach, M., Imfeld, T., and Imfeld, C. (2009). Cannabis and caries – does regular cannabis use increase the risk of caries in cigarette smokers? *Schweizer Monatsschrift für Zahnmedizin* 119 (6): 576–583.

Sheridan, J., Aggleton, M., and Carson, T. (2001). Dental health and access to dental treatment: a comparison of drug users and non-drug users attending community pharmacies. *Brit. Dent. J.* 191 (8): 453–457.

Shetty, V., Mooney, L.J., Zigler, C.M. et al. (2010). The relationship between methamphetamine use and increased dental disease. *J. Am. Dent. Assoc.* 141 (3): 307–318.

Shetty, V., Harrell, L., Murphy, D.A. et al. (2015). Dental disease patterns in methamphetamine users: findings in a large urban sample. *J. Am. Dent. Assoc.* 146 (12): 875–885. Cited in: Rossow, I., 2021. Illicit drug use and oral health. *Addiction,* 116(11), pp.3235-3242.

Shetty, V., Harrell, L., Clague, J. et al. (2016). Methamphetamine users have increased dental disease: a propensity score analysis. *J. Dent. Res.* 95 (7): 814–821.

Smit, D.A. and Naidoo, S. (2015). Oral health effects, brushing habits and management of methamphetamine users for the general dental practitioner. *Bri. Dent. J.* 218 (9): 531–536. Cited in: Rossow, I., 2021. Illicit drug use and oral health. *Addiction*, 116(11), pp.3235-3242.

Titsas, A. and Ferguson, M.M. (2002). Impact of opioid use on dentistry. *Aust. Dent. J.* 47 (2): 94–98.

Truong, A., Higgs, P., Cogger, S. et al. (2015). Oral health-related quality of life among an Australian sample of people who inject drugs. *J. Public Health Dent.* 75 (3): 218–224.

Van Boekel, L.C., Brouwers, E.P., Van Weeghel, J., and Garretsen, H.F. (2013). Stigma among health professionals towards patients with substance use disorders and its consequences for healthcare delivery: systematic review. *Drug Alcohol Depend.* 131 (1–2): 23–35.

Versteeg, P.A., Slot, D.E., Van Der Velden, U., and Van Der Weijden, G.A. (2008). Effect of cannabis usage on the oral environment: a review. *Int. J. Dent. Hyg.* 6 (4): 315–320.

World Health Organization (2022a). ICD-11 for mortality and morbidity statistics. https://icd.who.int/browse11/l-m/en#/http://id.who.int/icd/entity/1934475925 (accessed 30 March 2022).

World Health Organization (2022b). Drugs (psychoactive). https://www.who.int/health-topics/drugs-psychoactive#tab=tab_1about:blank - tab=tab_1 (accessed 30 March 2022).

Ye, T., Sun, D., Dong, G. et al. (2018). The effect of methamphetamine abuse on dental caries and periodontal diseases in an Eastern China city. *BMC Oral. Health. 18* (1): 1–6. Cited in: Rossow, I., 2021. Illicit drug use and oral health. Addiction, 116(11), pp.3235–3242.

6

Human Papillomavirus as a Risk Factor for Oropharyngeal Squamous Cell Carcinoma

Elizabeth Marsh

University of Derby, Derby, UK

Human papillomaviruses are small DNA viruses of the *Papillomaviridae* family that cause a number of papillomas, including common warts, verrucae, and genital warts. They are found across the world, and more than 160 different viruses (viral types) have been described (Burk et al. 2013). Most human papillomavirus (HPV) infections are low risk; some are even asymptomatic, whilst others cause benign papillomas, although these papillomas can persist over time and can be challenging to limit in immunocompromised individuals (Doorbar et al. 2012). However, 15 viral types are considered high-risk or cancer-causing HPVs. These high-risk viruses, which include two of the types the current UK vaccine protects against (HPV16 and HPV18), are predominantly known for causing cervical cancer as well as other genital cancers; they are reviewed in Doorbar et al. (2012).

Most infections – even with high-risk viruses – will be naturally cleared by the immune system and will not develop into cancer. However, in instances where infections are not cleared, the persistence of high-risk viral infections allows viral proteins that drive oncogenesis to interfere with normal cell function, leading to transformation and, ultimately, cancer (Doorbar et al. 2012). HPVs cause 99% of cervical cancers, with HPV16 and HPV18 the most prevalent types (about 70% of these) (Castle and Maza 2016).

HPV in Head and Neck Cancer

For the past 20 years or so, the incidence of a subset of head and neck cancers (HNCs), oropharyngeal squamous cell carcinoma (OPSCC), primarily in the palatine and lingual tonsils, has been increasing in the UK and across the world (Chaturvedi et al. 2013). We now know that these cancers are associated with oral HPV infection, and the WHO formally recognised HPV as a distinct cause of OPSCC in 2017 (World Health Organization 2017). This association is dominated by the presence of high-risk type HPV16 in 90% of HPV-positive OPSCC (Kreimer et al. 2005). Individuals presenting with HPV-positive OPSCC are generally much younger than those with HPV-negative HNC; they tend to be healthy individuals, male, and the prognosis is often better than for HPV-negative HNC (Chaturvedi et al. 2013; Ang et al. 2010). It was predicted that the incidence of HPV-positive OPSCC was due to overtake that of cervical cancer in 2020 (Chaturvedi et al. 2011; Mourad et al. 2017); however, other studies have suggested that the incidence has now stabilised (Nulton et al. 2018). The clinical burden of HPV-mediated oropharyngeal disease is estimated to be more than 29 000 cases a year, about a third of the global cancers at this site (de Martel et al. 2017).

The incidence rates of HPV-positive OPSCC, and the prevalence levels of oral HPV infections, vary significantly across the literature; there are considerable worldwide differences in distribution as well as reporting differences based upon the method used to detect the virus. In the healthy community (those without OPSCC), HPV prevalence ranges from 0% in the populations sampled to 23.2% (do Sacramento et al. 2006; D'Souza et al. 2009; Esquenazi et al. 2010; Pickard et al. 2012; Tristao et al. 2012; Gillison et al. 2012; Matos et al. 2015; Knight et al. 2016; Conway et al. 2016; Mehanna et al. 2019a, D'Souza et al. 2014; Kreimer et al. 2013; Lupato et al. 2017; Antonsson et al. 2021; Sonawane et al. 2017). Studies examining the persistence of HPV in the oropharynx suggest that infections are generally transient with most, but not all, infections undetectable within two years (Pickard et al. 2012; Edelstein et al. 2012; Kreimer et al. 2013; Kero et al. 2014; Zhang

Care of Head and Neck Cancer Patients for Dental Hygienists and Dental Therapists, First Edition. Edited by Jocelyn J. Harding.

et al. 2017; Wood et al. 2017; Antonsson et al. 2021; D'Souza et al. 2020). Interestingly, changes in the oral mucosa were observed in 50.1% of participants at the final follow-up in one of the persistence studies (Kero et al. 2014), suggestive of potential HPV-associated lesions, although the appearance of such lesions in the oropharynx is contested by others (Palmer et al. 2014).

The viral lifecycle within the oral mucosa is relatively unknown. Most HPV-positive tumours originate within the tonsillar crypt: deep, specialised, pocket-like structures of stratified epithelium that offer an interface with the immune system (Tang et al. 1995). It is therefore believed that this is where HPV infections also establish, and HPV has been shown to be localised to the biofilm of the tonsillar crypt (Rieth et al. 2018), though this association of HPV DNA within the tonsillar crypt is believed to be very rare (Palmer et al. 2014). The tonsil is an unusual area to host an HPV infection as its cell biology is not seen as fully permissible to host a 'normal' HPV viral infection; it is proposed that this unusual cell biology could be the reason why HPV is more likely to persist and cause cancer (rather than be a benign and cleared infection) in this region of the mouth, as is the case for cervical HPV cancers (Roberts et al. 2019).

The pathogenesis of oral HPV within the healthy (noncancerous) population is largely undetermined, and what we know is from retrospective studies, although *in vitro* model systems are being developed to elucidate viral pathogenesis in mediating OPSCC prospectively (Israr et al. 2016; Evans et al. 2017; Engelmann et al. 2020; Facompre et al. 2020). Active transcription of the viral oncogenes E6, E6*, and E7 is clinically relevant within HPV-positive OPSCC (Jung et al. 2010; Bishop et al. 2012; Nulton et al. 2017), and integration of the viral episome into the host genome (an established step for the development of cervical cancer (McBride and Warburton 2017)) is found in HPV-positive OPSCC and associated with a poor clinical outcome (Nulton et al. 2018). However, there is also evidence for the viral episome to remain extrachromosomal as well as form a 'viral-human DNA hybrid episome' in some tumours, where the viral genome has integrated into the human genome but subsequently been excised to form an episomal structure consisting of both human and viral DNA (Nulton et al. 2017). The clinical implications of this new viral state are yet to be established.

Recent work examining HPV-positive OPSCC at different stages of disease has described potential biomarkers that may inform clinical prognosis and influence treatment strategies, including differential expression of epidermal growth factor receptor (EGFR, a protein involved in tumorigenesis), p16 (a tumour suppressor involved in the cell cycle), yes-associated protein 1 (YAP1) (another oncogene involved in cell growth and apoptosis), programmed cell death protein 1 (PD-1)/programmed death-ligand 1 (PD-L1) (involved in the immune response to tumours), various micro-RNAs (involved in regulating gene expression), and HPV DNA itself (Badoual et al. 2013; Quabius et al. 2017; Eun et al. 2017; Lu et al. 2017; Camacho et al. 2018; Taberna et al. 2018; Koenigs et al. 2019; Mena et al. 2018; Hong et al. 2019). However, there have been very few investigations examining the prospective value of biomarkers for the transformation and development of OPSCC within precancerous tissues (Gultekin et al. 2015; Nankivell et al. 2014; Mooren et al. 2014).

Ultimately, unlike for cervical cancer, we simply do not know how HPV causes OPSCC, and there is a limited understanding of the natural history (prevalence, pathogenesis, and persistence) of HPV infections within the oropharynx. Research is urgently needed to address this shortfall in our knowledge and improve disease outcomes for individuals.

Risk Factors for HPV-Positive OPSCC

Whilst oral HPV is, in itself, a significant risk factor for HNC, there are other lifestyle factors that are associated with oral HPV infections and may also influence the persistence and oncogenic potential of the virus, thereby mediating the development of HPV-positive OPSCC.

Gender

The most significant risk factor for HPV-mediated OPSCC is gender: men have a higher incidence of oral HPV (Chaturvedi et al. 2008) and are six times more likely to be infected with the high-risk viral type HPV16 (Sonawane et al. 2017). The prevalence of oral HPV infection in men and women was reported to be 11.5% and 3.2%, respectively, within the large-scale National Health and Nutritional Examination Survey 2011–2014 population study in the US (Sonawane et al. 2017). These data therefore suggest a fundamental difference in the pathogenesis of oropharyngeal HPV infections between men and women, or that previous genital infections offer systemic protection in women (Safaeian et al. 2010) but not in men (Lu et al. 2012; Windon et al. 2019).

We do not know whether gender is associated with the pathogenesis and persistence of oral infection. No significant difference in viral load of high-risk HPV infections (a prognostic indicator for the development of HPV-associated cervical cancer (Schlecht et al. 2003)) between men and women has been observed (Chaturvedi et al. 2014), suggesting that viral load alone cannot explain the increased prevalence of HPV-positive OPSCC in men. Interestingly, men have lower circulating HPV antibodies than women, despite higher infections, but this is likely to reflect vaccination status (Brouwer et al. 2015).

Sexual Behaviours

As with genital HPV, oral HPV infections are believed to be sexually transmitted (D'Souza and Dempsey 2011). Several studies have suggested that the practice of oral sex increases the risk of transmission, as well as the prevalence, of oral HPV (D'Souza et al. 2009; D'Souza et al. 2014; D'Souza et al. 2016; Knight et al. 2016; Dalla Torre et al. 2016; Sánchez-Vargas et al. 2010; Oliver et al. 2018; Drake et al. 2021). Oral HPV is also believed to be transmitted during open-mouth, or deep, kissing (D'Souza et al. 2009), with saliva able to carry HPV particles (Pickard et al. 2012).

Smoking

Smoking is independently associated with oral HPV infection upon multivariable analysis (D'Souza et al. 2009; Kreimer et al. 2011; Kreimer et al. 2013; Gillison et al. 2012; Pickard et al. 2012; Sonawane et al. 2017; Dalla Torre et al. 2016), potentially as a result of its immunosuppressive activity (Arnson et al. 2010), the loss of the protective function of the epithelial-barrier due to cigarette smoke damage (Olivera et al. 2007), or a direct synergy between smoke and viral activity (Aguayo et al. 2020). Smoking also contributes to malignant transformation of oral tissues (Jethwa and Khariwala 2017) and may therefore directly influence HPV-mediated OPSCC. In HPV-positive OPSCC, smoking has a detrimental impact upon an individual's response to treatment (Ang et al. 2010; Elhalawani et al. 2020).

Alcohol Use

Similarly, drinking behaviours are also associated with oral HPV infection and HPV-positive OPSCC, although the picture isn't as clear as it is for smoking, with some studies supporting the association, whilst others do not find a link (Gillison et al. 2012; Farsi et al. 2017; Sonawane et al. 2017; Pickard et al. 2012; D'Souza et al. 2009). Potentially, there may be a direct effect of alcohol use upon oral HPV infections, or instead drinking behaviours may correlate with other risk-taking behaviours, including sexual risks.

HPV-Positive OPSCC

HPV infections occur when young and then persist for many years, so there is a considerable delay between the infection and the onset of OPSCC years, or even decades, later. The presentation of HPV-mediated OPSCC is typically in younger men who do not drink or smoke excessively (Gillison et al. 2014). There is no screening practice for oral HPV (as there is for cervical cancer), and this disease is often diagnosed late as cystic metastases, with significant morbidity and mortality (Paver et al. 2020).

Implications for Treatment

Individuals with HPV-mediated OPSCC respond much better to treatment than those with HPV-negative OPSCC, and, survival outcomes are much improved (Ang et al. 2010). This could be because of their younger age and better general health, and because the activity of key tumour-suppressor genes such as *p53* are suppressed by the virus and therefore wild-type, not mutated as they are in HPV-negative HNC. There is, therefore, a strong case for the de-intensification of treatment for HPV-mediated OPSCC given the improved responses of these individuals to therapies that are highly toxic and result in significant morbidity. Clinical trials examining radiation dose reduction are showing promising results (Rosenberg and Vokes 2021). Immunotherapies are also being tested for efficacy, but recent reports have actually shown that de-escalating treatment with the EGFR inhibitor, cetuximab, over the usual regimen of cisplatin chemotherapy, results in worse, not better, tumour control (Gillison et al. 2019; Mehanna et al. 2019b). There is a clear need for a better understanding of how HPV causes OPSCC, and the pathophysiology of disease, to inform targeted therapies and predict treatment response for patient stratification.

The Role of Vaccination

The HPV vaccination programme for adolescent girls to reduce the incidence of cervical cancer was introduced across the world from 2007 and into the UK in 2008. A quadrivalent vaccine protecting against two low-risk HPV types, 6 and 11, which cause genital warts, as well as high further risk types HPV16 and 18 (Merck) is currently used in the UK, and Merck have now licensed a 9-valent vaccine that offers further protection against other high-risk HPV strains.

The HPV vaccination programme has proved to be highly efficacious for reducing cervical HPV infection and cancer worldwide (Drolet et al. 2019; Porras et al. 2020). Interestingly, a number of countries (including the UK from 2019) have adopted gender-neutral vaccination programmes in recent years, with other countries recommending vaccination of adolescent boys as HPV vaccines offer protection to male genital infections, with increasing evidence suggesting protection for oral HPV infections (Herrero et al. 2013; Handisurya et al. 2016; Mehanna et al. 2019a; Castillo et al. 2019). The impact of vaccination on oral HPV infection within the healthy population will become clearer with time; however, there is a significant proportion of the global population who remain at risk of HPV-positive OPSCC (mechanisms and risk factors summarized in Figure 6.1).

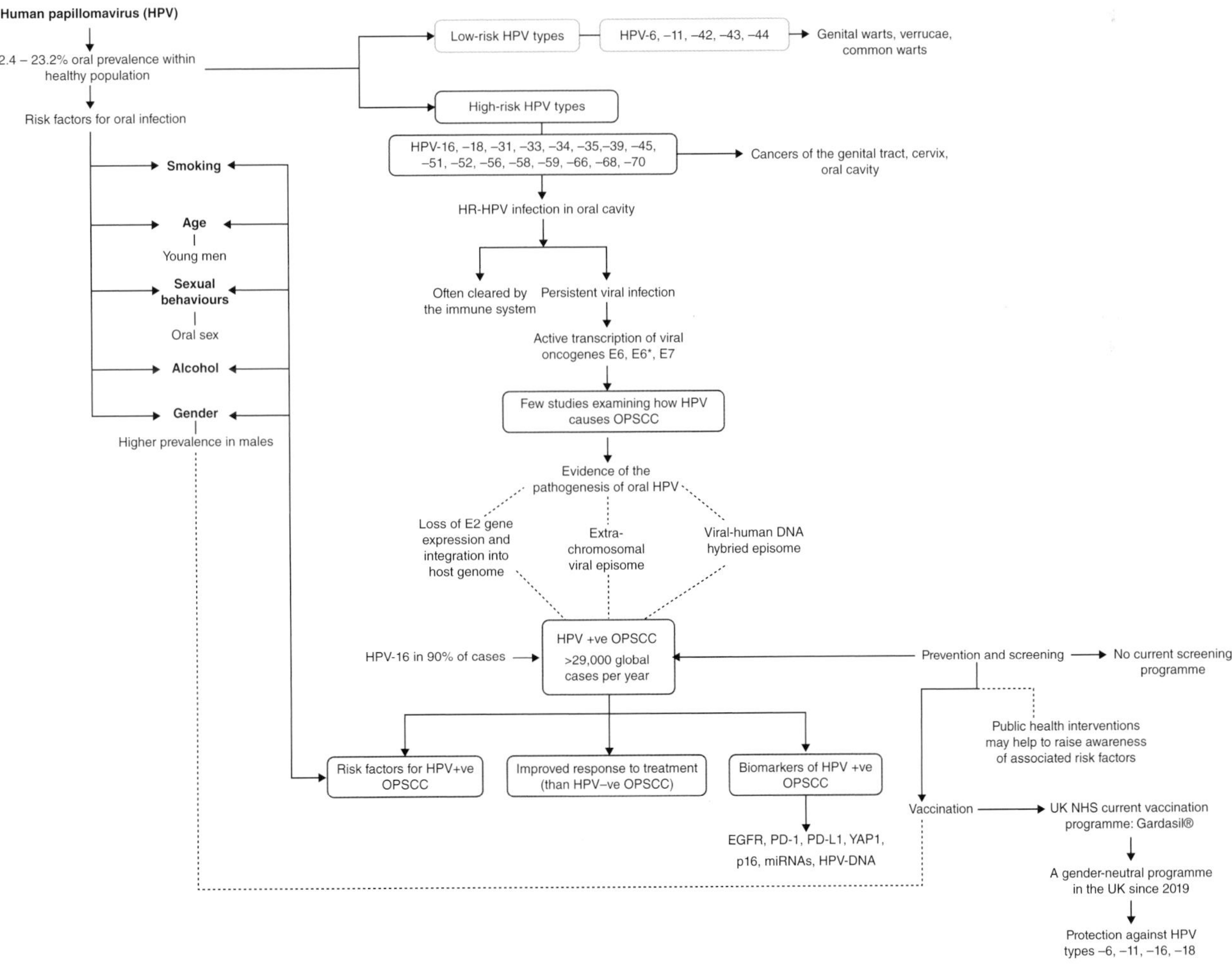

Figure 6.1 Oral HPV infection and its clinical relevance in cancer of the head and neck. A flowchart outlining the risk factors of oral HPV infection, low-risk and high-risk-HPV viral types, current pathogenesis knowledge, salient points of HPV-positive OPSCC, and preventative measures against infection. Dotted lines indicate potential relationships; solid lines show greater confidence in associations. HPV, human papillomavirus; OPSCC, oropharyngeal squamous cell carcinoma; EGFR, epidermal growth factor receptor; PD-1, programmed cell death protein 1; PD-L1, programmed death-ligand 1; YAP1, yes-associated protein 1, miRNA, microRNA; HR-HPV, high-risk human papillomavirus. *Source:* Courtesy of Mary-Anne Freckleton 2021.

References

World Health Organization (2017). *WHO Classification of Head and Neck Tumours*. Lyon: IARC Publications.

Aguayo, F., Muñoz, J.P., Perez-Dominguez, F. et al. (2020). High-risk human papillomavirus and tobacco smoke interactions in epithelial carcinogenesis. *Cancers (Basel)* 12: 2201.

Ang, K.K., Harris, J., Wheeler, R. et al. (2010). Human papillomavirus and survival of patients with oropharyngeal cancer. *N. Engl. J. Med.* 363: 24–35.

Antonsson, A., De Souza, M., Wood, Z.C. et al. (2021). Natural history of oral HPV infection: longitudinal analyses in prospective cohorts from Australia. *Int. J. Cancer* 148: 1964–1972.

Arnson, Y., Shoenfeld, Y., and Amital, H. (2010). Effects of tobacco smoke on immunity, inflammation and autoimmunity. *J. Autoimmun.* 34: J258–J265.

Badoual, C., Hans, S., Merillon, N. et al. (2013). PD-1-expressing tumor-infiltrating T cells are a favorable prognostic biomarker in HPV-associated head and neck cancer. *Cancer Res.* 73: 128–138.

Bishop, J.A., Ma, X.J., Wang, H. et al. (2012). Detection of transcriptionally active high-risk HPV in patients with head and neck squamous cell carcinoma as visualized by a novel E6/E7 mRNA in situ hybridization method. *Am. J. Surg. Pathol.* 36: 1874–1882.

Brouwer, A.F., Eisenberg, M.C., Carey, T.E., and Meza, R. (2015). Trends in HPV cervical and seroprevalence and associations between oral and genital infection and serum antibodies in NHANES 2003–2012. *BMC Infect. Dis.* 15: 575.

Burk, R.D., Harari, A., and Chen, Z. (2013). Human papillomavirus genome variants. *Virology* 445: 232–243.

Camacho, M., Aguero, A., Sumarroca, A. et al. (2018). Prognostic value of CD45 transcriptional expression in head and neck cancer. *Eur. Arch. Otorhinolaryngol.* 275: 225–232.

Castillo, A., Osorio, J.C., Fernández, A. et al. (2019). Effect of vaccination against oral HPV-16 infection in high school students in the city of Cali, Colombia. *Papillomavirus Res.* 7: 112–117.

Castle, P.E. and Maza, M. (2016). Prophylactic HPV vaccination: past, present, and future. *Epidemiol. Infect.* 144: 449–468.

Chaturvedi, A.K., Anderson, W.F., Lortet-Tieulent, J. et al. (2013). Worldwide trends in incidence rates for oral cavity and oropharyngeal cancers. *J. Clin. Oncol.* 31: 4550–4559.

Chaturvedi, A.K., Engels, E.A., Anderson, W.F., and Gillison, M.L. (2008). Incidence trends for human papillomavirus-related and -unrelated oral squamous cell carcinomas in the United States. *J. Clin. Oncol.* 26: 612–619.

Chaturvedi, A.K., Engels, E.A., Pfeiffer, R.M. et al. (2011). Human papillomavirus and rising oropharyngeal cancer incidence in the United States. *J. Clin. Oncol.* 29: 4294–4301.

Chaturvedi, A.K., Graubard, B.I., Pickard, R.K. et al. (2014). High-risk oral human papillomavirus load in the US population, National Health and Nutrition Examination Survey 2009–2010. *J. Infect. Dis.* 210: 441–447.

Conway, D.I., Robertson, C., Gray, H. et al. (2016). Human papilloma virus (HPV) oral prevalence in Scotland (HOPSCOTCH): a feasibility study in dental settings. *PLoS One* 11: e0165847.

D'Souza, G., Agrawal, Y., Halpern, J. et al. (2009). Oral sexual behaviors associated with prevalent oral human papillomavirus infection. *J. Infect. Dis.* 199: 1263–1269.

D'Souza, G., Clemens, G., Strickler, H.D. et al. (2020). Long-term persistence of oral HPV over 7 years of follow-up. *JNCI Cancer Spectr.* 4: pkaa047.

D'Souza, G. and Dempsey, A. (2011). The role of HPV in head and neck cancer and review of the HPV vaccine. *Prev. Med.* 53 (Suppl 1): S5–s11.

D'Souza, G., Gross, N.D., Pai, S.I. et al. (2014). Oral human papillomavirus (HPV) infection in HPV-positive patients with oropharyngeal cancer and their partners. *J. Clin. Oncol.* 32: 2408–2415.

D'Souza, G., Wentz, A., Kluz, N. et al. (2016). Sex differences in risk factors and natural history of oral human papillomavirus infection. *J. Infect. Dis.* 213: 1893–1896.

Dalla Torre, D., Burtscher, D., Sölder, E. et al. (2016). The impact of sexual behavior on oral HPV infections in young unvaccinated adults. *Clin. Oral Investig.* 20: 1551–1557.

De Martel, C., Plummer, M., Vignat, J., and Franceschi, S. (2017). Worldwide burden of cancer attributable to HPV by site, country and HPV type. *Int. J. Cancer* 141: 664–670.

Do Sacramento, P.R., Babeto, E., Colombo, J. et al. (2006). The prevalence of human papillomavirus in the oropharynx in healthy individuals in a Brazilian population. *J. Med. Virol.* 78: 614–618.

Doorbar, J., Quint, W., Banks, L. et al. (2012). The biology and life-cycle of human papillomaviruses. *Vaccine* 30 (Suppl 5): F55–F70.

Drake, V.E., Fakhry, C., Windon, M.J. et al. (2021). Timing, number, and type of sexual partners associated with risk of oropharyngeal cancer. *Cancer* 127: 1029–1038.

Drolet, M., Bénard, É., Pérez, N., and Brisson, M. (2019). Population-level impact and herd effects following the introduction of human papillomavirus vaccination programmes: updated systematic review and meta-analysis. *Lancet* 394: 497–509.

Edelstein, Z.R., Schwartz, S.M., Hawes, S. et al. (2012). Rates and determinants of oral human papillomavirus infection in young men. *Sex. Transm. Dis.* 39: 860–867.

Elhalawani, H., Mohamed, A.S.R., Elgohari, B. et al. (2020). Tobacco exposure as a major modifier of oncologic outcomes in human papillomavirus (HPV) associated oropharyngeal squamous cell carcinoma. *BMC Cancer* 20: 912.

Engelmann, L., Thierauf, J., Koerich Laureano, N. et al. (2020). Organotypic co-cultures as a novel 3D model for head and neck squamous cell carcinoma. *Cancers (Basel)* 12: 2330.

Esquenazi, D., Bussoloti Filho, I., Carvalho, M., and Barros, F.S. (2010). The frequency of human papillomavirus findings in normal oral mucosa of healthy people by PCR. *Braz. J. Otorhinolaryngol.* 76: 78–84.

Eun, Y.G., Lee, D., Lee, Y.C. et al. (2017). Clinical significance of YAP1 activation in head and neck squamous cell carcinoma. *Oncotarget* 8: 111130–111143.

Evans, M.R., James, C.D., Loughran, O. et al. (2017). An oral keratinocyte life cycle model identifies novel host genome regulation by human papillomavirus 16 relevant to HPV positive head and neck cancer. *Oncotarget* 8: 81892–81909.

Facompre, N.D., Rajagopalan, P., Sahu, V. et al. (2020). Identifying predictors of HPV-related head and neck squamous cell carcinoma progression and survival through patient-derived models. *Int. J. Cancer* 147: 3236–3249.

Farsi, N.J., Rousseau, M.C., Schlecht, N. et al. (2017). Aetiological heterogeneity of head and neck squamous cell carcinomas: the role of human papillomavirus infections, smoking and alcohol. *Carcinogenesis* 38: 1188–1195.

Gillison, M.L., Broutian, T., Pickard, R.K. et al. (2012). Prevalence of oral HPV infection in the United States, 2009-2010. *JAMA* 307: 693–703.

Gillison, M.L., Castellsague, X., Chaturvedi, A. et al. (2014). EUROGIN roadmap: comparative epidemiology of HPV infection and associated cancers of the head and neck and cervix. *Int. J. Cancer* 134: 497–507.

Gillison, M.L., Trotti, A.M., Harris, J. et al. (2019). Radiotherapy plus cetuximab or cisplatin in human papillomavirus-positive oropharyngeal cancer (NRG Oncology RTOG 1016): a randomised, multicentre, non-inferiority trial. *Lancet* 393: 40–50.

Gultekin, S.E., Senguven, B., Klussmann, J.P., and Dienes, H.P. (2015). P16(INK 4a) and Ki-67 expression in human papilloma virus-related head and neck mucosal lesions. *Investig. Clin.* 56: 47–59.

Handisurya, A., Schellenbacher, C., Haitel, A. et al. (2016). Human papillomavirus vaccination induces neutralising antibodies in oral mucosal fluids. *Br. J. Cancer* 114: 409–416.

Herrero, R., Quint, W., Hildesheim, A. et al. (2013). Reduced prevalence of oral human papillomavirus (HPV) 4 years after bivalent HPV vaccination in a randomized clinical trial in Costa Rica. *PLoS One* 8: e68329.

Hong, A.M., Ferguson, P., Dodds, T. et al. (2019). Significant association of PD-L1 expression with human papillomavirus positivity and its prognostic impact in oropharyngeal cancer. *Oral Oncol.* 92: 33–39.

Israr, M., Biryukov, J., Ryndock, E.J. et al. (2016). Comparison of human papillomavirus type 16 replication in tonsil and foreskin epithelia. *Virology* 499: 82–90.

Jethwa, A.R. and Khariwala, S.S. (2017). Tobacco-related carcinogenesis in head and neck cancer. *Cancer Metastasis Rev.* 36: 411–423.

Jung, A.C., Briolat, J., Millon, R. et al. (2010). Biological and clinical relevance of transcriptionally active human papillomavirus (HPV) infection in oropharynx squamous cell carcinoma. *Int. J. Cancer* 126: 1882–1894.

Kero, K., Rautava, J., Syrjanen, K. et al. (2014). Smoking increases oral HPV persistence among men: 7-year follow-up study. *Eur. J. Clin. Microbiol. Infect. Dis.* 33: 123–133.

Knight, G.L., Needham, L., Ward, D., and Roberts, S. (2016). Pilot study investigating the prevalence of oral human papilloma viral (HPV) infection in young adults. *Public Health* 132: 105–107.

Koenigs, M.B., Lefranc-Torres, A., Bonilla-Velez, J. et al. (2019). Association of estrogen receptor alpha expression with survival in oropharyngeal cancer following chemoradiation therapy. *J. Natl. Cancer Inst.* 111: 933–942.

Kreimer, A.R., Clifford, G.M., Boyle, P., and Franceschi, S. (2005). Human papillomavirus types in head and neck squamous cell carcinomas worldwide: a systematic review. *Cancer Epidemiol. Biomark. Prev.* 14: 467–475.

Kreimer, A.R., Pierce Campbell, C.M., Lin, H.Y. et al. (2013). Incidence and clearance of oral human papillomavirus infection in men: the HIM cohort study. *Lancet* 382: 877–887.

Kreimer, A.R., Villa, A., Nyitray, A.G. et al. (2011). The epidemiology of oral HPV infection among a multinational sample of healthy men. *Cancer Epidemiol. Biomark. Prev.* 20: 172–182.

Lu, B., Viscidi, R.P., Wu, Y. et al. (2012). Seroprevalence of human papillomavirus (HPV) type 6 and 16 vary by anatomic site of HPV infection in men. *Cancer Epidemiol. Biomark. Prev.* 21: 1542–1546.

Lu, Z., Zhang, H., Tao, Y. et al. (2017). MDM4 genetic variants predict HPV16-positive tumors of patients with squamous cell carcinoma of the oropharynx. *Oncotarget* 8: 86710–86717.

Lupato, V., Holzinger, D., Höfler, D. et al. (2017). Prevalence and determinants of oral human papillomavirus infection in 500 young adults from Italy. *PLoS One* 12: e0170091.

Matos, L.L., Miranda, G.A., and Cernea, C.R. (2015). Prevalence of oral and oropharyngeal human papillomavirus infection in Brazilian population studies: a systematic review. *Braz. J. Otorhinolaryngol.* 81: 554–567.

McBride, A.A. and Warburton, A. (2017). The role of integration in oncogenic progression of HPV-associated cancers. *PLoS Pathog.* 13: e1006211.

Mehanna, H., Bryant, T.S., Babrah, J. et al. (2019a). Human papillomavirus (HPV) vaccine effectiveness and potential herd immunity for reducing oncogenic oropharyngeal HPV-16 prevalence in the United Kingdom: a cross-sectional study. *Clin. Infect. Dis.* 69: 1296–1302.

Mehanna, H., Robinson, M., Hartley, A. et al. (2019b). Radiotherapy plus cisplatin or cetuximab in low-risk human papillomavirus-positive oropharyngeal cancer (De-ESCALaTE HPV): an open-label randomised controlled phase 3 trial. *Lancet* 393: 51–60.

Mena, M., Taberna, M., Tous, S. et al. (2018). Double positivity for HPV-DNA/p16(ink4a) is the biomarker with strongest diagnostic accuracy and prognostic value for human papillomavirus related oropharyngeal cancer patients. *Oral Oncol.* 78: 137–144.

Mooren, J.J., Gultekin, S.E., Straetmans, J.M. et al. (2014). P16(INK4A) immunostaining is a strong indicator for high-risk-HPV-associated oropharyngeal carcinomas and dysplasias, but is unreliable to predict low-risk-HPV-infection in head and neck papillomas and laryngeal dysplasias. *Int. J. Cancer* 134: 2108–2117.

Mourad, M., Jetmore, T., Jategaonkar, A.A. et al. (2017). Epidemiological trends of head and neck cancer in the United States: a SEER population study. *J. Oral Maxillofac. Surg.* 75: 2562–2572.

Nankivell, P., Williams, H., Webster, K. et al. (2014). Investigation of p16(INK4a) as a prognostic biomarker in oral epithelial dysplasia. *J. Oral Pathol. Med.* 43: 245–249.

Nulton, T.J., Kim, N.K., Dinardo, L.J. et al. (2018). Patients with integrated HPV16 in head and neck cancer show poor survival. *Oral Oncol.* 80: 52–55.

Nulton, T.J., Olex, A.L., Dozmorov, M. et al. (2017). Analysis of the cancer genome atlas sequencing data reveals novel properties of the human papillomavirus 16 genome in head and neck squamous cell carcinoma. *Oncotarget* 8: 17684–17699.

Oliver, S.E., Gorbach, P.M., Gratzer, B. et al. (2018). Risk factors for oral human papillomavirus infection among young men who have sex with men—2 cities, United States, 2012–2014. *Sex. Transm. Dis.* 45: 660–665.

Olivera, D.S., Boggs, S.E., Beenhouwer, C. et al. (2007). Cellular mechanisms of mainstream cigarette smoke-induced lung epithelial tight junction permeability changes in vitro. *Inhal. Toxicol.* 19: 13–22.

Palmer, E., Newcombe, R.G., Green, A.C. et al. (2014). Human papillomavirus infection is rare in nonmalignant tonsil tissue in the UK: implications for tonsil cancer precursor lesions. *Int. J. Cancer* 135: 2437–2443.

Paver, E.C., Currie, A.M., Gupta, R., and Dahlstrom, J.E. (2020). Human papilloma virus related squamous cell carcinomas of the head and neck: diagnosis, clinical implications and detection of HPV. *Pathology* 52: 179–191.

Pickard, R.K., Xiao, W., Broutian, T.R. et al. (2012). The prevalence and incidence of oral human papillomavirus infection among young men and women, aged 18–30 years. *Sex. Transm. Dis.* 39: 559–566.

Porras, C., Tsang, S.H., Herrero, R. et al. (2020). Efficacy of the bivalent HPV vaccine against HPV 16/18-associated precancer: long-term follow-up results from the Costa Rica vaccine trial. *Lancet Oncol.* 21: 1643–1652.

Quabius, E.S., Merz, I., Gorogh, T. et al. (2017). miRNA-expression in tonsillar squamous cell carcinomas in relation to HPV infection and expression of the antileukoproteinase SLPI. *Papillomavirus Res* 4: 26–34.

Rieth, K.K.S., Gill, S.R., Lott-Limbach, A.A. et al. (2018). Prevalence of high-risk human papillomavirus in tonsil tissue in healthy adults and colocalization in biofilm of tonsillar crypts. *JAMA Otolaryngol. Head Neck Surg.* 144: 231–237.

Roberts, S., Evans, D., Mehanna, H., and Parish, J.L. (2019). Modelling human papillomavirus biology in oropharyngeal keratinocytes. *Philos. Trans. R. Soc. Lond. Ser. B Biol. Sci.* 374: 20180289.

Rosenberg, A.J. and Vokes, E.E. (2021). Optimizing treatment de-escalation in head and neck cancer: current and future perspectives. *Oncologist* 26: 40–48.

Safaeian, M., Porras, C., Schiffman, M. et al. (2010). Epidemiological study of anti-HPV16/18 seropositivity and subsequent risk of HPV16 and -18 infections. *J. Natl. Cancer Inst.* 102: 1653–1662.

Sánchez-Vargas, L.O., Díaz-Hernández, C., and Martinez-Martinez, A. (2010). Detection of human papilloma virus (HPV) in oral mucosa of women with cervical lesions and their relation to oral sex practices. *Infect. Agent Cancer* 5: 25.

Schlecht, N.F., Trevisan, A., Duarte-Franco, E. et al. (2003). Viral load as a predictor of the risk of cervical intraepithelial neoplasia. *Int. J. Cancer* 103: 519–524.

Sonawane, K., Suk, R., Chiao, E.Y. et al. (2017). Oral human papillomavirus infection: differences in prevalence between sexes and concordance with genital human papillomavirus infection, NHANES 2011 to 2014. *Ann. Intern. Med.* 167: 714–724.

Taberna, M., Torres, M., Alejo, M. et al. (2018). The use of HPV16-E5, EGFR, and pEGFR as prognostic biomarkers for oropharyngeal cancer patients. *Front. Oncol.* 8: 589.

Tang, X., Hori, S., Osamura, R.Y., and Tsutsumi, Y. (1995). Reticular crypt epithelium and intra-epithelial lymphoid cells in the hyperplastic human palatine tonsil: an immunohistochemical analysis. *Pathol. Int.* 45: 34–44.

Tristao, W., Ribeiro, R.M., Oliveira, C.A. et al. (2012). Epidemiological study of HPV in oral mucosa through PCR. *Braz. J. Otorhinolaryngol.* 78: 66–70.

Windon, M.J., Waterboer, T., Hillel, A.T. et al. (2019). Sex differences in HPV immunity among adults without cancer. *Hum. Vaccin. Immunother.* 15: 1935–1941.

Wood, Z.C., Bain, C.J., Smith, D.D. et al. (2017). Oral human papillomavirus infection incidence and clearance: a systematic review of the literature. *J. Gen. Virol.* 98: 519–526.

Zhang, C., Liu, F., Pan, Y. et al. (2017). Incidence and clearance of oral human papillomavirus infection: a population-based cohort study in rural China. *Oncotarget* 8: 59831–59844.

Further Reading and Resources

European Research Organisation on Genital Infection and Neoplasia (EUROGIN): www.eurogin.com, @EUROGINHPV
Head and Neck Cancer Alliance: www.headandneck.org, @hncalliance
HPV Action Network: www.europeancancer.org/topic-networks/1:hpv-action.html, @HPVAction
HPV and Me: hpvandme.org, @hpvandmeorg
HPV Roundtable: www.headandneck.org, @HPVRoundtable
HPV World: www.hpvworld.com, @hpv_world
Jabs for the Boys: jabsfortheboys.uk, @HPVjabsforboys
NOMAN is an Island: www.nomancampaign.org, @NOMANCampaign
Oracle Cancer Trust: oraclecancertrust.org, @Oracle_Cancer
Superman HPV: www.supermanhpv.com, @SupermanHPV
Swallows Head and Neck Cancer Charity: www.theswallows.org.uk, @swallowsgroup
Throat Cancer Foundation: www.throatcancerfoundation.org, @TCF_Foundation

7

Pathologists: The Cornerstone of Head and Neck Cancer Diagnosis and Treatment

Paul Hankinson[1] *and Syed Ali Khurram*[2]

[1] *University of Sheffield, Sheffield, UK*
[2] *Unit of Oral and Maxillofacial Pathology, School of Clinical Dentistry, University of Sheffield, Sheffield, UK*

Introduction

Pathologists are one of the many members of the team caring for patients with HNC. They are either doctors or dentists who have completed specialist training in the histological diagnosis of diseases. Depending on the location where patients are treated, the pathologists aiding their care may be a general pathologist (a doctor who has completed specialist training in pathology), a general pathologist specialising in head and neck pathology (a pathologist who maintains competence in head and neck pathology), or an oral and maxillofacial pathologist (a dentist who has completed specialist training in pathology).

The pathologist is involved in the care of HNC patients at three main stages: the initial diagnosis, analysis of cancer resection specimens following surgery, and in the posttreatment monitoring to diagnose disease recurrence. There are several forms of cancer that may be diagnosed in the head and neck, including: squamous cell carcinomas (SCCs) of the mucosa, salivary gland cancers, cancers of the soft tissues and bones, lymphomas, and metastases from other sites. The majority of HNCs are SCCs of the mucosa lining the upper aerodigestive tract. Pathologists are also involved in the diagnosis of benign and 'premalignant' diseases as well as malignant ones. Of particular relevance are the potentially malignant disorders (PMDs), which are lesions with a risk of transforming into cancer and often display dysplasia on biopsy.

The Initial Diagnosis

Journey of a Cancer Biopsy

The first step of pathologist involvement is diagnosis of the initial biopsy. The laboratory will receive a biopsy of a clinically suspected cancer or a PMD. Usually, dependent on the clinical presentation, this is a piece of mucosa, though the first sign of cancer may well be a metastasis to the lymph nodes in the neck. In the latter, the tissue received is likely be a needle core biopsy (a small cylinder of tissue from a lymph node or other deep structure) or a fine needle aspirate. The tissue is received in formalin (formaldehyde in aqueous solution), which preserves it in a life-like state, preventing tissue decay and making it firm and easier to work with. The pathologist or a trained biomedical scientist (BMS) will describe the biopsy, measuring the tissue and making a note of any abnormality of the tissue visible to the naked eye. The biopsy may then be trimmed as required. Following the naked-eye description and dissection, the specimen is sent for processing (Figure 7.1).

Tissue Processing

There are several stages to processing of the tissue. First, the tissue is dehydrated and then embedded in wax to make it rigid. Following this, it is cut into very thin (usually 3–4 μm) slices, which are laid onto a glass slide before being rehydrated and then stained with haematoxylin (stains the cell nuclei blue) and eosin (stains cell cytoplasm pink) (H&E). The outcome of this process is a stained, thin section of tissue on a glass slide for viewing using a light microscope (Figure 7.1).

Care of Head and Neck Cancer Patients for Dental Hygienists and Dental Therapists, First Edition. Edited by Jocelyn J. Harding.

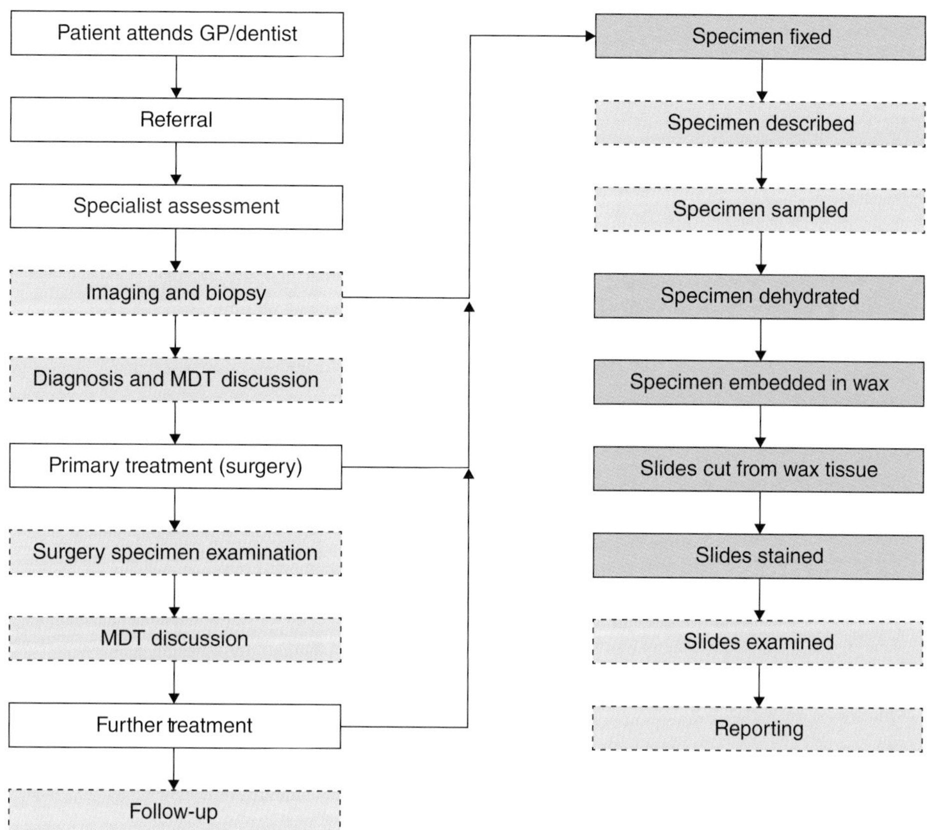

Figure 7.1 A flow diagram showing the patient (left) and specimen (right) journeys. The stages of pathologist involvement have dashed-line boxes in blue. Red boxes indicate the pathology laboratory processes. MDT, multidisciplinary team.

The pathologist can examine this tissue under a microscope at a very high magnification (usually ×20–×400) and identify any features within the tissue that may lead to the diagnosis.

Examination and Diagnosis

The main feature used to identify SCC is invasion into the tissues deep to the mucosa (Figure 7.2a). The cancer cells can show a range of abnormal appearances including variation in cell and nuclei shape and size, enlarged and dark staining nuclei, dark staining and prominent nucleoli, and abundant as well as abnormal-looking mitotic figures. Dysplastic cells also exhibit abnormal features but do not show invasion into the underlying tissues (Figure 7.2b).

Further special tests may be requested to identify features not evident on routine H&E examination. For example, p16 immunohistochemistry (IHC) is now routinely employed to determine presence of HPV infection in oropharyngeal and tonsillar cancers where it impacts staging, prognosis, and treatment decisions (Figure 7.3a). IHC can highlight and identify markers within cells and tissues that are not visible using routine H&E examination. Additionally, molecular markers of disease using fluorescence in situ hybridisation (FISH) and/or polymerase chain reaction (PCR) can be utilised. Recently, IHC for PD-L1 expression has also seen utilisation for directing treatment in recurrent and metastatic HNCs (National Institute for Care Excellence 2020) (Figure 7.3b).

Potentially Malignant Lesions

PMDs have many different clinical appearances microscopically, but most will display changes termed *dysplasia* under a microscope. The main difference between dysplasia and cancers is that the abnormal features are limited to the epithelium and there is no invasion into the underlying tissues (Figure 7.2). In addition to changes in the cells previously described, changes in the architecture of epithelium are also evaluated by a pathologist for diagnosis of dysplasia. Some common

(a)

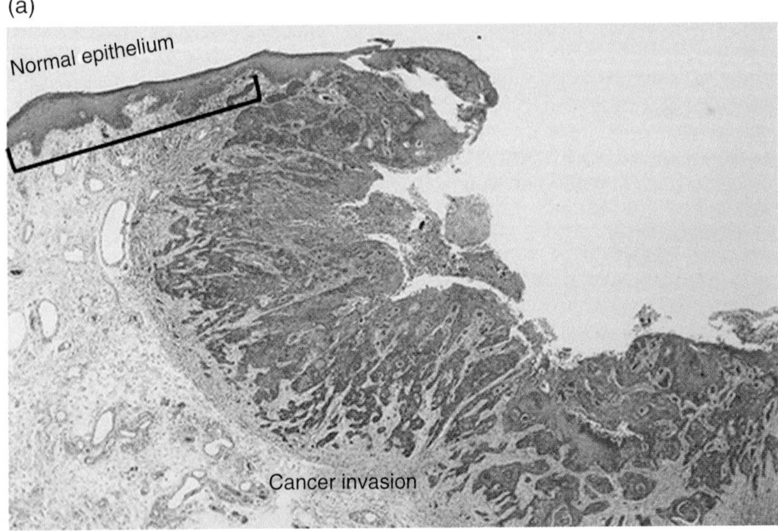

(b)

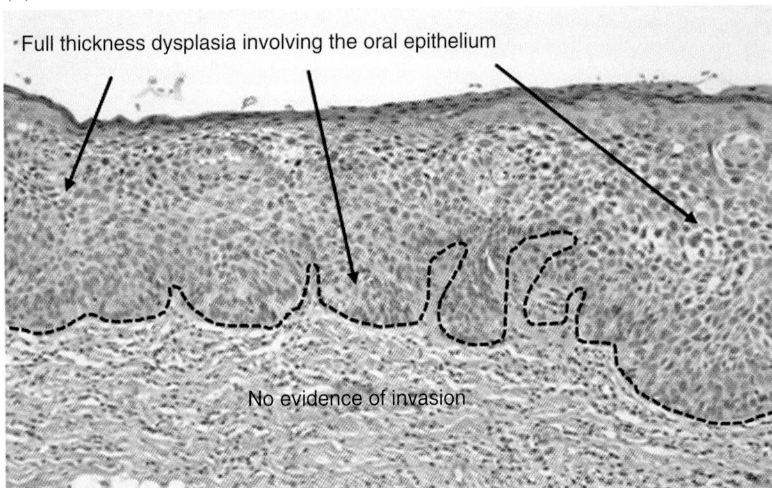

Figure 7.2 (a) Normal epithelium, left, with evidence of invasive cancer on the right. (b) Severe dysplasia with abnormal cells extending throughout the epithelium but no evidence of invasion (dotted line indicates intact epithelial basement membrane).

architectural changes include bulbous rete processes, abnormal stratification of the epithelium, and abnormal keratinisation. Oral epithelial dysplasia is usually graded using the WHO classification (Reibel et al. 2017). This splits dysplasia into three grades: mild, moderate, and severe. Mild dysplasia is characterised by abnormal cells in the deepest (basal) third of the epithelium, while in moderate and severe dysplasia the atypical features extend to the middle and superficial third of the epithelium, respectively (Figure 7.4). However, numerous studies have suggested that dysplasia grading can be subjective, with low inter- and intraobserver reliability (Kujan et al. 2006), which has led to the development of other grading systems. A dysplasia diagnosis is important, as higher-grade dysplasia in a PMD is more likely to progress to cancer (Speight et al. 2018), and patients with a higher (or severe) grade are more likely to have a closer follow-up or excision of the lesion.

Multidisciplinary Team Meeting

Once a patient has a diagnosis of HNC, they will be discussed at the multidisciplinary team meeting (MDTM), where specialists from many different clinical specialties and backgrounds involved in a patient's care come together to discuss the diagnosis, prognosis, treatment, and any issues specific to the patient such as personal, social, and health circumstances. Some of the people attending the MDTM include pathologists, oncologists, surgeons, radiologists, specialist nurses, speech and language therapists, dentists, and dieticians. In light of the pathology and radiology information, an

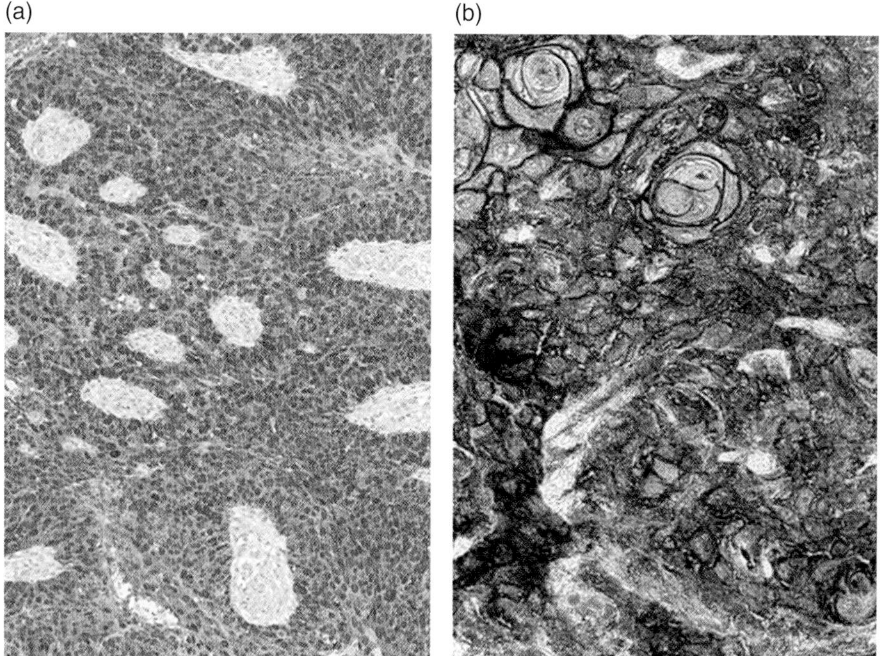

Figure 7.3 Representative immunohistochemistry images showing (a) p16 and (b) PD-L1 staining in head and neck cancers. Brown colour indicates positive staining that would guide patient treatment.

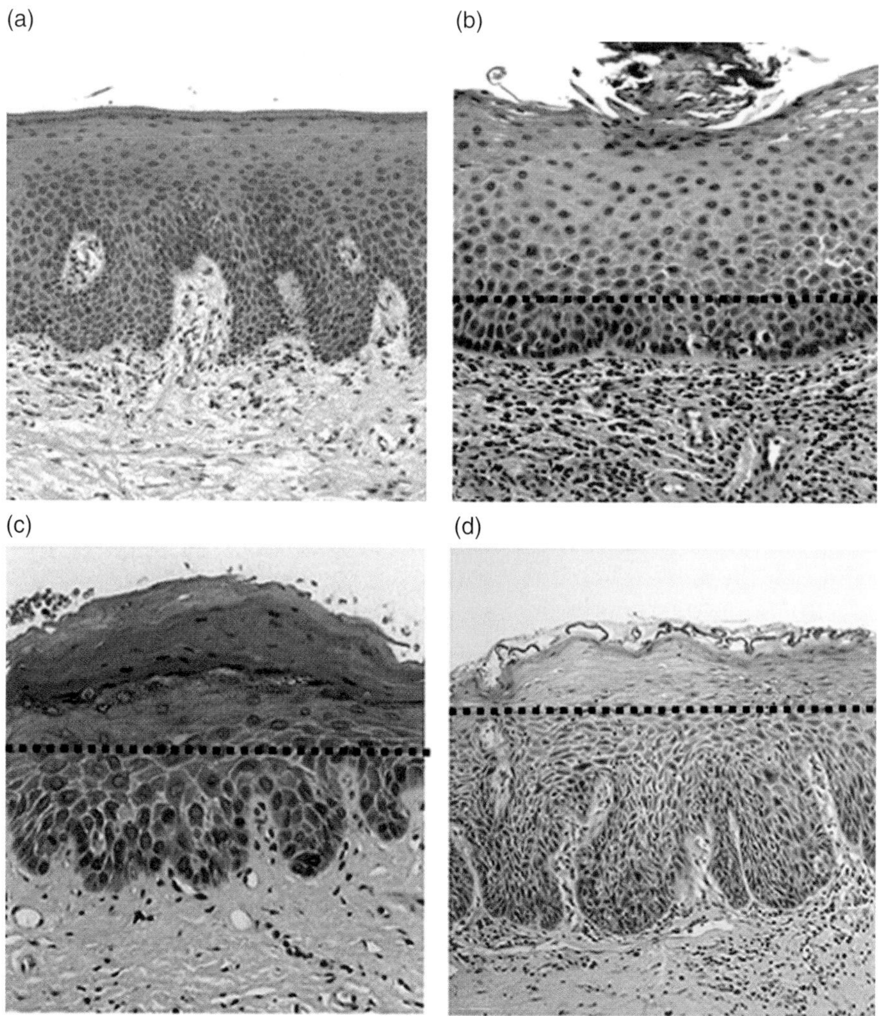

Figure 7.4 Representative histological images showing (a) normal oral mucosa, (b) mild dysplasia, (c) moderate dysplasia, and (d) severe dysplasia.

optimal treatment plan is agreed to be discussed with each patient individually. Finally, a preliminary presurgical stage is decided using the TNM (tumour, node, metastasis) system (Brierly et al. 2017). Often (especially to those with an oral cavity cancer), surgery to remove the cancer will be offered as a first line of treatment. This is routinely accompanied by a neck dissection to remove the lymph nodes from the patient's neck, allowing simultaneous detection and treatment of any regional metastasis.

Cancer Resection Specimen

Primary Tumour

Once the tumour is surgically removed or excised, the pathologist undertakes a detailed macroscopic (naked-eye) analysis and samples it appropriately. The sampled tissue slices are then thoroughly examined using a light microscope. The objectives of this evaluation include confirmation of diagnosis, accumulation of prognostic information (such as tumour size, depth, etc.), determination of the tumour proximity to surgical margins, and provision of pathological staging. Adverse features such as invasion into blood or lymphatic vessels, nerves, and bone are also documented. Tumour proximity to surgical margins (i.e. clear, close, or involved) has an impact on patient survival (Woolgar 2006), recurrence (Anderson et al. 2015), and future treatment. If residual tumour is present, it may inform a decision for further surgery or radiotherapy.

Lymph Nodes

For neck dissection specimens, the pathologist will look and feel through the fat and tissue of the neck to identify and retrieve the lymph nodes for microscopic examination. Counts of both the number of lymph nodes containing metastatic tumour and the total number of lymph nodes are tallied. The metastases are carefully examined to determine if any metastatic tumour has 'escaped' from the lymph node and shows extranodal extension (ENE) by invading into the surrounding tissues. The presence of ENE has a significant adverse impact on prognosis (Shaw et al. 2010).

The Pathology Report

All of the information collected between the initial biopsy, primary resection, and neck dissection is written into a report that must contain a minimum amount of data as per recommendations by the Royal College of Pathologists (Helliwell and Woolgar 2013a,b). This includes details of the specimen, histological features, tumour size, adverse features, metastases, and distance to surgical margins as well as tumour grade.

Postoperative Care

The pathologist remains involved in patient care, follow-up, and surveillance for disease recurrence. Where a clinician or radiologist suspects recurrent or residual disease, a tissue biopsy is taken and diagnosed by the pathologist in the same way as discussed previously. This diagnosis aids future treatment planning for that patient or provides reassurance that no recurrence has occurred.

Digital Pathology and Artificial Intelligence

In addition to the traditional approach of viewing glass slides using a light microscope and ancillary techniques such as IHC and molecular tests, there has been a more recent uptake of the use of digital pathology (DP). This is where specialised scanners are utilised to capture a high-resolution digital image of the tissue on a slide, enabling examination on a computer. DP has several benefits over traditional glass slide use including access to remote viewing, easier storage, the option of automated analysis, and no requirement of having a microscope. Remote viewing allows easy access to the images by pathologists from any location as well as rapid sharing of images for both second opinions and teaching. However, there are some disadvantages to this process, including high initial cost of scanners, validation, and digital

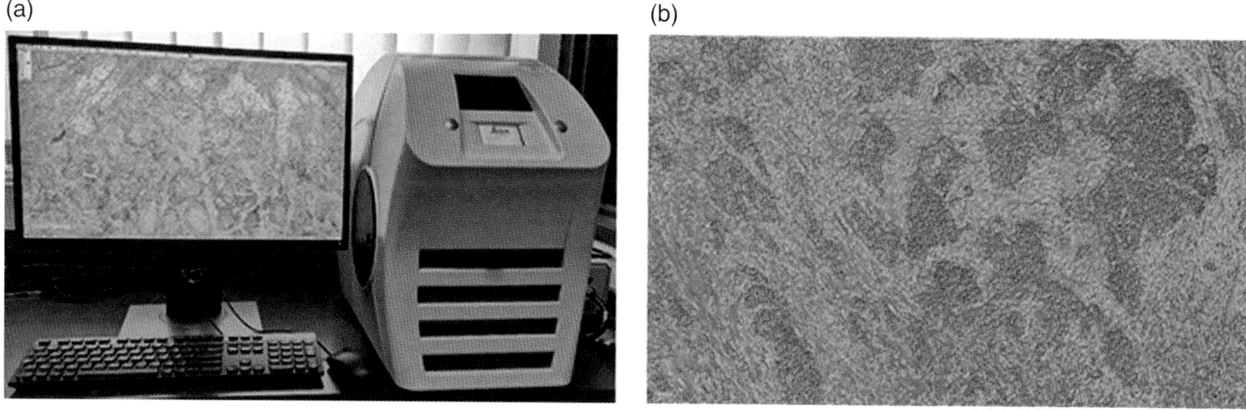

Figure 7.5 (a) A digital slide scanner with connected display and computer. (b) Automated detection of tumour, stroma, and immune cells where tumour = red, stroma = blue, and immune cells = green.

infrastructure to allow storage and retrieval of large image files (Griffin and Treanor 2017). The advent of digital pathology and acquisition of tissue slides as data has proven to be an exciting breakthrough that is allowing development of image analysis and artificial intelligence (AI) algorithms to aid pathologists. The whole slide images which are obtained from scanning tissue slides are large information rich multi-gigapixel images which can be utilised to aid diagnosis and provide prognostic information based on a digital analysis of pathological features (Figure 7.5). AI algorithms allow computers to learn from human experience and in some instances have been shown to be as (if not more) accurate than experienced pathologists, in addition to providing objective and quantifiable assessment scores of histological features (Bera et al. 2019).

In summary, the pathologist is involved in patient care at several stages, from the initial diagnosis and treatment planning through to staging and determination of further treatment following primary treatment and the diagnosis of recurrence during a patient's follow-up period. The key role of the pathologist is in the examination of tissue both macroscopically and microscopically to determine the nature of a tumour and convert this into clinically useful information, such as a diagnosis and prognosis, and therefore allow informed treatment decisions.

References

Anderson, C.R., Sisson, K., and Moncrieff, M. (2015). A meta-analysis of margin size and local recurrence in oral squamous cell carcinoma. *Oral Oncol.* 51 (5): 464–469.

Bera, K., Schalper, K.A., Rimm, D.L. et al. (2019). Artificial intelligence in digital pathology – new tools for diagnosis and precision oncology. *Nat. Rev. Clin. Oncol.* 16 (11): 703–715.

Brierly, J., Gospodarowicz, M.K., and Wittekind, C. (2017). *TNM Classification of Malignant Tumours*, 8e. Oxford, UK; Hoboken, NJ: Wiley.

Griffin, J. and Treanor, D. (2017). Digital pathology in clinical use: where are we now and what is holding us back? *Histopathology* 70 (1): 134–145.

Helliwell, T. and Woolgar, J. (2013a). *Dataset for Histopathology Reporting of Mucosal Malignancies of the Oral Cavity*. London, UK: The Royal College of Pathologists.

Helliwell, T. and Woolgar, J. (2013b). *Dataset for Histopathology Reporting of Nodal Excisions and Neck Dissection Specimens Associated with Head and Neck Carcinomas*. London, UK: The Royal College of Pathologists.

Kujan, O., Oliver, R.J., Khattab, A. et al. (2006). Evaluation of a new binary system of grading oral epithelial dysplasia for prediction of malignant transformation. *Oral Oncol.* 42 (10): 987–993.

National Institute for Health and Care Excellence (2020). Pembrolizumab for untreated metastatic or unresectable recurrent head and neck squamous cell cerainoma (TA661). https://www.nice.org.uk/guidance/ta661 (accessed 20 February 2021).

Reibel, J., Gale, N., Hille, J. et al. (2017). Oral potentially malignant disorders and oral epithelial dysplasia. In: *WHO Classification of Head and Neck Tumours*, 4e (ed. A.K. El-Naggar, J.K.C. Chan, J.R. Grandis, et al.), 112–114. Lyon: IARC.

Shaw, R.J., Lowe, D., Woolgar, J.A. et al. (2010). Extracapsular spread in oral squamous cell carcinoma. *Head Neck* 32 (6): 714–722.

Speight, P.M., Khurram, S.A., and Kujan, O. (2018). Oral potentially malignant disorders: risk of progression to malignancy. *Oral Surg. Oral Med. Oral Pathol. Oral Radiol.* 125 (6): 612–627.

Woolgar, J.A. (2006). Histopathological prognosticators in oral and oropharyngeal squamous cell carcinoma. *Oral Oncol.* 42 (3): 229–239.

8

Mental Health and Well-Being Pretreatment

Lauren Barry

York and Scarborough Teaching Hospitals NHS Foundation Trust, York, UK

Any cancer diagnosis has a far-reaching impact on people's lives and the lives of those around them. Given that *every two minutes someone in the UK is diagnosed with cancer* (Cancer research UK 2021), it is safe to assume that most people have some experience of cancer. This could be a friend, loved one, colleague, or their personal experience.

Cancer conjures up many images and feelings. It is important to remember that the emotional experience of one individual diagnosed with cancer will not always be the same as another. It may be helpful to think along the lines of 'every journey might have a different route, but there are likely some common paths shared'. Being aware of the common themes places dental hygienists and dental therapists in a good position to listen to and support our patients. However, in supporting our patients, it is not expected that we are to solve their problems or undertake any formal method of psychological support. It can be too easy to feel a need to fulfil this role when our patients come with emotional difficulties, a natural consequence of working in a caring profession. Simply being there for these patients, being able to listen, and in some cases signposting to helpful services can be important.

In psychology, a bio-psycho-social model helps practitioners to assess and understand the effects of life on an individual. This approach considers biology (our physical and physiological state and all of the processes that go with it), psychology (the emotional state and its processes), and finally the social aspects of life (a person's place in society, those that surround them, work, play, socioeconomic status, to name but a few aspects). Using this model allows practitioners to look past the single moment, in this case of a cancer diagnosis, and consider the whole person and the world the person lives in.

At the point of diagnosis, patients can feel a whirlwind of unsettling emotions. There is often a shock at diagnosis, even though it may have been expected. There may also be fear, some denial, perhaps anger, sadness, a loss of control – a whole list of unsettling emotions. It is important to remember that these are normal reactions to an incredibly stressful and life-changing situation. For this reason, a formal method of psychological support, such as referral to a therapist or psychologist, is not common. Instead, time is given to the patient to process thoughts and emotions. Jumping in too quickly with professional services can take away from this normal process.

Different people have a diverse range of coping strategies, sometimes helpful to think of as their toolkit. This is likely to be influenced by their general personality. Those who are naturally anxious and/or depressed are unfortunately liable to feel this more acutely during this time. Some patients cope by speaking to those around them and may have good social networks ready to step up and support them. Others may close down and retreat into their own world.

Some patients will seek out all of the information possible, speak to professionals, scour the Internet, find charities and support groups, and read academic papers. Others prefer not to know the full story; this is simply too much or not for them.

This pretreatment phase is often a busy time for the mind. There is a lot of information to take in at a time where doing so is likely to be very difficult. There are many decisions to be made, with long-term impacts that are difficult to imagine. It is also demanding in time, going to appointments, having tests, planning the future.

The cancer diagnosis itself and the treatment will have a wider-reaching impact than just the individual. Those around the patient will often share in the worries and fears of their loved one. The high level of emotion can put stress and strain on relationships, but it can also strengthen them.

Care of Head and Neck Cancer Patients for Dental Hygienists and Dental Therapists, First Edition. Edited by Jocelyn J. Harding.

Patients will have to stop working, at least for a period during treatment and recovery, and some may not be able to return to their regular employment long term. This has financial implications as well as the psychological impact of having to stop work or change careers. Often our employment is part of our identity.

The physical impacts of the cancer itself cannot be ignored. For some patients they may have no symptoms at all. This in itself can be confusing to patients. 'What do you mean I have cancer? I don't even feel unwell'. Those who do experience symptoms may find that these already affect their psychological state.

Lethargy, pain, and emotional stress can cloud the mind, making things that seem difficult already sometimes seem impossible. This may affect memory, at a time where the person is taking in a lot of information. The patient's ability to cope with the emotions of others may also be impaired, at a time when those around them may well be more emotional. These low-energy states impact on what a person is able to do, taking away the natural structure of day-to-day life.

It cannot be ignored that for some patients there is no pretreatment phase, as there may not be a treatment option available to them; their route is one of palliative care. This will bring with it its own psychological challenges.

A multidisciplinary team approach is required to give patients the best support possible. Throughout this book there will be an exploration of the roles of the many professionals involved in patient care. In terms of mental health and well-being, some patients will be lucky enough to have a clinical nurse specialist. They will often undertake a holistic needs assessment, using the biopsychosocial approach, and signpost the patient to reliable support services or to the information they need.

As dental hygienists and dental therapists we may see the patient during this phase. As always, listening is an important skill. An important lesson to learn as a professional is never to assume; patients often surprise us. Some will ask for a lot of detailed information, and having written information that they can take away and process later is a good option. Samples of useful oral hygiene tools (covered in later chapters) can offer practical reassurance. Most importantly, we are in a good position to encourage patients to be kind to themselves. The consequences of the treatment may impede their ability to carry out normal oral hygiene routines, and dental professionals should be realistic and understanding. Providing contact details for your service, should they need advice, is also a good step. They may not call, but you have potentially added to their coping toolkit.

Useful organisations and websites are also listed below.

Reference

Cancer Research UK (2021). Cancer incidence statistics. https://www.cancerresearchuk.org/health-professional/cancer-statistics/incidence/age%23heading-Zero (accessed 21 March 2021).

Further Reading and Resources

Cancer Research UK: https://www.cancerresearchuk.org/. General cancer support and care website with very specific information on different types of head and neck cancer.

Macmillan Cancer Support, head and neck cancer: https://www.macmillan.org.uk/cancer-information-and-support/head-and-neck-cancer. General cancer support and care website with specific information on head and neck cancer.

maxfacts: https://maxfacts.uk/. A database aimed at providing accurate information about conditions, treatment, and managing the aftereffects of treatment in the mouth, jaws, and face.

9

Flowchart

Stephanie Wright

Stephanie Wright Gloucestershire Hospitals NHS Foundation Trust Gloucester, UK

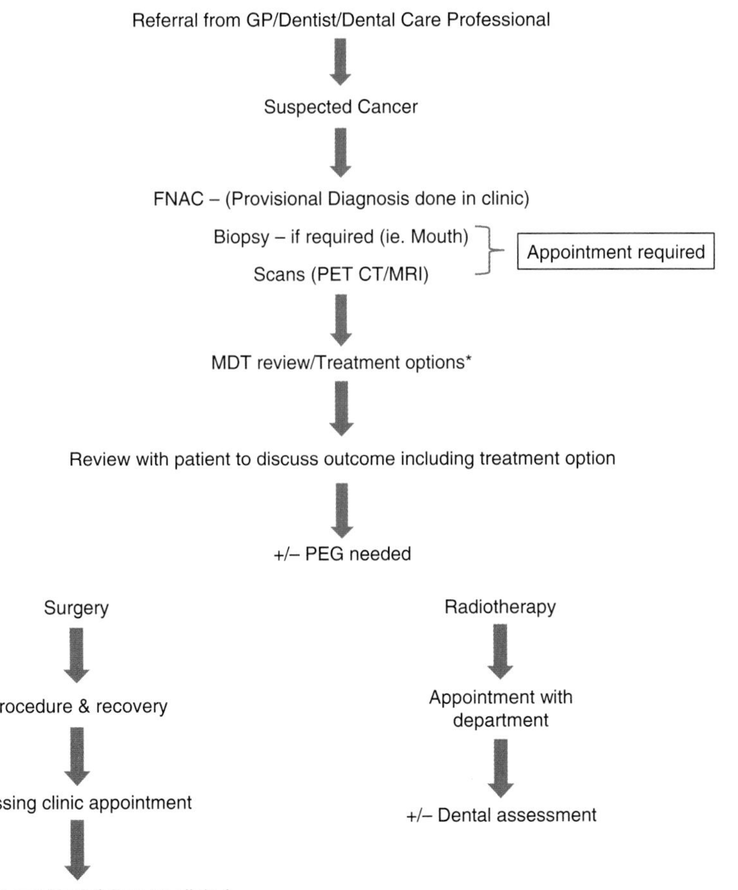

Image by Stephanie Wright.

Care of Head and Neck Cancer Patients for Dental Hygienists and Dental Therapists, First Edition. Edited by Jocelyn J. Harding.

Section 2

Specialists, Roles, and Departments

10

The Multidisciplinary Team

Lucy Baker

Portsmouth Hospitals University NHS Trust, Portsmouth, UK

Due to the complexities of treating HNC, implementation of a multidisciplinary team (MDT) approach to care is required. This approach combines an integrated team of health care professionals, from multiple specialities, collaborating on an individual's diagnosis, staging, treatment planning, management, and support (Licitra et al. 2016, 73).

This combination of expertise, knowledge, and skills offers patient-centric coordinated care, improving health and well-being outcomes for individuals whilst providing the best delivery of patient care. The MDT is an essential component of oncologic disease management. Treatment is carried out within a head and neck department in a hospital setting.

The MDT will be involved with the management of all new cases of HNC, newly identified recurrent/metastatic disease, the review following initial surgery, and cases other team members feel need MDT oversight and input (National Institute for Health and Care Excellence [NICE] 2004). Patient cases are discussed with a core team meeting, with referrals to a wider extended team of specialists depending on individual treatment needs.

The MDT will provide (Shellenberger and Weber 2018, 436):

- A complete evaluation of patients prior to commencing treatment
- Accuracy of diagnosis and staging on which to base the most appropriate treatment
- Improve outcomes of treatment with clinical experience, highest available evidence, adhering to clinical practice guidelines and treatment algorithms. Participating in clinical research trials is also considered.

The Team

Individual patient cases are discussed within the core team. The composition of the core team can vary. Guidelines will provide specific recommendations regarding the specialist that should be involved in the MDT (NICE 2004).

Although it is not compulsory for the MDT to include all types of specialist, all members should be specialised in HNC and include the range of skills required to comprehensively plan treatment for the complex treatment needs of this group of patients (NICE 2004). The intention of this team approach is to provide all patients with a comprehensive individual treatment plan, focusing on delivering the most effective care possible (Licitra et al. 2016, 75). The integration of specialties involved in a patient's care aims to reduce time to diagnosis and/or commencement of treatment.

Care of Head and Neck Cancer Patients for Dental Hygienists and Dental Therapists, First Edition. Edited by Jocelyn J. Harding.

The MDT team

Core team	
Speciality	**Role**
Head and neck surgeons/oral and maxillofacial surgeons/ear, nose, and throat surgeons	Surgical specialists proficient in the removal and reconstruction of head and neck disease.
Clinical oncologists	Clinical oncologists specialise in treating patients with head and neck cancer and are primarily responsible for radiation treatment, chemotherapy, and immunosuppressants. Involved in staging, selection of appropriate treatment options, and supervision of the treatment.
Pathologists	Assist surgeons in making an accurate diagnosis and evaluation of resection margins.
Clinical nurse specialists (CNSs)	Essential members of the MDT. Provide full support and coordination of care, acting as the patient's 'key worker' throughout the whole diagnostic and treatment process, offering continuity of care.
Radiologists	Imaging is important to assist with identifying and monitoring the diseased site when staging the extent of malignancy. The radiologist can offer discussion in case of doubt or any variation in clinical presentation, whilst imaging can determine a treatment plan.
Restorative dental consultants	Expert dental treatment is required, with dental assessments during each stage of the oncologic process. Involved in the complex needs during the oral rehabilitation of patients. Consultants are experienced in maxillofacial prosthetics and implantology.
Dieticians	Close nutritional management during treatment is important to prevent malnutrition and to adjust nutritional support. HNC patients can have complex and unique challenges due to surgery and treatment. Offer a supportive role through the individual cancer journey.
Speech and language therapists	Vocal rehabilitation, adaptation, and readjustment to aid communication and quality of life to individuals where their treatment affects communication or swallowing.
MDT meeting coordinators	Responsible for organising the MDT meetings. Ensure relevant patient documentation is available when required, with an effective system in place to track the patient journey.
Team secretaries/data managers	May also be the MDT coordinator. Assists in the organisation of the MDT weekly meeting, ensuring details, care plans, and other data are available. The secretary provides clerical support, recording, and communicating team discussions. Involved in clinical audit.

Extended team	
Speciality	**Role**
Dental hygienists/therapists	Support patients with oral hygiene and preventative advice throughout treatment and with the long-term effects of surgery/radiotherapy. Work closely with the restorative consultant during the rehabilitation process and liaise with primary dental care services.
Clinical psychologists	Profound functional and physical changes result from treatment and disease, often having a psychological impact on individuals and family. Work closely with CNS.
Dental technicians	Assist the dental restorative team in facial and oral rehabilitation with construction of maxillofacial prosthetics and implantology.
Anaesthesiologists	Aid decision-making for guiding the operative management of patients with complex head and neck pathology.
Pain management specialists	Provides advice on management of pain during treatment.
Gastroenterologists/health care professionals with expertise in gastrostomy placement	Prophylactic feeding tube percutaneous endoscopic gastrostomy (PEG) may be required to reduce the risk of malnutrition disruptions in treatment, improving quality of life and survival.
Palliative care	Provide palliative care services in the community.
Benefits advisors	The benefits advisor assists with a range of grants from Macmillan and other organisations for those experiencing financial difficulties because of their illness.
Dermatologists	Provide specialist advice to the team regarding skin cancers.

Extended team	
Speciality	**Role**
Physiotherapists/occupational therapists	Provide support with patients returning to independence following treatment. Patients may have reduced mobility of neck and shoulder after surgery.
Social workers	Clinical social workers are involved in the assessment and interventions for managing a patient's psychosocial distress.
Counsellors	Profound functional and physical changes result from treatment and disease, often having a psychological impact on individuals and family.

Based on NICE (2004).

The MDT becomes involved in the patient journey during the initial diagnosis and treatment planning stage. A treatment plan is devised dependent on the individual's disease, comorbidities, health performance status, and treatment goals. The suitability for relevant clinical trials is also explored (Licitra et al. 2016, 75).

The MDT will be involved throughout the management of disease, recovery, or when a new management plan is required due to relapse or new disease. Objectives, outcomes, and side effects of treatment will be discussed.

The MDT have weekly sessional meetings chaired by a lead clinician. The MDT coordinator arranges and ensures all of the relevant patient information is available to the team, including diagnostic imaging and pathology. It is important all team members are allocated sessions beforehand to prepare, resulting in an efficient and succinct meeting outcome.

Established protocols for documenting patient outcomes and the capture of decisions made at the MDT meeting, alongside comprehensible communication with primary care providers, are essential. Regular data collection for audit is required to confirm MDTs are providing fully comprehensive, effective, and consistent care whist adhering to relevant guidelines. Teams are also reviewed to ensure they have the appropriately trained professionals involved in the decision process.

Evidence suggests this MDT approach to patient care positively impacts both the patients and team members, resulting in a higher quality of decision-making and improved clinical outcomes. The MDT provides a suitable setting to collect, collate and review each patient's progress. This approach also reduces time to treatment (Bradley 2012, 2451).

References

Bradley, P. (2012). Multidisciplinary clinical approach to the management of head and neck cancer. *Eur. Arch. Otorhinolaryngol.* 2451–2454. https://doi.org/10.1007/s00405-012-2209-y.

Licitra, L., Keilholz, U., Thara, M. et al. (2016). Evaluation of the benefit and use of multidisciplinary teams in the treatment of head and neck cancer. *Oral Oncol.* 59: 73–79. https://doi.org/10.1016/joraloncology.2016.06.002.

National Institute for Health and Care Excellence. (2004). Improving outcomes in head and neck cancers [NICE cancer service guideline CSG6]. https://www.nice.org.uk/guidance/csg6

Shellenberger, T.D. and Weber, R.S. (2018). Multidisciplinary team planning for patients with head and neck cancer. *Oral Maxillofac. Surg. Clin. North Am.* 30 (4): 435–444. https://doi.org/10.1016/j.coms.2018.06.005.

11

History of Oral and Maxillofacial Surgery

Mahesh Kumar

Northwick Park Hospital and the Hillingdon Hospitals NHS Trusts, London, UK

Oral and maxillofacial surgery (OMFS) is a medical specialty involved in the diagnosis and management of conditions of the mouth, jaws, face, and neck. It is unique as a specialty as it requires dual registerable qualifications in both dentistry and medicine. The majority of practitioners started with the dental pathway and then proceeded to a medical qualification. However, since recently becoming a medical specialty, many trainees are pursuing the dental degree after medicine. OMFS appeals to many surgical trainees who previously would have considered plastic and reconstructive and ear, nose, and throat (ENT) surgery, as it offers both the hard and soft tissue aspects in the anatomical area of the head and neck, with a huge variety of subspecialty interests. OMFS covers areas including oral surgery, craniofacial trauma, head and neck cancer, reconstructive, facial deformity, salivary gland, skin cancer, facial aesthetic/cosmetics, temporomandibular joint, skull base, cleft lip, and palate surgery.

Historically, OMFS arose from oral surgery. Dental surgeons with an interest in the injuries and deformities caused during two world wars developed new skills in the specialty of oral surgery alongside modern plastic and reconstructive surgery. Many surgeons were dentally qualified and worked with their medical colleagues developing their techniques fixing fractures of the jaws and facial skeleton in injured servicemen. The dexterity of the oral surgeons allowed the injured to recover some function of their jaws and reduced the resulting deformities.

Following the Second World War, it became clear that a medical qualification would be advantageous to the future of the specialty. With the advent of the motor vehicle and the rapid growth in number and speeds, it became commonplace to see high-velocity road traffic collisions involving cars and motorcycles presenting to accident and emergency departments across the UK. Although front seat belts were installed into cars in the UK from 1968, it did not become compulsory to wear a seat belt until 1983. Almost overnight this reduced the numbers of panfacial fractures across the country. The number and severity of injures has also reduced since the use of rear seat belts and air bags.

In the 1980s, many dentally qualified surgeons who went back to medical school completed the full Fellowship of the Royal College of Surgeons Certificate in General Surgery. This meant that after basic surgical training, they had experience in specialties such as ENT surgery, plastics and reconstructive, and neurosurgery. This allowed OMFS to surgically manage head and neck patients who were previously being treated by our ENT head and neck colleagues.

OMFS and the Multidisciplinary Team

Modern-day care of HNC patients is truly multidisciplinary. The MDT involves, MDT coordinators, surgeons, radiation and medical oncologists, radiologists, cytopathologists, histopathologists, restorative dental surgeons, clinical nurse specialists (CNSs), dietitians, speech and language therapists (SLTs), and dental hygienists and therapists, although many MDTs do not have funding for dental-allied health professionals.

In the UK, head and neck cancer is managed by maxillofacial and otolaryngologist (ENT) specialist surgeons with input from plastic and reconstructive and neurosurgeons. Skull base cancers will often involve neurosurgeons, especially if the tumour invades the into the meninges or brain.

Care of Head and Neck Cancer Patients for Dental Hygienists and Dental Therapists, First Edition. Edited by Jocelyn J. Harding.

The otolaryngologist in cancer surgery within an MDT will manage the oropharyngeal cancers, that is, tonsils and tongue base disease and laryngeal disease as well as thyroid cancers. The larynx is subdivided into supraglottic (above the vocal cords), glottic (involves the cords), and infraglottic (below the cords). With the advent of minimal access surgery, many of the procedures are carried out with endoscopes, e.g. transoral laser microsurgery (TLM) and transoral robotic surgery (TORS). These novel procedures reduce the morbidity (patient complications) and length of stay in hospital.

Where the larger cancers of the throat and voice box have failed primary treatment such as radiotherapy (RT) and chemotherapy, or if the disease has involved the cartilage of the voice box, major surgery may be required. The removal of the voice box (larynx) is known as a *laryngectomy*. The removal of the voice box and part of the throat is a laryngopharyngectomy. The voice can be reconstructed artificially with an electronic device or substituted with air being diverted with a valve through the oesophagus (gullet) into the throat. Where the throat is removed, the tissue may require replacement with a flap. This may be local or regional skin (deltopectoral flap from the shoulder) or a pedicled flap from the chest wall muscle (a pectoralis major flap from the front of the chest). Free flaps can also be used where skin and fascia is taken from a donor site such as the thigh or the small bowel (jejunal flap) and transferred to reconstruct the throat.

Plastic and reconstructive surgeons are often involved in these cases where complex reconstructions are needed within the MDT. However, many head and neck surgeons are now trained in microvascular surgical techniques, with the reconstruction carried out themselves in two-team operating.

Although the NHS has set up a two-week pathway for referral of suspected cancer patients, many patients still present through routine referrals and via the accident and emergency department. The rapid access pathway is available for general medical and dental practitioners. The value of the urgent two-week suspected cancer pathway is that the NHS has funded this appropriately, so it is adequately resourced with staffing and administrative support.

The Cancer Patient's Journey: Clinical History and Examination, Imaging, and Biopsy

The patient attends an outpatient clinic and is consulted by a senior clinician. A full history and head and neck examination are carried out. Often a specialist will visualise the back of the throat with a nasendoscope, using a flexible endoscope with direct visualisation either via an eyepiece or a monitor screen (see Figure 11.1). This allows inspection of tumours that

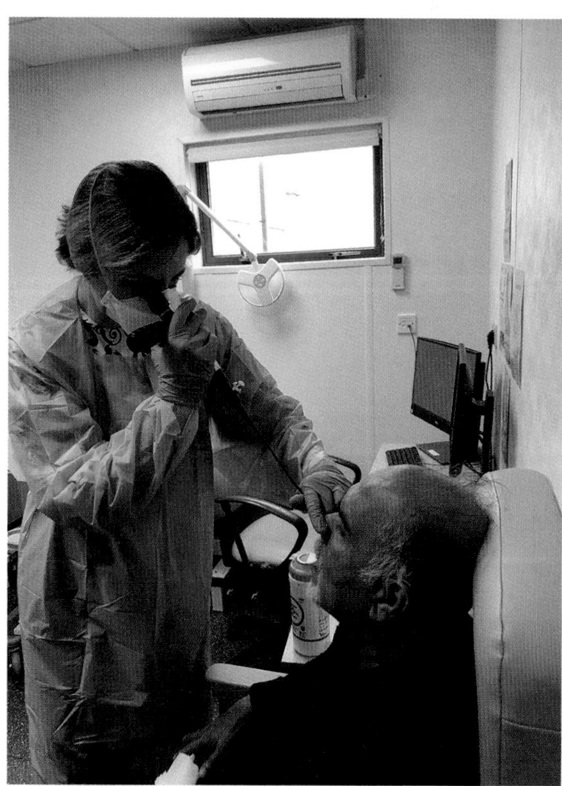

Figure 11.1 Nasendoscopy shows a direct view of the posterior nasal, oral, and laryngopharynx spaces.

arise from or extend into the pharynx (throat) or larynx (voice box). If there is an obvious tumour, then often the imaging is arranged first before the biopsy is carried out. This is so that there is no distortion of the area with stigmata of the biopsy affecting the interpretation of the head and neck images.

Many two-week wait clinics offer a one-stop service where the patient is offered an ultrasound scan (USS) to assess if there is neck disease. The USS is very sensitive to show changes in the anatomy of lymph nodes, which can be changes in size, shape, and internal texture such as loss of their normal fatty hilum through which the blood supply and lymphatic drainage of the node occurs. Lymph nodes are generally enlarged with cancer or inflammation. However, smaller lymph nodes can have metastatic cancer and appear more solid and rounded. If abnormality is detected, the ultrasonographer can either collect a needle sample of cell known as a *fine needle aspirate cytology/fine needle aspirate biopsy* (FNAC/FNAB) or take a core tissue sample (core biopsy). The benefit of the core biopsy is that it can provide more information on the cells within the tissues rather than just identify cancer cells or not. However, core biopsies require more patient compliance and risk increase of discomfort and complications.

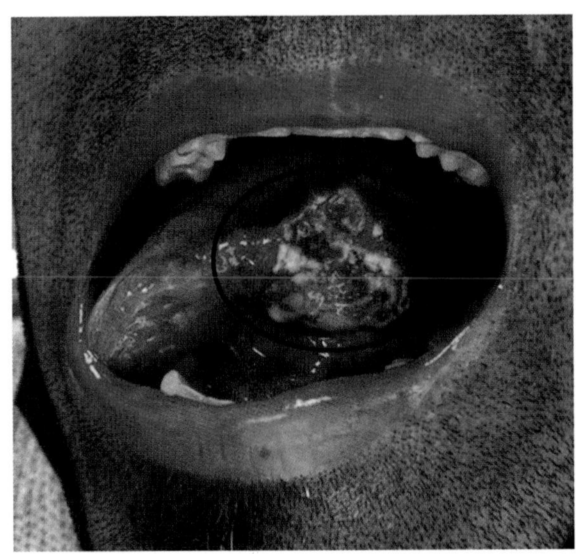

Figure 11.2 Left lateral carcinoma of the tongue (black outline).

Most units (depending on resources) arrange for magnetic resonance (MR) for the head and neck primary and locoregional neck disease and computerised tomography (CT) for distant disease in the chest or for bony skeletal involvement (see Figures 11.2 and 11.3). An orthopantomogram (OPG) is useful if there is suspicion of tumour involvement in the jaw bones; however, this will be further evaluated with both MR and CT scans. The OPG will allow for dental assessment prior to surgical and RT planning. Teeth with pathology or extensive restorations in

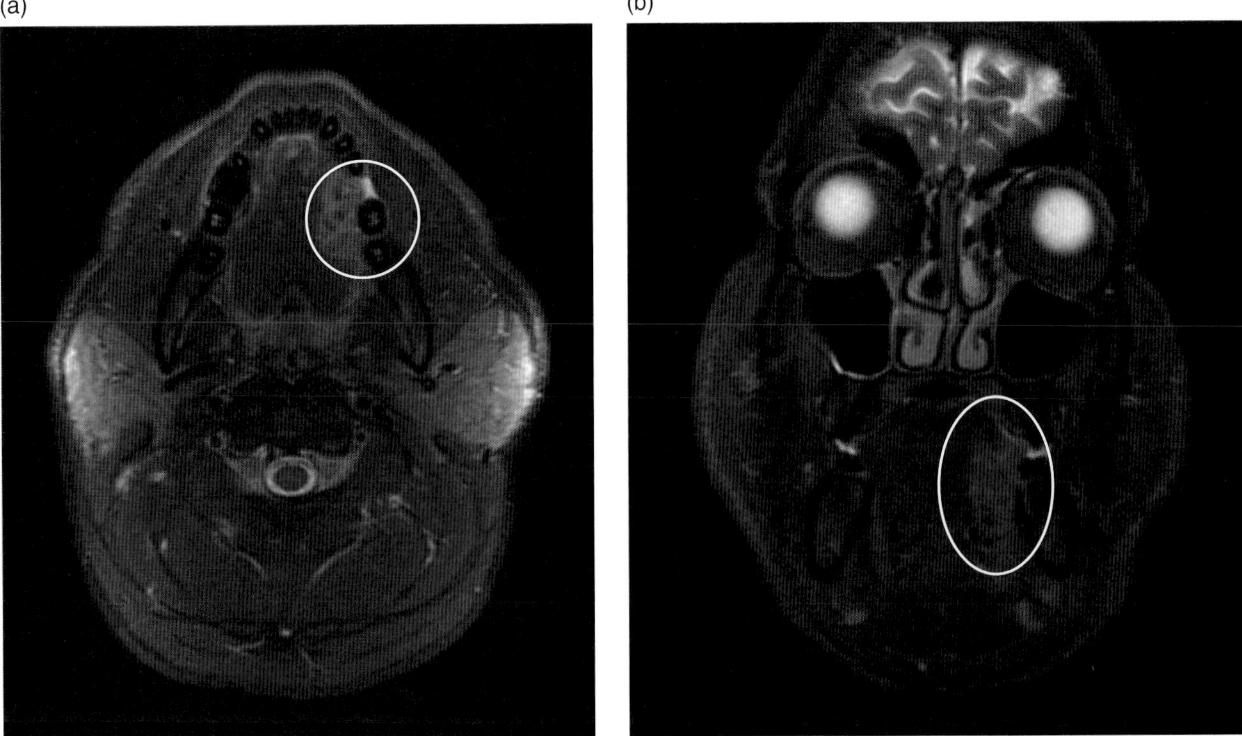

Figure 11.3 The MR scan showing the same tumour on the left side of the tongue (white outline). (a) Axial and (b) coronal views.

the RT fields are at increased risk of damage post-RT. If the teeth then become pathological or symptomatic, there is a risk of osteoradionecrosis (ORN). ORN is most commonly in the mandible (lower jaw) and may result in exposed dead bone and possible chronically discharging pus intraorally or extraorally via sinuses onto the skin. In severe cases pathological fracture of the jaw can ensue.

Further specialised investigation known as a *PET CT* (positron emission tomography fused with the CT) scan is carried out for further evaluation if there is a large tumour or if there is suspicion of distant spread and to rule out other synchronous pathologies. The PET scan component involves injection of a radionucleotide of glucose known as *FDG* (fluorodeoxyglucose F18) into the blood stream. Glucose is taken up in all metabolically active cells and tissues including and often preferentially by active cancer cells. This lights up on the PET scan as 'hotspots', and these images can be fused with the CT scans, giving a precise indication anatomically where metabolically active areas are in the head and neck or throughout the body.

The MDT Discussion

Once the initial investigations are carried out and the biopsy confirmed as a malignancy, the patient's case is discussed at the head and neck MDT. The senior clinician presents the case to the MDT involving the clinical photographs, scans and histo, and cytopathology. This allows for the patient's stage of cancer to be confirmed based on the TNM classification.

The American Joint Committee on Cancer (AJCC) produced the TMN classification, now in its 8th edition. In the head and neck it is subdivided anatomically into oral cavity (mouth), oropharynx (throat), and larynx (voice box). In the oral cavity, tumour size (T) and its depth of invasion (more than or less than 5 mm depth) are classified from T1 to T4. Nodal status (N) is the number of lymph nodes that are involved with cancer (N1–N3) less than or more than 3 cm and with or without extra nodal extension. Metastasis (presence or absence of metastatic disease) is classified as M0 or M1. This allows for staging of the cancer from I to IV depending on the TNM; that is, a T1N0M0 cancer is stage I. A T4N0M0 or a T1N1M1 is a stage IV cancer with various different intervening permutations of TNM reflecting different stages. Generally, the higher the stage the poorer the prognosis and survival. There is a different TNM classification for cancers of the oropharynx that have HPV-positive status. These HPV-driven cancers have a better prognostic outcome and generally respond better to treatment, which is usually chemoradiotherapy (CRT) or RT, despite often being larger in tumour size and with nodal disease compared with nonvirally driven cancers.

Following on from the MDT, the patients are reviewed at the oncology clinic to break the bad news and discuss treatment options. This appointment must include a CNS to support patients through their cancer journey. Often the CNS is present at the initial meeting if there is suspicion of cancer, and we advise patients to bring a relative or close friend with them for support. It is important to provide as much information as they wish for or need and head and neck cancer literature to read later with contact details of the CNS and agencies that can advise – for example, psychologist and counselling, income support, patient groups, and additional therapies.

If the management requires CRT, RT, chemotherapy, or immunotherapy, patients will referred onto the specialist service after a comprehensive dental assessment.

Head and Neck Surgery: Removal of the Cancer

More than 70% of mouth cancers occur in the tongue and floor of the mouth (see Figures 11.4–11.6). It is thought had carcinogens within tobacco, betel nut, and alcohol pool in the sump area of the mouth and affect the adjacent mucosa. If the primary modality of treatment is surgery, then the patient will be prepared for the surgical journey.

Preoperative assessments are carried out on all major cases prior to surgery. This is often nurse lead with an anaesthetic review, in case of cardiorespiratory or any other issues that need to be identified and the patient possibly optimised prior to surgery. An assessment of the patient's nutritional status and needs before and

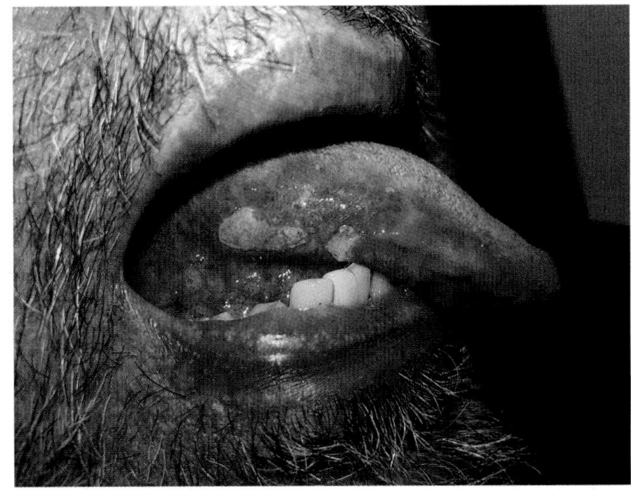

Figure 11.4 Early right-sided tongue cancer.

after treatment is included. The patient will be reviewed by a speech and language therapist and advised on how the surgery may affect the ability to communicate and eat and swallow. A dental assessment will be carried out to ascertain the likelihood of extractions and if remedial dental treatment will need to be carried out. The dental team will focus on oral health and hygiene, and the patient's dental practitioner will be apprised of the treatment plan. The CNS together with the surgical team, as mentioned, will link the patient to the various agencies to support the patient through the cancer journey. There is also an enhanced recovery programme that encourages early mobilisation with a view to early postoperative discharge of the patient.

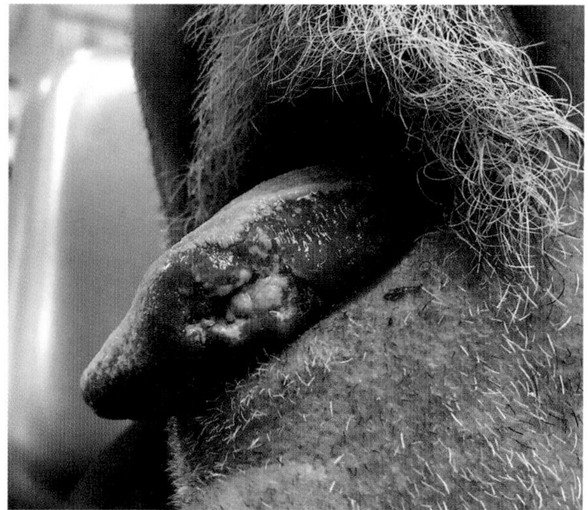

Figure 11.5 Deeply invading left tongue cancer.

The surgical plan for the patient will depend on the aim of the surgery (see Figure 11.7). Surgery will be either with curative or palliative intent. Most surgical procedures will be with the aim of a cure; however, a few advanced cases may aim to alleviate the patient of the distress of a fungating tumour or risk of a fatal uncontrolled bleed.

The aim of curative surgery is to remove or resect the index tumour with a cuff of normal tissue surrounding the lesion. Histopathologically a tumour with a margin of 5 mm or more is declared a completely excised specimen. If the margin is between less than 5 mm but more than 1 mm, it is known as a *close margin*. If it is less than 1 mm, then it is called a *positive margin*. A positive resection margin indicates the worst prognostic outcome with other adverse features including a discohesive (disordered) tumour front with presence of skip lesions, perineural, lymphovascular invasion, and degree of cell differentiation.

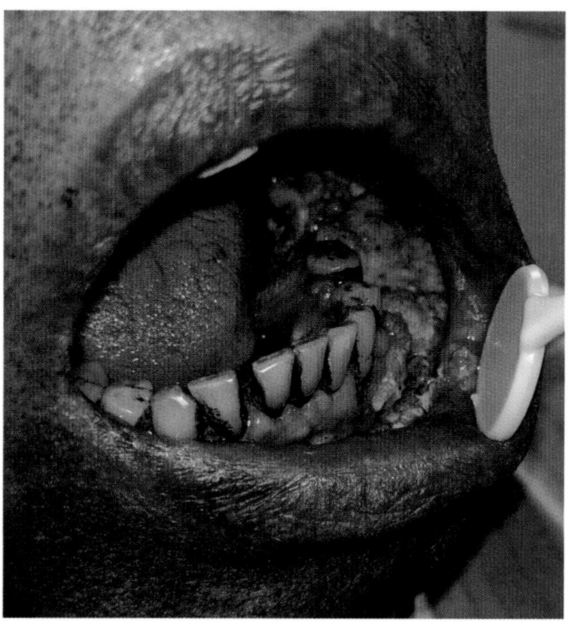

Figure 11.6 Locally advanced left jaw carcinoma.

The mucosal changes with cancer and abnormalities such as dysplasia can be used and highlighted with special stains such as Lugol's iodine. Although not routinely used, the iodine is not taken up by cancer and dysplastic cells, as they lose the ability to metabolise glycogen. The normal tissues therefore stain brown, whereas abnormal and cancerous tissue stays pale (see Figures 11.8 and 11.9).

The tumour resection is often accompanied with a neck dissection. This is to remove the possible draining lymph nodes of the cancer to allow further information to clarify its staging; that is, the size and number of cancer-involved lymph nodes and the presence or absence of ENE, where the tumour metastasis spreads outside the capsule of the lymph node. ENE is a poor prognostic factor and recognised as such in the new 8th edition TMN classification. There are various types of neck dissection, and the one chosen depends on the site of the primary tumour, stage of the tumour, and whether neck metastasis has been confirmed (see Figures 11.10–11.12).

The cervical nodes (lymph nodes of the neck) are located around the internal jugular vein from the skull base posteriorly, the lower jaw anteriorly to the clavicle inferiorly. They are designated different levels I–V (excluding the central neck nodes) depending on their anatomical position.

Most oral cavity cancer will involve anatomically the nearest draining lymph nodes first before draining further down the chain of nodes. For instance, a tongue or a floor-of-mouth cancer may drain to the submandibular and submental nodes and the jugulodigastric (upper cervical) lymph nodes and before spreading down to the jugulo-omohyoid and lower cervical nodes.

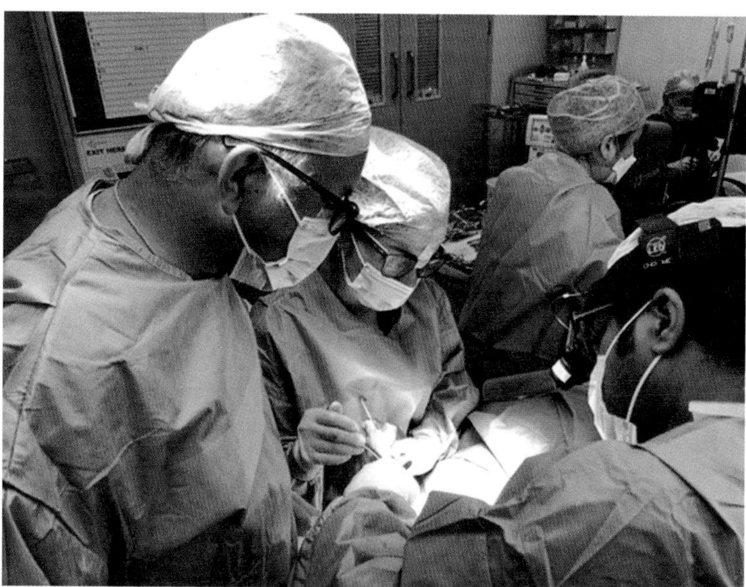

Figure 11.7 The surgical team.

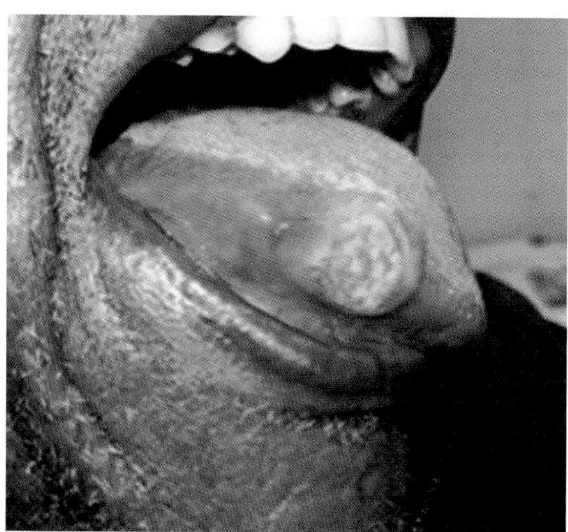

Figure 11.8 The tongue cancer in vivo.

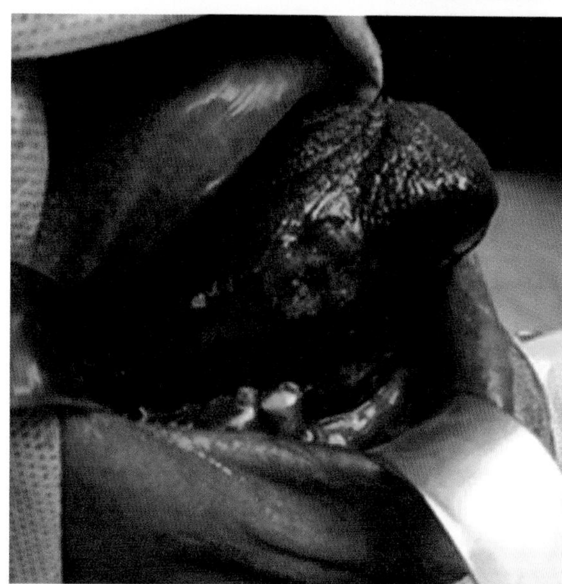

Figure 11.9 The same lesion with iodine staining.

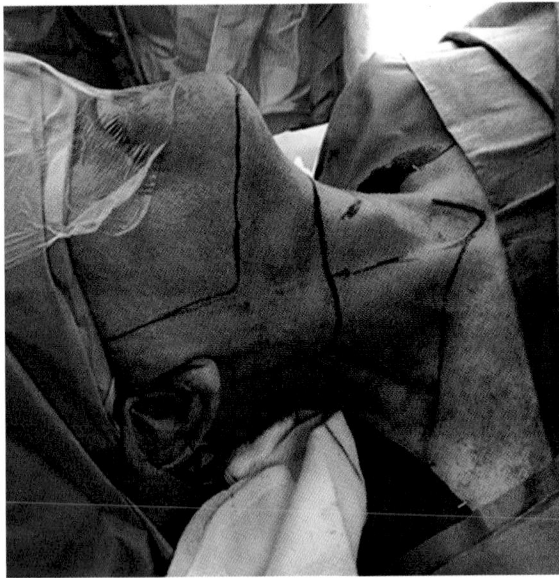

Figure 11.10 Preparation for a right neck dissection with markings.

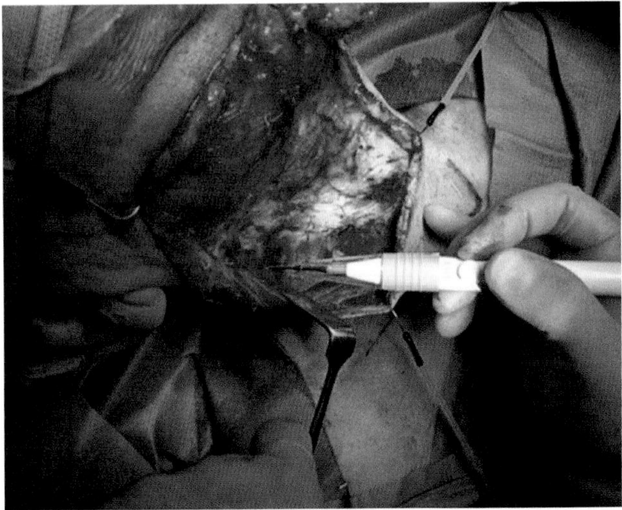

Figure 11.11 The skin flaps raised with a diathermy needle.

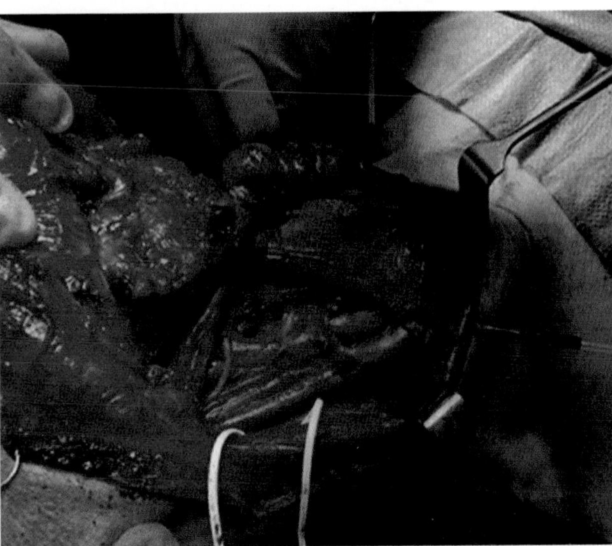

Figure 11.12 The selective neck dissection completed in continuity with the main specimen.

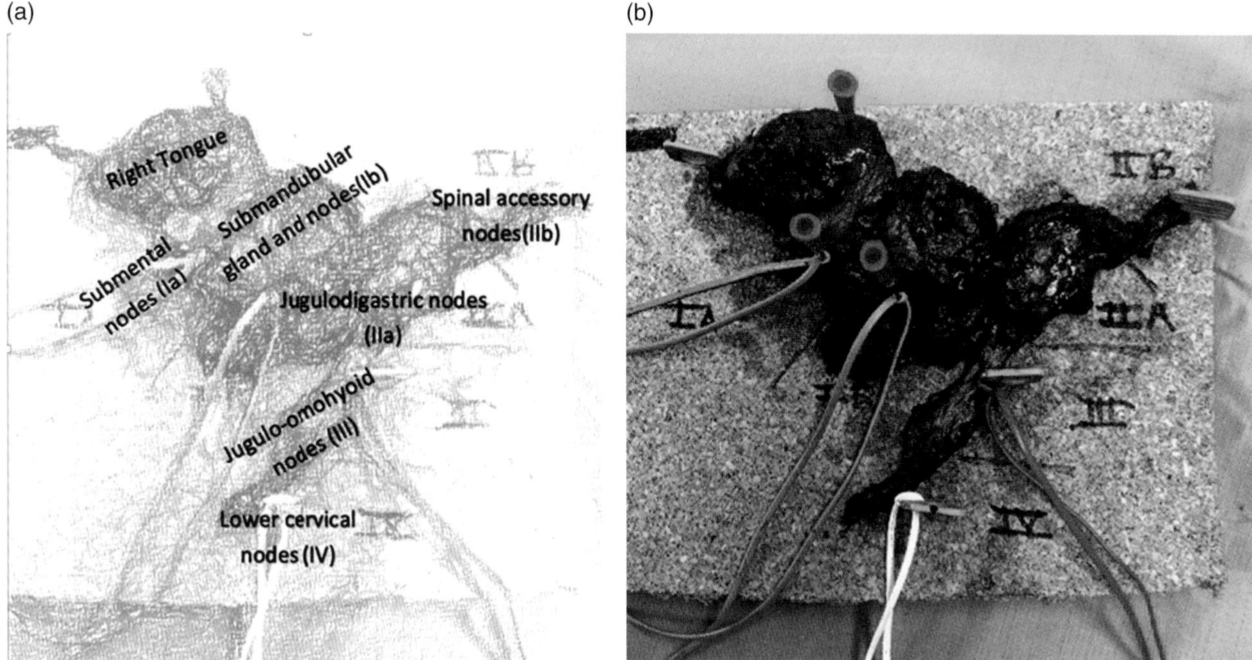

Figure 11.13 (a and b) The above tongue cancer (shown in Figures 11.8–11.12) was resected in continuity with the left neck dissection as illustrated.

In the case shown in Figure 11.13, the cancer was completely excised with good margins (greater than 5 mm histological clearance) and did involve two lymph nodes. Due to the size of the tongue cancer and adverse tumour biology including the spread to the lymph nodes, it was recommended by the MDT that the patient should have adjuvant RT.

Historically, a radical neck dissection involved clearing all of the lymph nodes on one side of the neck with surrounding structures including the sternocleidomastoid muscle, the internal jugular vein, and the spinal accessory nerve. This resulted in significant morbidity with a large scar, a visible deformity, and shoulder dysfunction. Over the years it has been shown that we can mostly preserve the above adjacent structures with no adverse effect on long-term survival.

Modern neck dissections are known as *functional* and *selective*. Functional refers to preservation of adjacent structures and selective means removing only certain levels depending on the extent of the disease. They can also be classified as therapeutic or for staging purposes. A therapeutic neck dissection is one where it is known that there is malignant disease in the neck, and this is removed along with the other required levels. A staging neck dissection is where it is thought that there is no known malignant disease in the neck; however, the final histopathological specimen may show microscopic disease or a node not discernible on preoperative imaging.

Highly selective neck procedures known as *sentinel node* (SEN) biopsies are being trialled to see if one can remove just the most likely involved nodes and check if they have cancer. If at operation the sentinel lymph nodes (i.e. the first draining lymph nodes) are positive for metastatic cancer, then the surgeon will proceed to a completion neck dissection. This decreases the morbidity (the length of scar, risk of injuries to adjacent structures, and duration of operating time and length of stay in hospital) for the SEN-negative patients. The SEN procedures do require significant support both financially and with staff, including the preparation and injection of the radionucleotide from the nuclear medicine department. The operating surgeon injects the radionucleotide solution into the lesion in the mouth the day before or morning of the procedure. Simultaneously a visible dye, methylene blue, can also be injected into the lesion to follow the lymphatic fluid into the cervical nodes. On table the surgeon can then identify the radioactive tracer (and dye) and the SEN(s) with a gamma probe and selectively remove for rapid testing for disease. This rapid testing is known as *frozen section*, where the lymph node sample is frozen in liquid nitrogen, sectioned, and examined by a histopathologist in real time with the patient in theatre.

As discussed, for early cancers involving soft tissues, simple wide excision is carried out. The tools and instruments used vary on the cost, availability, and access. The commonest modalities are cold steel (scalpel), diathermy (thermal energy), laser (CO_2 laser; see Figures 11.14 and 11.15), and ultrasonic devices (Harmonic scalpel by Ethicon). Smaller resections may not need reconstructions and are allowed to heal by primary closure or secondary intention. Some surgeons cover the wound with a dressing; for example, antiseptic-impregnated ribbon gauze, cellulose (absorbable oxidised cellulose), or even full or split thickness skin graft. A graft is a tissue used to reconstruct a defect and relying on the local blood supply to survive. Larger resections or anatomically critical areas will be better served by a reconstruction.

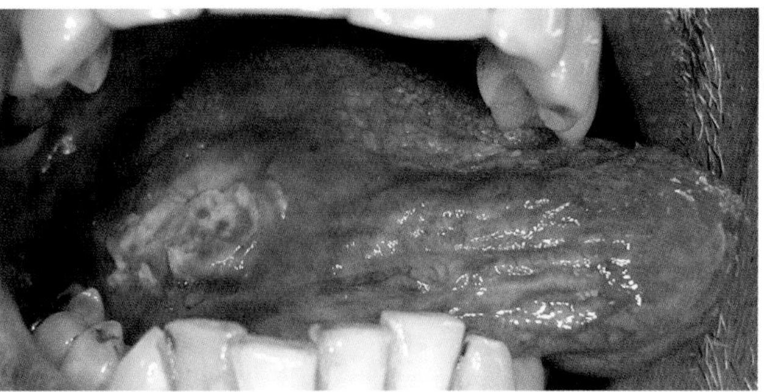

Figure 11.14 Right-sided tongue cancer.

Head and Neck Surgery: Reconstruction of the Defect

Following removal of the tumour the surgeon may need to reconstruct the defect. The reconstruction will depend on the extent and site of the tumour resection. A small cancer – for example, T1 of the lateral tongue – can be excised and primarily closed with no reconstruction. A large tumour of the maxilla (upper jaw) may be removed and the resulting defect reconstructed with an obturator and denture prosthesis.

In general, the most convenient local flap (reconstruction) with the least morbidity (damage to the patient) is often chosen to repair the defect. Larger resections may require distant flaps either pedicled (attached to a blood supply) or free flap (transplanted from one part of the patient's body to another part, such as the head and neck). In the free flap, the blood supply is cut when it is raised (from the donor site) but reattached with the aid of a microscope and fine sutures to the site in the head and neck (the recipient site).

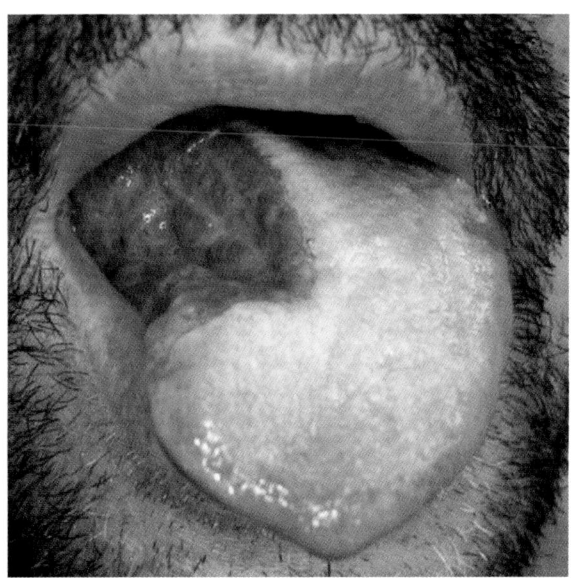

Figure 11.15 Two weeks after laser excision of tongue cancer. The base of the wound is granulating.

Commonly an area of skin and fascia (subcutaneous tissue) is raised from the forearm along with the radial artery and associated veins to reconstruct the tongue or floor of the mouth following cancer surgery. Similarly, the fibular bone (supporting from the leg) can be removed along with a small patch of skin and used to reconstruct a jaw bone. These technically difficult procedures often take 8–10 hours of time in the operating theatre using a microscope for the microvascular anastomosis (reconnecting the small blood vessels of the free flap).

Head and Neck Procedures

Reconstruction restores form and function to the tissue or organ resected. Reconstructions follow a ladder of increasing complexity and can be either local or distant flaps. A flap is tissue used for reconstruction of a defect and survives with its own blood supply. It can be from a donor site locally or a distant site remote from the head and neck region.

Common local flaps for the oral cavity include buccal fat pad, nasolabial, and facial artery musculo-mucosal flaps. Distant flaps can be either pedicled (taken with an intact blood supply) or free flap, where the blood supply is detached from the donor site and then reanastomosed to vessels near the recipient site.

Common pedicled flaps to the head and neck area are the pectoralis major and latissimus dorsi myocutaneous flaps. Common free flaps used to reconstruct the head and neck region are the radial forearm, anterolateral thigh, rectus, and medial sural artery perforator (MSAP) and thoracodorsal artery perforator (TDAP) flaps.

The workhorse soft tissue free flap is the *radial forearm flap*, also known as the *Chinese flap* due to its origins. This is ideal for the head and neck (especially the mouth), as the skin of the forearm is thin, pliable, and soft. The flap is based on the radial artery, and invariably the anatomy of the forearm and hand allows for removal of this vessel without any significant harm to the limb following surgery. The radial artery has two small veins that run along this, known as *venae comitantes*, which drain the flap (although some operators prefer to raise it with the cephalic vein, which passes nearby) (see Figures 11.16–11.20).

The commonest bony free flap used is the fibula bone. This reconstruction is mainly used when a segment of the mandible is resected for cancer (or occasionally for ORN) and sometimes for maxillary reconstruction. The fibula flap is only raised once it has been established that the lower leg has a normal blood supply and removal of the fibula bone and its accompanying vasculature will not compromise the leg. This is usually done with a preoperative CT (or MR) angiogram or duplex USS depending on local protocols. The fibula flap is often raised with the overlying skin paddle, which will help restore the soft tissue element of the resection (i.e. the mucosal component) (see Figures 11.21–11.24).

A skin graft is often required to repair the defect from the donor site. This can be a split or full-thickness skin graft usually from the abdominal wall (where there is usually redundant skin) or from the thigh.

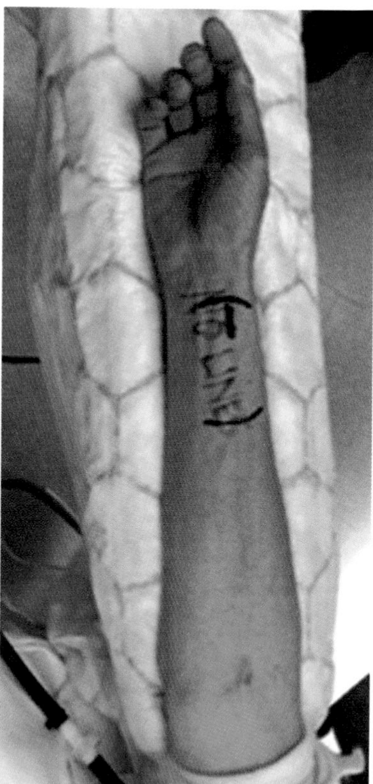

Figure 11.16 The right forearm positioned for flap harvesting with a tourniquet placed above the elbow.

Patient Recovery

The length of stay of the patient is dependent on the type of procedure and patient factors (see Figures 11.25–11.32). The smaller resections with primary closure may be performed as a day case procedure if the patient is fit to go home. Following a major procedure, the patient is often recovered in a high-dependency unit or, if kept intubated overnight, transferred to the intensive care unit. For more complex larger resections and free flap reconstructions, the patient may remain an inpatient for two to three weeks. Continued input from the CNS, SLT, and dietetic is required. The patient may have a temporary tracheostomy and need nasogastric feeding for the initial few days.

Limiting factors for discharge of a patient may be medical comorbidities, postoperative complications, and social factors. A safe discharge home may need an occupational therapist visit and assessment with modifications in the home, social care support in the home environment, and GP and district nurse review. Following the surgery and discharge home, the patient is reviewed in clinic to discuss the postoperative histology (see Figure 11.33). This can take several weeks if bone has to be decalcified prior to staining and examining.

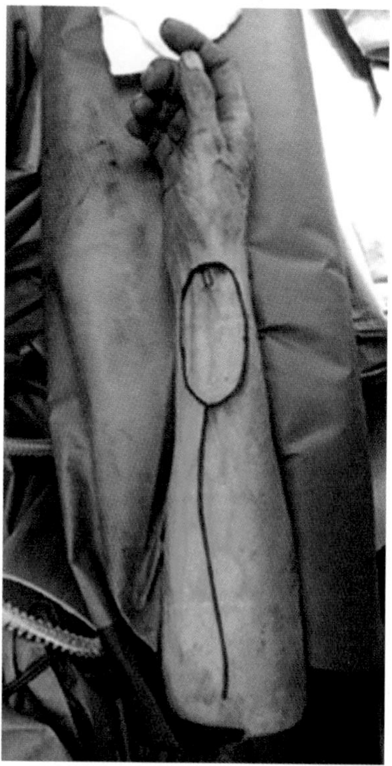

Figure 11.17 The incisions marked for the flap.

Adjuvant Treatment for Cancer

If tumour is involved in the surgical margins or there are adverse features in the cancer such as ENE or more than two lymph nodes involved with cancer, then adjuvant treatment may be recommended. This may require RT, chemotherapy, CRT, or immunotherapy. The main adjuvant treatment is radiation treatment (RT), which is normally started six to eight weeks following the surgery. This time allows the swelling and bruising to settle and the wounds to heal.

A radiation oncologist will assess the patient with a planning CT, and a mask fitting is arranged. The mask allows the radiation to be targeted to the same area consistently, maximising its effect with reduced surrounding tissue toxicity. A radical dose of RT may be a six-week course of treatment from Monday to Friday (often 30 sessions). Newer linear accelerators (RT machines) can bend the x-ray beams using magnets to spare certain important structures; for example, the salivary gland, mandible, spinal cord, and eyes. This is known as *intensity-modulated RT* (IMRT). RT is generally carried out as an outpatient; however, occasionally patients may need admission with acute toxicities.

If the nutritional status is of concern, a gastrostomy tube may be inserted prior to treatment. This is a day case procedure or one overnight stay.

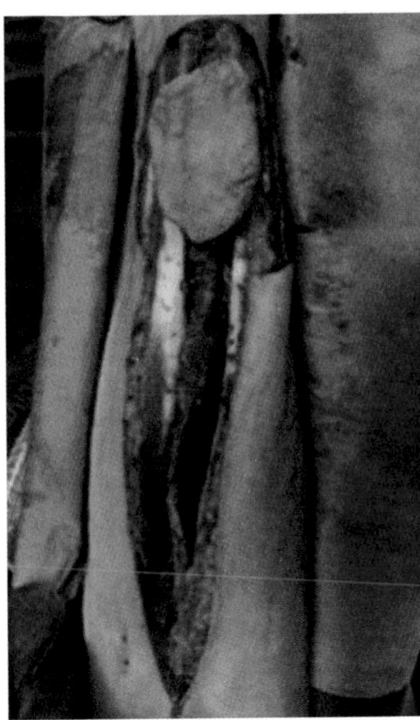

Figure 11.18 The radial forearm flap raised with the radial artery and venae comitantes.

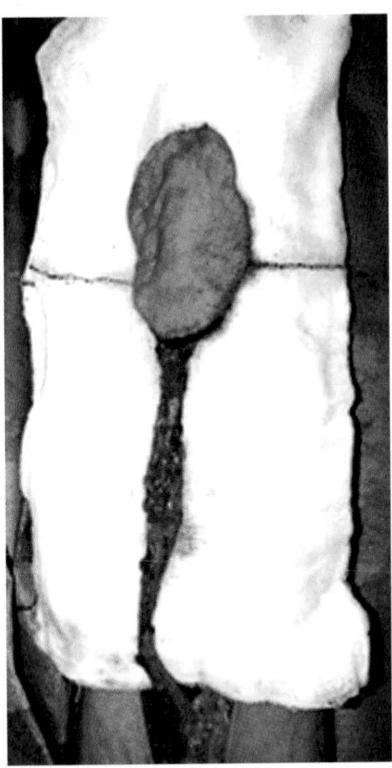

Figure 11.19 The flap raised prior to disconnection and transfer.

Cancer Patient Follow-Up

Following successful cancer treatment, the patient is followed up over the subsequent five years. As each year passes, the review intervals will increase. In the first year the patient may be seen every four to six weeks and in the final year just twice if there are no concerns. With the advent of virtual clinics, some reviews may be carried out remotely; however, this will have to be validated.

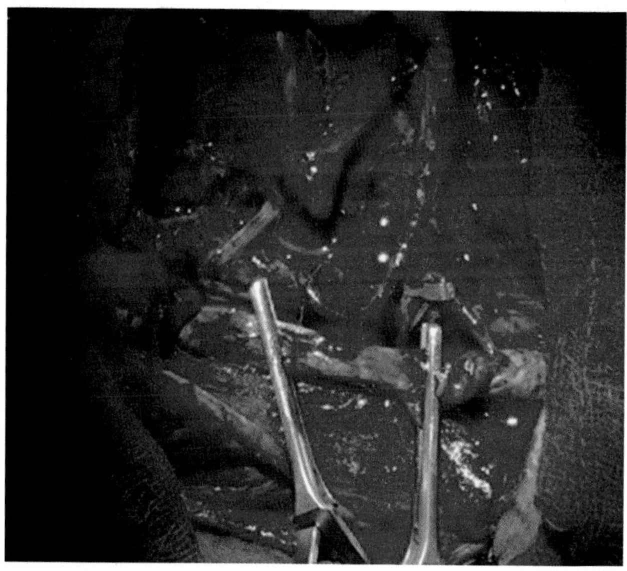

Figure 11.20 The microscopic anastomosis of the artery and vein. Here the artery and a single vein have been anastomosed and prepared to anastomose (join) the second vein to the internal jugular vein (shown temporarily clamped).

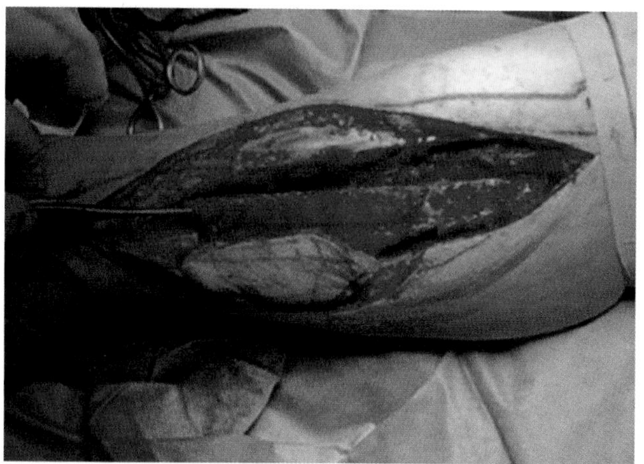

Figure 11.21 A fibula flap with skin raised.

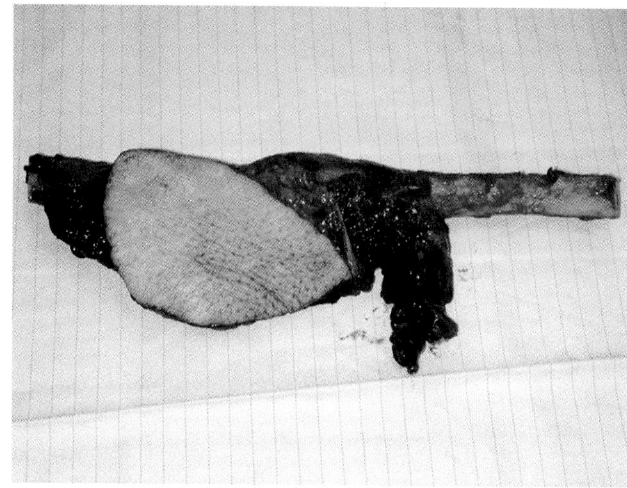

Figure 11.22 The fibula flap is detached and then shaped to fit the defect, with the skin to line inside the mouth.

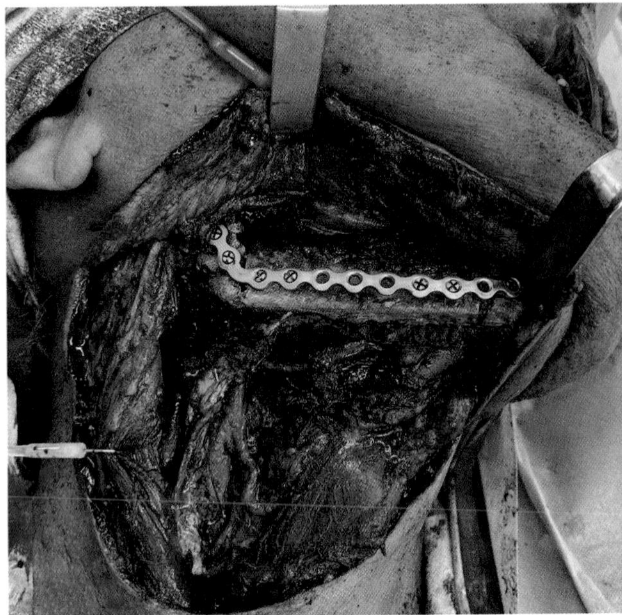

Figure 11.23 The fibula flap reconstructing the right mandible.

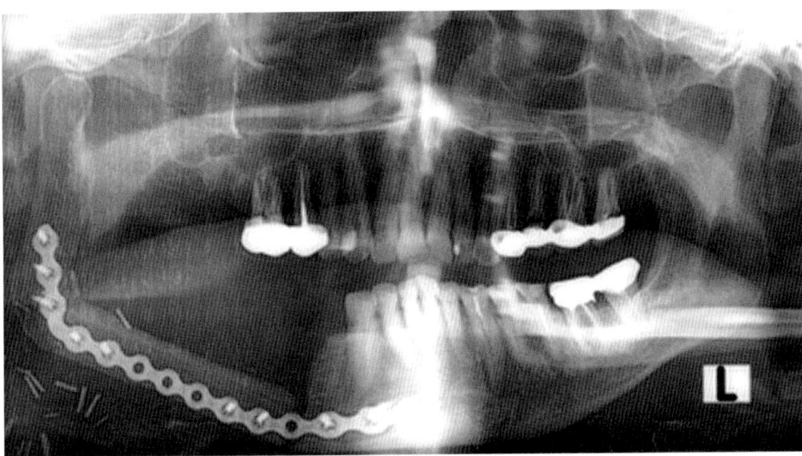

Figure 11.24 The reconstruction shown on the OPG radiograph.

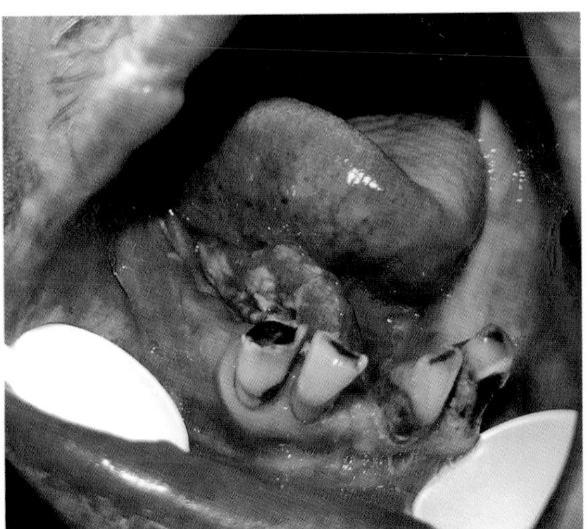

Figure 11.25 The cancer seen on the right floor of the mouth.

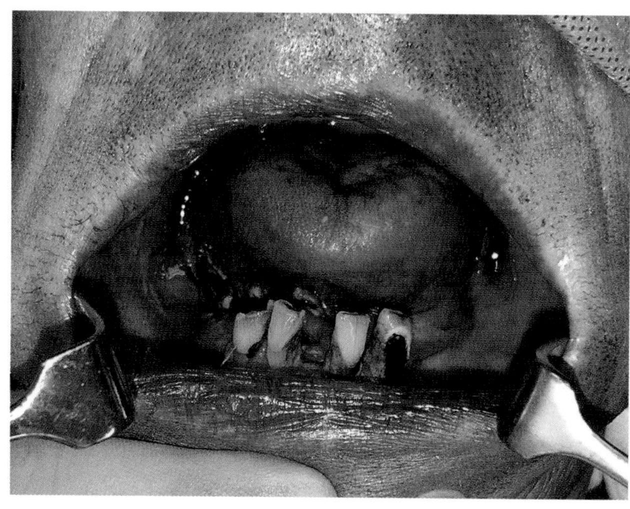

Figure 11.26 At operation the patient is prepared.

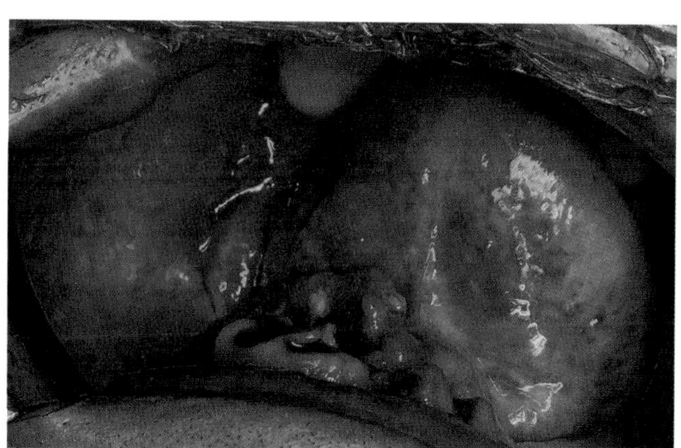

Figure 11.27 The teeth removed, showing the tumour extending into the retromolar trigone.

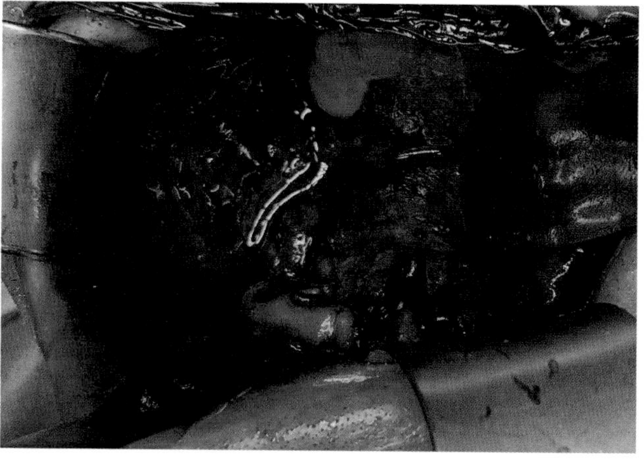

Figure 11.28 Staining the mouth with iodine to identify the suspicious areas.

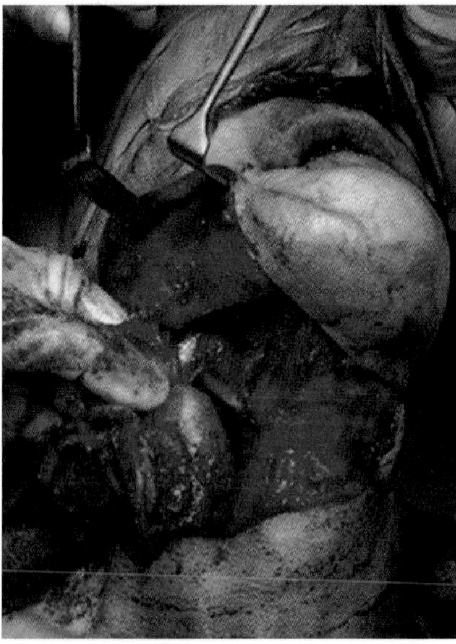

Figure 11.29 Removal of the cancer in continuity with the neck dissection, dropping the tumour down into the neck.

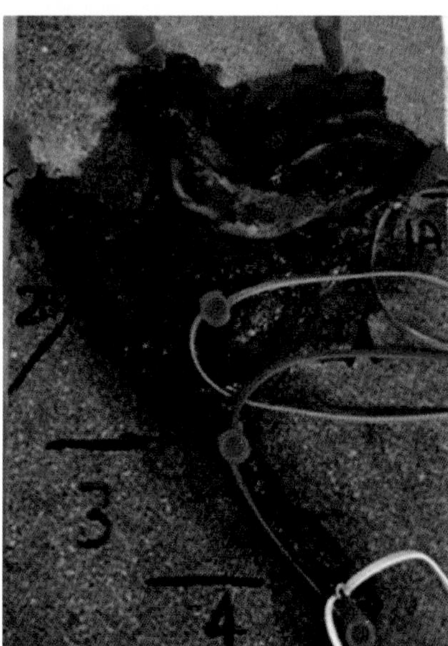

Figure 11.30 The specimen pinned out and labelled on the cork board.

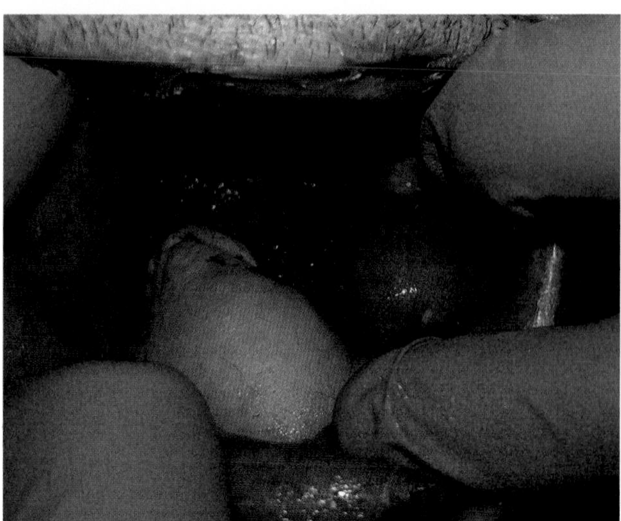

Figure 11.31 The radial forearm free flap reconstruction reviewed the next day on the ward.

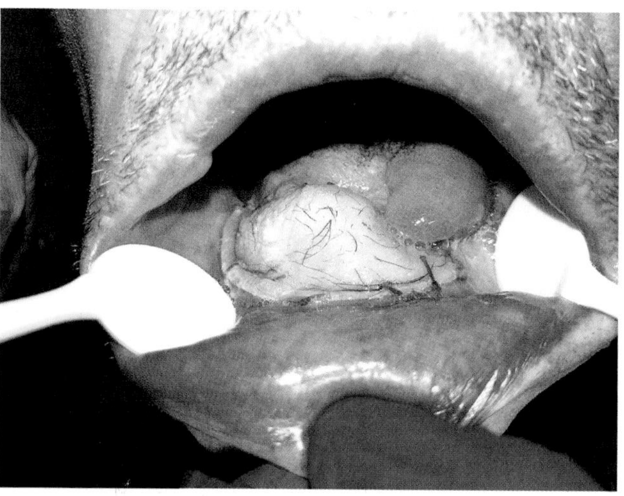

Figure 11.32 The patient two weeks after the swelling settling in clinic.

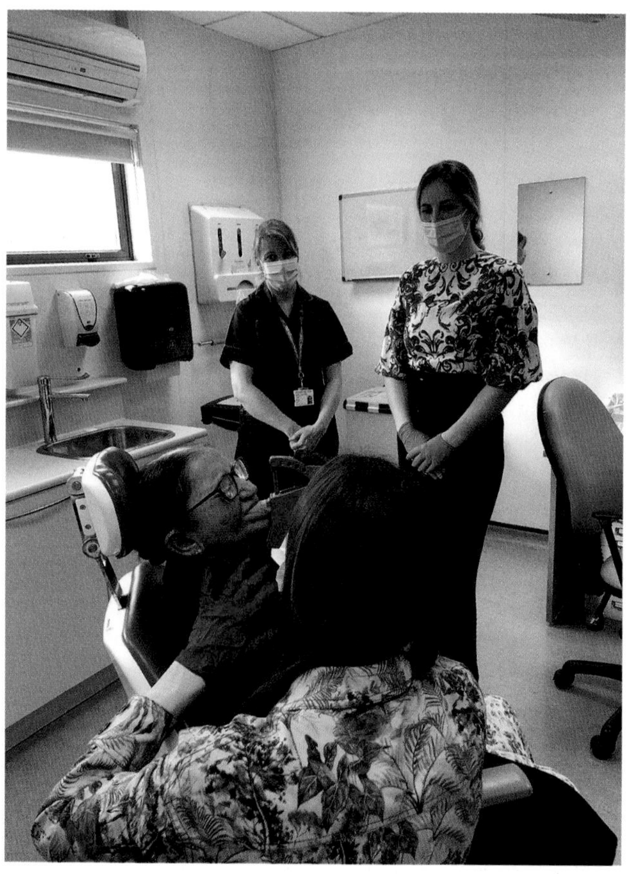

Figure 11.33 Patient reviewed by surgeon, speech and language therapist, and CNS.

In the UK surveillance is usually clinical monitoring and imaging only requested if there is a suspicion of disease. Initially, an MR scan may be requested if local recurrence is suspected and a CT or PET CT for distant metastasis. The patient is then rediscussed on the MDT.

The follow-up appointments give reassurance to the patients and allow a detailed examination to be performed, including nasendoscopy if required. Patients who have primary CRT follow a different protocol and have PET CT scans at six weeks and three to six months following treatment.

12

Head and Neck Cancer: Clinical Nurse Specialist Role

Sonja Hoy and Joanna Rydon

The Royal Marsden NHS Foundation Trust, London, UK

A clinical nurse specialist (CNS) is a clinical expert in evidence-based nursing practice within a specialty, in this instance head and neck cancer. The term *CNS* refers to a registered nurse who is educated to at least graduate level, if not master's. As nursing has evolved, many CNSs have additional qualifications – including physical assessment, medical prescribers, and nonmedical referrers for imaging requests – that further increase their autonomy (Royal College of Nursing 2021).

The role of the CNS within head and neck oncology is to provide individuals with support, information, education, and specialist knowledge. The CNS is involved with the patient from diagnosis through treatment, rehabilitation, and long-term recovery or supporting patients with a noncurative diagnosis. The role is instrumental in providing information and coordinating with primary and secondary health care providers, as well as other members of the wider MDT such as speech therapists, dietitians, and medics, to ensure the patient is cared for holistically. The term *key worker* is used to identify the health care professional who is, with the patient's consent, the person taking on the key role in coordinating the patient's journey through the head and neck cancer pathway (National Cancer Action Team 2010); the key worker is usually the head and neck cancer CNS (Macmillan 2015).

Diagnosis, treatment, and potential recovery from a head and neck cancer is complex and extremely distressing for patients and their family, friends, and carers. Through involvement of the CNS, patients and family are supported through the cancer pathway with clear information, at the relevant time and onwards. The use of holistic needs assessments helps the CNS coordinate and plan care with individual patients so that their needs are addressed physically, psychologically, spiritually, culturally, and socially. Through building rapport with the patient, the CNS is uniquely placed to be the advocate on the patient's behalf, helping liaise back to the MDT about the patient's wishes with treatment plans (British Association of Head & Neck Oncologists 2020).

The role of the head and neck cancer CNS has been shown to improve the experience of the cancer pathway for patients and carers through clear, individualised care plans giving as much information as the patient needs to make informed choices. The *Cancer Reform Strategy* (Department of Health 2007), *Improving Outcomes in Head and Neck Cancer* (National Institute for Health and Care Excellence 2004), and other sources (Dempsey et al. 2016) clearly state that patients value the role and impact CNSs have through their cancer treatment pathway.

Patients are referred to the CNS via the MDT meetings when each patient's diagnosis and treatment plan is discussed. The named CNS will then meet patients when they are informed of their diagnosis and follow them through the pathway alongside the other health care professionals. Patients are seen regularly throughout their treatment; specialist head and neck units will have dedicated pathways that are followed. Once treatment is completed for a patient, the CNS still maintains a role as key worker. Patients require as much, if not more, support after completing treatment; in particular, psychological support to navigate their rehabilitation and living with long-term side effects of treatment. Referrals to appropriate support are essential, and the CNS, being key worker, is often the first person accessed by patients or family for this ongoing referral. Centres such as Maggie's and online support through Macmillan and Cancer Research are all able to provide ongoing support for patients. Many hospitals will also have their own psychological support departments and rehabilitation services.

Care of Head and Neck Cancer Patients for Dental Hygienists and Dental Therapists, First Edition. Edited by Jocelyn J. Harding.

The National Institute for Health and Care Excellence *Improving Outcomes* guidance (2004) stated that CNSs are an integral member of the MDT and provide psychological support, coordination of care, and advocacy on behalf of patients. This fundamental role of the CNS has not changed in the 18 years since this guidance was published, as the British Association of Head & Neck Oncologists standards (2020) states the role of the CNS is essential within the multiprofessional head and neck oncology team.

Head and neck oncology CNSs are not solely clinical; the role also helps evaluate and steer service provision through audit and clinic research and share knowledge with junior colleagues through formal and informal teaching at ward, trust, national, and international levels. The CNS can be described as a lynch pin for patients and for the MDT, through leadership, advocacy, navigation, a holistic approach, compassion, and individualised care.

References

British Association of Head & Neck Oncologists (2020). British Association of Head & Neck Oncologists standards. https://bahno.org.uk/_userfiles/pages/files/final_bahno_standards_2020.pdf.

Dempsey, L., Orr, S., Lane, S., and Scott, A. (2016). The clinical nurse specialist's role in head and neck cancer care: United Kingdom national multidisciplinary guidelines. *J. Laryngol. Otol.* 130 (Suppl. S2): S212–S215.

Department of Health. (2007). Cancer reform strategy. https://www.nhs.uk/NHSEngland/NSF/Documents/Cancer%20Reform%20Strategy.pdf.

Macmillan (2015). Cancer clinical nurse specialist: impact brief. https://www.macmillan.org.uk/documents/aboutus/research/impactbriefs/clinicalnursespecialists2015new.pdf.

National Cancer Action Team (2010). Excellence in cancer care: the contribution of the clinical nurse specialist. https://www.lcnuk.org/system/files/ExcellenceinCancerCaretheContributionoftheClinicalNurseSpecialist.pdf.

National Institute for Health and Care Excellence (2004). Improving outcomes in head and neck cancers. https://www.nice.org.uk/guidance/csg6/resources/improving-outcomes-in-head-and-neck-cancers-update-pdf-773377597.

Royal College of Nursing. Clinical: exploring roles within the clinical practice arm of nursing (2021). https://www.rcn.org.uk/professional-development/your-career/nurse/career-crossroads/career-ideas-and-inspiration/clinical. Scroll down and click on 'Considering a specialist role?'

13

The Role of the Dietitian in the Care of Head and Neck Cancer Patients

Laura Kent and Hannah Cook

Gloucestershire NHS Foundation Trust, Gloucester, UK

Nutrition is an essential aspect of the management of head and neck cancer due to the high prevalence of malnutrition within this patient population. Patients can be malnourished at the point of diagnosis or experience nutritional losses caused by multimodal treatment side effects, tumour position, disease burden, or lifestyle factors (Findlay et al. 2014). Consequently, this can lead to poor health outcomes and a reduced quality of life from loss of muscle mass, psychosocial stress, impaired healing and immunity, and treatment toxicity. This can affect treatment tolerance and result in unplanned hospital admissions (Arends et al. 2017). Therefore, UK guidance is that a specialist head and neck oncology dietitian should be part of the MDT for treating patients throughout the continuum of their care, with frequent contact, which has demonstrated improved patient outcomes (Talwar et al. 2016).

What Is a Dietitian?

A dietitian is a health care professional who holds a degree in dietetics and is registered with the British Dietetic Association (BDA) and the Health and Care Professions Council (HCPC). An undergraduate degree in dietetics takes three to four years or two in a postgraduate setting. A dietetic course covers a variety of topics including biochemistry, human nutrition and physiology, pharmacology, and incorporates practical placements (BDA 2021). Dietitians differ from nutritionists as dietitians are qualified to practise in clinical settings and are the only nutrition professionals regulated by law and have a protected title (HCPC 2021).

What Is the Role of a Head and Neck Oncology Dietitian?

A dietitian will assess the patients' nutritional status throughout their care pathway. Evidence-based advice is provided to ensure the right balance of nutrients and adequate nutritional intake can be maintained. Each assessment is personalised to fit with the individual's lifestyle, routine, and comorbidities, considering the patient's holistic needs, with quality of life a top priority (National Institute for Health and Care Excellence 2004).

Day to day, dietitians work alongside SLTs, CNSs, oncologists, ear nose and throat (ENT) surgeons and oral and maxillofacial (OMF) surgeons and are involved in the weekly MDT meetings. During a patient's inpatient stay, dietitians work alongside the ward doctors, registered nurses, and other allied health professionals to ensure that nutritional status can be maximised. The following are some examples of the dietitian's role throughout a head and neck cancer patient's care pathway:

Care of Head and Neck Cancer Patients for Dental Hygienists and Dental Therapists, First Edition. Edited by Jocelyn J. Harding.

Dietetic Review Pathway For Individuals With Head And Neck Cancer

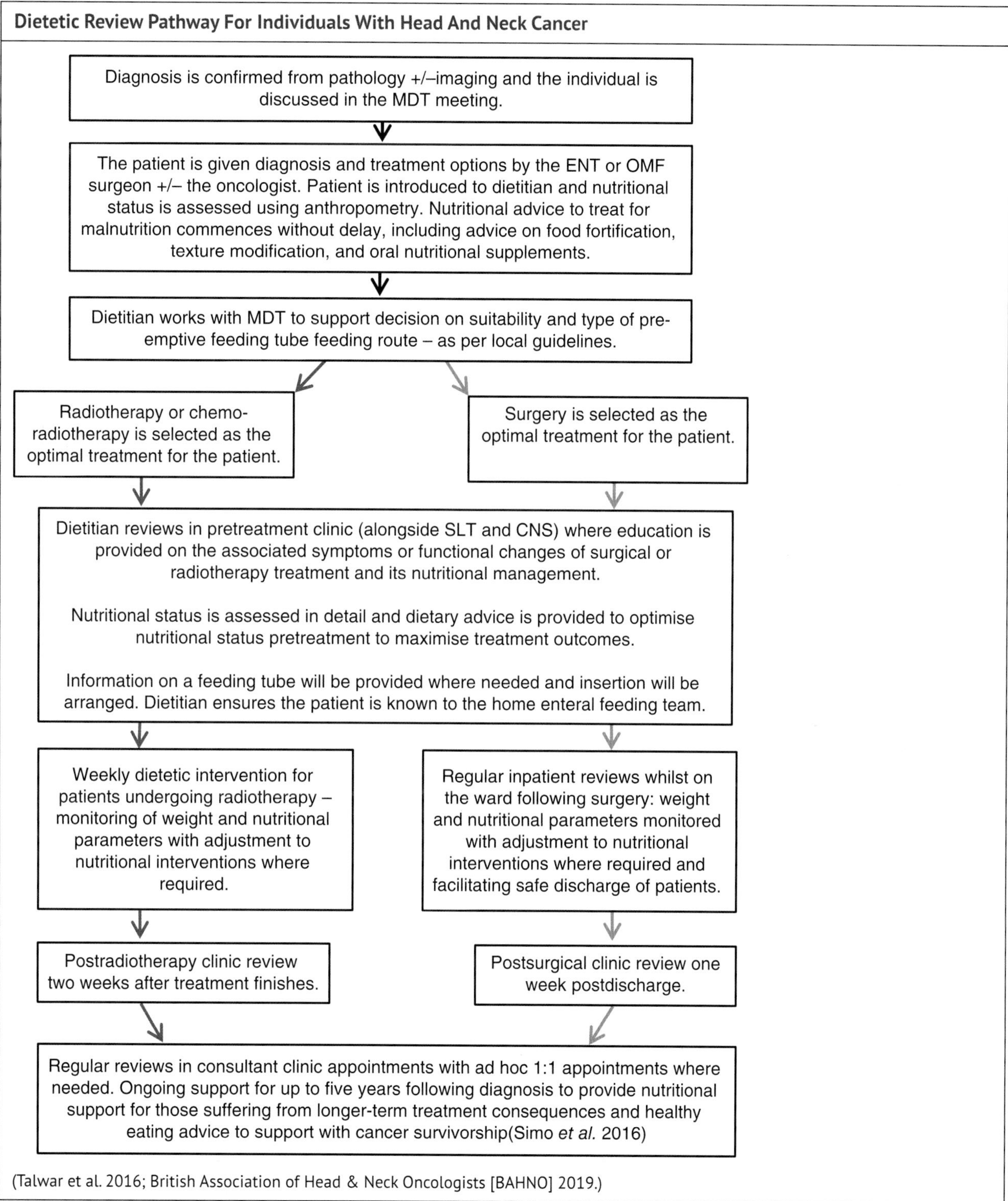

Diagnosis is confirmed from pathology +/–imaging and the individual is discussed in the MDT meeting.
The patient is given diagnosis and treatment options by the ENT or OMF surgeon +/– the oncologist. Patient is introduced to dietitian and nutritional status is assessed using anthropometry. Nutritional advice to treat for malnutrition commences without delay, including advice on food fortification, texture modification, and oral nutritional supplements.
Dietitian works with MDT to support decision on suitability and type of pre-emptive feeding tube feeding route – as per local guidelines.
Radiotherapy or chemo-radiotherapy is selected as the optimal treatment for the patient.
Surgery is selected as the optimal treatment for the patient.
Dietitian reviews in pretreatment clinic (alongside SLT and CNS) where education is provided on the associated symptoms or functional changes of surgical or radiotherapy treatment and its nutritional management.
Nutritional status is assessed in detail and dietary advice is provided to optimise nutritional status pretreatment to maximise treatment outcomes.
Information on a feeding tube will be provided where needed and insertion will be arranged. Dietitian ensures the patient is known to the home enteral feeding team.
Weekly dietetic intervention for patients undergoing radiotherapy – monitoring of weight and nutritional parameters with adjustment to nutritional interventions where required.
Regular inpatient reviews whilst on the ward following surgery: weight and nutritional parameters monitored with adjustment to nutritional interventions where required and facilitating safe discharge of patients.
Postradiotherapy clinic review two weeks after treatment finishes.
Postsurgical clinic review one week postdischarge.
Regular reviews in consultant clinic appointments with ad hoc 1:1 appointments where needed. Ongoing support for up to five years following diagnosis to provide nutritional support for those suffering from longer-term treatment consequences and healthy eating advice to support with cancer survivorship(Simo et al. 2016)

(Talwar et al. 2016; British Association of Head & Neck Oncologists [BAHNO] 2019.)

Dietitians also support patients who have untreatable disease with the aim of improving their symptoms and potential anxieties and helping to achieve the patient's own nutrition-related goals to maximise their quality of life (Cocks et al. 2016).

Alongside patient support, dietitians are also involved with:

- Education and resource provision for MDT colleagues on all aspects of the nutritional management of patients with head and neck cancer

- Regular audit, service evaluation, and research to develop and contribute to evidence-based practice and national guidelines
- Contribution to data collection for head and neck cancer databases (BAHNO 2019).

Barriers to Implementing Dietetic Advice

Whilst dietitians endeavour to support and encourage patients to eat and drink (where safe), there are a number of symptoms related to head and neck cancer treatments that can act as barriers to implementing dietetic advice:

Barrier	Cause	Impact	Management
Odynophagia	Postsurgical inflammation and swelling, radiotherapy-induced mucositis, or tumour position	Avoidance of oral intake due to associated pain	• Optimising pain relief • Modifying dietary textures • Oral nutritional supplements • Enteral nutrition
Mucositis	Radiotherapy side effect	Avoidance of oral intake due to ulceration of the oral mucosa and associated pain	• Optimising pain relief • Modifying dietary textures • Avoiding spicy/citrus foods • Good oral care • Oral nutritional supplements • Enteral nutrition
Altered secretions	Postoperative swelling, altered airway, or radiotherapy treatment	Swallowing difficulties, taste changes, and regurgitation that reduces oral intake	• Altering dietary patterns and meal timings • Steam inhalation or the use of nebulisers • Hydration • Carbonated drinks • Good oral care
Nausea	Anaesthetic, chemotherapy drugs, or treatment-related side effects and anxiety	Reduction in nutritional intake due to nausea or fear of being sick	• Altering dietary patterns and food types • Secretion management • Optimising the use of antiemetics or bowel care • Relaxation and distraction techniques
Reflux	Altered gastric motility, exacerbated by treatment and its side effects	Associated discomfort, nausea, and unpleasant taste impacting on the tolerance of dietary intake	• Altering dietary patterns and meal timings • Avoiding trigger foods • Optimising use of antacids and motility agents
Taste changes	Anosmia or damage and alteration to taste buds following surgery, chemotherapy, or radiotherapy	Lack of pleasure in eating, reducing oral intake	• Advice on alternative food choices • Good oral care • Support on viewing foods as necessity as opposed to pleasure
Altered gastrointestinal transit	Chemotherapy treatment and a side effect of symptom control medications (e.g. opioids or some types of antiemetics)	Sensation of early satiety or an aversion to food to minimise gastric upset, causing inadequate dietary intake	• Altering proportion of fibre • Adequate hydration • Change of dietary pattern • Bowel care medications and motility agents
Reduced appetite	Consequence of cancer and its treatment side effects. Emotional and lifestyle factors	Reduction in volume of food eaten	• Altering dietary patterns • Identifying and managing cause of reduced intake • Food fortification • Oral nutritional supplements • Enteral nutrition

Trismus, xerostomia, and dysphagia also have a significant impact on a patient's ability to implement dietetic advice. All three topics are covered elsewhere in this publication.

Dietitians can support by augmenting the patient's diet and providing practical tips to minimise the impact of the above barriers on nutritional intake. Liaising with other members of the MDT such as GPs, physiotherapists, social workers, clinical psychologists, specialist diabetes nurses, and district nurses is imperative for symptom management.

Reducing the symptom burden of a patient with head and neck cancer can prevent nutritional losses, which in turn can help maximise quality of life and treatment outcomes (Gorenc et al. 2015).

Should Patients Be Eating Sugar?

The myth: if cancer cells need lots of glucose, then cutting sugar out of our diet must help stop cancer growing and could even stop it developing in the first place.

Unfortunately, it's not that simple. All of our healthy cells need glucose too, and there's no way of telling our bodies to let healthy cells have the glucose they need but not give it to cancer cells. Our bodies will convert other types of food into glucose even if sugar is cut out of the diet.

Patients on active treatment have increased energy expenditure and nutritional losses as a result of the treatment and healing process. This means there is risk of rapid weight loss, metabolism of muscle mass, and deconditioning. Dietary intake of fats and simple carbohydrates can be a calorific way to supplement the diet in the short term to slow weight loss. Therefore, a low-sugar diet is not recommended during treatment.

A dietitian also ensures nutrients are absorbed and metabolised effectively within the body. If patients are on a steroid medication as part of their cancer treatment, a reduced utilisation of glucose and an increase in muscle breakdown can occur. This can be assessed through monitoring for high blood glucose levels.

In the long term, a reduction in high-sugar foods can help maintain a healthy body weight, which can in turn reduce the risk of some cancers.

Feeding Routes

Patients undergoing treatment for head and neck cancer will often not be able to meet their nutritional requirements via oral intake alone. This is usually determined by their tumour position, staging, and planned treatment. Patients receive counselling from the dietitian before their treatment begins about the potential need for artificial nutrition, and some also undergo a prophylactic gastrostomy placement. A gastrostomy tube is considered appropriate if enteral nutrition is required for more than 30 days (British Association for Parenteral and Enteral Nutrition 2019).

Different cancer centres offer patients different feeding tube options particularly for when patients are undergoing radiotherapy treatment, with no overall consensus on which tube is the most appropriate (Koyfman and Adelstein 2012). Some centres offer a 'reactive nasogastric tube insertion', where the tube is placed during their radiotherapy treatment at the point when the dietitian has identified enteral feed provision is required. Alternatively, other centres provide patients with a prophylactic gastrostomy placement prior to the commencement of their radiotherapy treatment and the tubes are used when required, with guidance by the dietitian.

Patients undergoing surgery may have gastrostomy tubes placed before their operation if it is known they will require longer-term enteral nutritional support, or a nasogastric tube can be placed in theatre for postoperative support.

Nasogastric Tubes

A nasogastric (NG) tube is a fine-bore tube passed through the nose and the oesophagus into the stomach (Figure 13.1); its lifespan is usually up to eight weeks depending on manufacturer (National Nurses Nutrition Group 2016). Before it is safe to use, confirmation that the tube is within

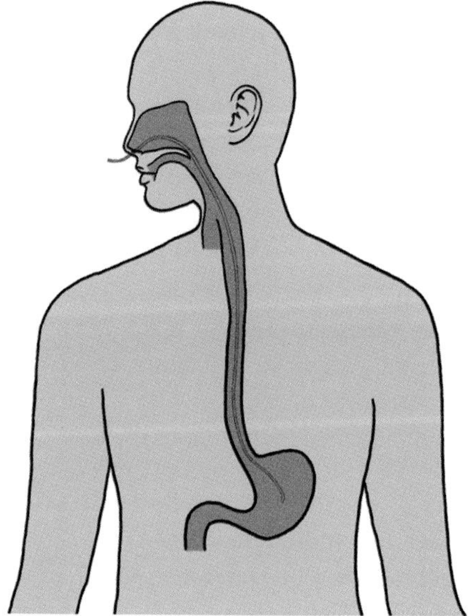

Figure 13.1 Nasogastric tube. *Source:* Courtesy of Emma Kent 2021.

the stomach is required, as there is risk it can be placed into the lungs. Correct positioning can be performed by testing an aspirate from the NG tube using pH paper. If the pH is below 5.5, the tube is safe to use. If a reading cannot be obtained or the pH is too high (which can occur if on antacids), a chest x-ray is required.

Care of the NG tube includes the following:
- Check tube length has not changed (length should be recorded at the nostril).
- Test the pH before each administration via the tube to ensure correct positioning is maintained.
- Monitor for pressure sores at nostril site.

Tracheoesophageal Tubes

If patients have had a laryngectomy, they can be fed via the fine-bore tube, known as a *TO tube*, that is placed through their laryngectomy stoma and a tracheoesophageal fistula directly down their oesophagus into their stomach (Figure 13.2). This can be a more comfortable tube than a NG tube, and it also helps keep the tracheoesophageal puncture open, which is then used for a speaking valve on recovery.

Care of the TO tube includes the following:
- Check tube length has not changed (length should be recorded at the stoma site).
- Test the pH before each administration via the tube to ensure correct positioning is maintained.
- Monitor for pressure sores at stoma site.

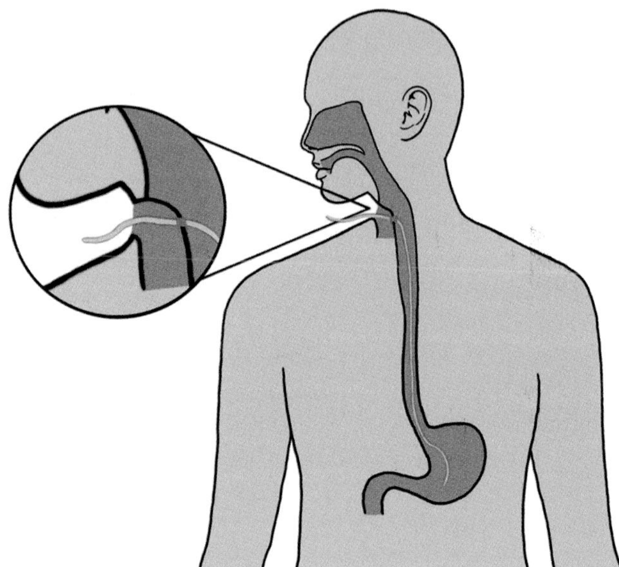

Figure 13.2 Tracheoesophageal tube. *Source:* Courtesy of Emma Kent 2021.

Gastrostomy Tube

A gastrostomy tube is placed directly into the patient's stomach (Figure 13.3). If it is placed by endoscopy it is called a percutaneous endoscopic gastrostomy (PEG); if it is placed with fluoroscopic x-ray guidance it is called a radiologically inserted gastrostomy (RIG).

These tubes can remain in situ for as long as required, with a lifespan of up to two years depending on manufacturer, and can be easier for patients to use in comparison to an NG or TO tube. Once the tube is no longer required it can be easily removed in a clinic setting or endoscopy by an appropriately trained health professional.

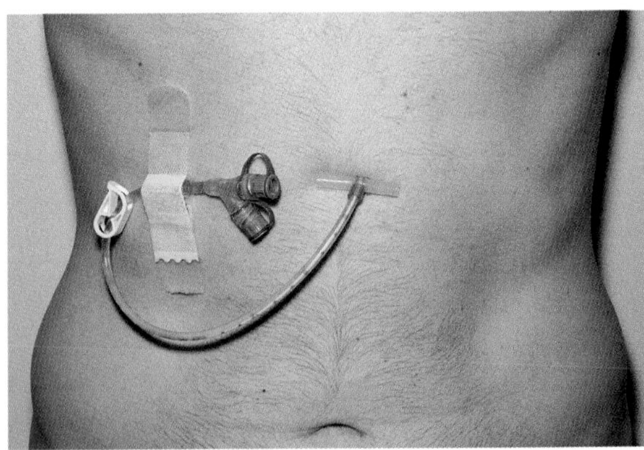

Figure 13.3 Gastrostomy tube. *Source:* Gloucestershire NHS Foundation Trust 2021.

PEG Tube

These tubes are held in place by an internal bumper. Externally they have a fixation device against the skin to keep the tube in position with a clamp and feeding connector attached to the end of the tube.

Care of the PEG tube includes the following:
- Clean around stoma site.
- Flush tube with water to keep patent when not in use.
- Advancement and rotation of tube minimum of weekly once tract has healed to prevent internal bumper becoming buried.

RIG Tube

These tubes are often held within the stomach with a balloon filled with water (balloon gastrostomy) or a flexible internal loop of the tube (pigtail). Both types of tubes also have an external fixation device to keep the tube in position against the skin and a feeding connector attached to the end. They do not have a clamp to help prevent leakage of gastric content on feed administration; however, an extension set to make the tube longer and provide a clamp can be used on the balloon gastrostomy tube.

Care of the RIG tube includes the following:

- Clean around stoma site.
- Flush tube with water to keep patent when not in use.
- Advancement and rotation of tube minimum of weekly once tract has healed to prevent internal bumper becoming buried.
- Water in the balloon needs to be checked and replaced every 7–10 days.
- Tube replacement every two to three months as required.

Jejunal Tube

Sometimes patients may require feeding into the first part of the small bowel due to anatomy or feed tolerance issues. Types of tubes can include:

- Jejunostomy (JEJ): surgically placed directly into the jejunum
- Percutaneous endoscopic gastro-jejunostomy (PEG-J): endoscopically placed PEG with a jejunal extension
- Radiologically inserted gastro-jejunostomy (RIG-J): radiologically placed PEG with jejunal extension
- Naso-jejunal (NJ): via the nasal passage, through the stomach into the jejunum.

Ways Enteral Nutrition Can be Given

The ways nutrition can be given include:

- Bolus feeding: This is an intermittent feeding pattern that can compare to set meal times and takes between 10 and 30 minutes. The feed can be injected from the syringe directly into the stomach using the plunger, or the feed can be poured into the syringe to drip through slowly, known as *gravity feeding*.
- Continuous feeding: A programmed pump delivers feed slowly into the stomach over a set number of hours.
- A combination of both types of feeding can also be used.

Home Enteral Feeding Team

Head and neck cancer patients with feeding tubes at home will also have the support of their local home enteral feeding team as well as their dedicated head and neck specialist dietitian. This team is made up of dietitians and nutrition nurses. The nurses can provide extra support for patients with respect to the care of their stoma sites and troubleshooting for tube issues.

Tube Removals

Individuals with head and neck cancer will all use their tubes for different lengths of time depending on their tumour site, treatment plan, and perseverance with the reintroduction of oral diet (Wiggenraad et al. 2007).

Some individuals may have lifelong dependence on their feeding tube if they are unable to maintain their nutritional intake orally. Some reasons for this are having an unsafe swallow; complications of treatment, for instance, a stricture or trismus; or major surgical procedures such as a total glossectomy.

Tube removal is usually authorised once all care providers agree the tube is no longer required and the following criteria have been met:

- Nutritional status can be consistently maintained with oral intake.
- The patient has a safe swallow.
- There is low risk of cancer recurrence and need for further treatment. A post treatment scan can help inform this decision.

The tube removal process varies between NHS hospitals and depends on the type of tube in situ.

Parenteral Nutrition

In rare cases parenteral nutrition is used to provide nutrition to patients. This is a last resort if the patient does not have suitable access for enteral feeding or has issues with digestion and absorption. This method of feeding is where nutrition is delivered directly into the veins.

References

Arends, J., Baracos, V., Bertz, H. et al. (2017). ESPEN expert group recommendations for action against cancer-related malnutrition. *Clin. Nutr.* 36 (5): 1187–1196. https://www.clinicalnutritionjournal.com/article/S0261-5614(17)30228-5/fulltext.

British Association for Parenteral and Enteral Nutrition (2019). Access routes/tube types. https://www.bapen.org.uk/nutrition-support/enteral-nutrition/access-routes-tube-types (accessed 14 May 2021)

British Association of Head & Neck Oncologists (2021). AHPs – dietitians. https://bahno.org.uk/ahps-dietitians.aspx (accessed 9 April 2021).

British Dietetic Association (2021). What is a dietitian? https://www.bda.uk.com/about-dietetics/what-is-dietitian.html (accessed 2 May 2021).

Cocks, H., Ah-See, K., Capel, M., and Taylor, P. (2016). Palliative and supportive care in head and neck cancer: United Kingdom multidisciplinary guidelines. *J. Laryngol. Otol.* 130 (2): 198–207. https://www.ncbi.nlm.nih.gov/pmc/articles/PMC4873917/.

Findlay, M., Bauer, J., Brown, T., and Head and Neck Guideline Steering Committee (2014). COSA: head and neck cancer nutrition guidelines/introduction. In: *Evidence-Based Practice Guidelines for the Nutritional Management of Adult Patients with Head and Neck Cancer*. Sydney: *Clinical Oncological Society of Australia*. https://wiki.cancer.org.au/australia/COSA:Head_and_neck_cancer_nutrition_guidelines.

Gorenc, M., Rotovnik-Kozjec, N., and Strojan, P. (2015). Malnutrition and cachexia in patients with head and neck cancer treated with (chemo) radiotherapy. *Rep. Pract. Oncol. Radi* 20 (4): 249–258. https://www.ncbi.nlm.nih.gov/pmc/articles/PMC4477124/.

Health and Care Professions Council (2021). Who we regulate. https://www.hcpc-uk.org/about-us/who-we-regulate/ (accessed 2 May 2021).

Koyfman, S.A. and Adelstein, D.J. (2012). Enteral feeding tubes in patients undergoing definitive chemoradiation therapy for head-and-neck cancer: a critical review. *Int. J. Rad. Oncol.* 84 (3): 581–589. https://www.redjournal.org/article/S0360-3016(12)00450-6/fulltext.

National Institute for Health and Care Excellence (2004). Improving outcomes in head and neck cancers. https://www.nice.org.uk/guidance/csg6 (accessed 1 May 2021).

National Nurses Nutrition Group (NNNG) (2016). Good practice guideline: safe insertion and ongoing care of nasogastric (NG) feeding tubes in adults. https://www.nnng.org.uk/download-guidelines/ (accessed 14 May 2021).

Simo, R., Homer, J., Clarke, P. et al. (2016). Follow-up after treatment for head and neck cancer: United Kingdom national multidisciplinary guidelines. *J. Laryngol. Otol.* 130 (S2): 208–211. https://www.ncbi.nlm.nih.gov/pmc/articles/PMC4873918/.

Talwar, B., Donnelly, R., Skelly, R., and Donaldson, M. (2016). Nutritional management in head and neck cancer: United Kingdom national multidisciplinary guidelines. *J. Laryngol. Otol.* 130 (2): 23–40. https://pubmed.ncbi.nlm.nih.gov/27841109/.

Wiggenraad, R., Flierman, L., Goossens, A. et al. (2007). Prophylactic gastrostomy placement and early tube feeding may limit loss of weight during chemoradiotherapy for advanced head and neck cancer, a preliminary study. *Clin. Otolaryngol.* 32 (5): 384–390. https://onlinelibrary.wiley.com/doi/abs/10.1111/j.1749-4486.2007.01533.x.

14

Speech and Language Therapy

Eve Ferguson[1] *and Sarah Hartigan*[2]

[1]*Clinical Lead Speech and Language Therapist in Head and Neck, Preston, UK*
[2]*Dental Hygienist, Dental Therapist, Manchester, UK*

Head and neck cancer and its treatment can result in communication and swallowing difficulties (National Institute for Health and Care Excellence [NICE] 2004). Communicating, eating, and drinking are integral parts of being human and can significantly impact quality of life, respiratory status, and oral health. Speech and language therapists (SLTs) are key members of the head and neck multidisciplinary team. SLTs are specialists in communication and swallowing and aim to optimise patients' function before, during, and after treatment.

Patient Pathway

Following diagnosis, patients attend a pretreatment head and neck clinic. This appointment gives the opportunity for the patient to meet an SLT, dietitian, and Clinical Nurse Specialist (CNS). The SLT completes a baseline assessment of communication and swallowing and provides counselling, management, or prehabilitation exercises as appropriate. Detailed discussions on the short and long-term impact of the patient's upcoming treatment are particularly important for patients (Brady et al. 2020). Psychoeducation on predicted communication and swallowing function is essential and promotes informed decision-making regarding treatment options.

Surgical patients are assessed postoperatively and continue to be supported by SLTs during their inpatient stay. Oncology patients also have access to assessment and therapy during their outpatient treatment. Patients are then reviewed at the posttreatment head and neck clinic. The SLT, dietitian, and CNS are all present to ensure holistic management of the post-treatment acute phase (NICE 2004).

If patients require ongoing rehabilitation of their communication and swallowing, they attend speech and language therapy appointments that may be via telephone, video consultation, or face to face. Communication and swallowing disorders can present months or even years following treatment, therefore long-term access to speech and language therapy services is essential (Patterson 2019).

Communication

Head and neck cancer can affect the production of voice (dysphonia) and speech, and patients may struggle to be understood. Difficulties vary depending on tumour location, extent, and treatment. Communication impairments can cause a high psychological burden and significantly impact quality of life (Elaldi et al. 2021).

Assessment

Assessment may include perceptual assessment of voice and speech intelligibility or articulation assessment and assessment of functional communication. SLTs also collect patient-reported outcome measures to capture the individuals' perceptions

Care of Head and Neck Cancer Patients for Dental Hygienists and Dental Therapists, First Edition. Edited by Jocelyn J. Harding.

of their communication. In cases where a more detailed assessment of voice is required, patients may have an endoscopic evaluation of the larynx (EEL) procedure (British Association of Head & Neck Oncologists [BAHNO] 2021a). EEL involves the insertion of a rigid endoscope into the mouth or a flexible endoscope into the nose. This allows detailed assessment of structure, movement, and function of the vocal cords at rest and during the production of voice (Carding et al. 2008).

Treatment

SLTs provide information and exercises to improve or maintain function, alongside support for communication partners. This may include breathing exercises, voice exercises, implementing use of strategies to improve intelligibility, and so forth. SLTs also assess and manage nonverbal communication, which may include written communication, charts, apps, or using other devices to support patients to express themselves. Patients with head and neck cancer rarely have language difficulties, though pre-existing cognitive impairment is more common (Williams et al. 2017). SLTs can differentially diagnose and treat a range of language impairments, including cognitive communication disorders.

Swallowing

Difficulty in swallowing (dysphagia) can result in food and drinks going down the wrong way (aspiration), which can lead to choking, chest infections, malnutrition, and dehydration. The lips, tongue, palate, larynx, pharynx, and oesophagus work closely together for safe and efficient swallowing. Head and neck cancers and their treatments can cause problems at different stages of the swallow, and dysphagia is often associated with other treatment side effects (Pezdirec et al. 2019).

Oral-stage dysphagia symptoms include difficulty in closing the lips, chewing, controlling food or drink in the mouth, nasal regurgitation, and difficulty clearing food or drink from the mouth (Royal College of Speech and Language Therapists [RCSLT] 2021). Pharyngeal-stage symptoms include difficulty triggering or a delayed swallow, sticking sensation, or difficulties clearing food or drink from the throat and regurgitation. Coughing, choking, breathlessness, or voice changes associated with eating and drinking can indicate dysphagia, though they may or may not be associated with aspiration (Farneti et al. 2018).

Assessment

SLTs evaluate the swallow function by assessing movement and sensation of oral and laryngeal structures (Villegas 2018). A detailed assessment of the oral structures, strength, range, and speed of movement can allow the SLT to predict likely difficulties. Patients may be asked to trial a variety of food and drink consistencies or strategies. For some people thicker or smoother textures can be easier and safer to swallow. However, for others thicker textures can accumulate in the throat and be difficult to clear. Some patients require chewy food textures or different temperatures to provide more sensory feedback during swallowing. SLTs may suggest the use of specialist spoons, cups, or straws to make eating and drinking easier. They may advise a range of different head positions and swallowing manoeuvres too (Clarke et al. 2016). Swallowing is a complex process that requires individualised specialist assessment and management.

In some cases, SLTs require further information about swallowing and carry out instrumental assessments. Videofluoroscopy is a swallowing x-ray (Figure 14.1). SLTs carry out the procedure with specialist radiographers who control the equipment in the x-ray department. Patients are given small amounts of food and drink to swallow, mixed with a contrast (e.g. barium), whilst x-ray images are being taken. Patients may be asked to carry out different swallowing strategies during the procedure. Videofluoroscopy aims to gather specific information on the anatomy and physiology of the swallow, identify possible solutions to reduce aspiration, guide therapy, educate patients, or inform further medical or surgical management (RCSLT 2013). The procedure takes approximately 20 minutes. Videofluoroscopy can also be helpful in troubleshooting problems with alaryngeal speech after total laryngectomy. As videofluoroscopy involves exposure to radiation, careful consideration of patients is required.

Fibreoptic endoscopic evaluation of swallowing (FEES) is a procedure that involves inserting a small camera into the nostril and passing it to the laryngopharynx. FEES allows direct assessment of the structures, movement, and function of the upper airway at rest and during voicing and swallowing. This procedure can be used to inform decisions about tracheostomy removal, secretions, voice, and swallowing management (RCSLT 2020b). Patients will be asked to do some short speech tasks to allow assessment of speech and voice structures. Patients may be asked to swallow small amounts of coloured food and drink or trial different strategies during the procedure. The procedure takes approximately 10–20 minutes

Figure 14.1 Aspiration of contrast with a tracheostomy.

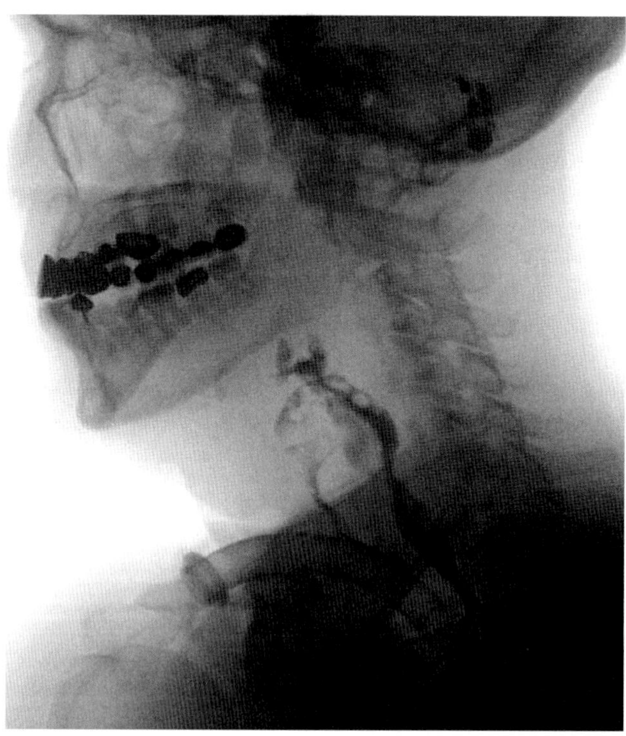

and can be done at bedside or in a clinic room. Although there is no radiation exposure, FEES is an invasive procedure, and patient selection requires consideration.

Both videofluoroscopy and FEES are possible for inpatients and outpatients, though services can vary locally.

Management

SLTs advise on food and fluid volumes, consistencies, and strategies to make swallowing safe and comfortable. This could include taking smaller sips or slowing the pace of eating and drinking. SLTs provide therapy plans based on the type of swallowing disorder patients present with and their goals and ability to participate in therapy. Common exercise examples may focus on improving the strength and range of movement of the tongue base, closure of the airway, cough strength, or relaxing of the muscle at the top of the oesophagus (cricopharyngeal sphincter). However, there may be particular exercises or strategies focusing on any part of swallowing or cough. Swallowing therapy may also include sensory rehabilitation, practicing swallowing by taking small amounts of food or drink to work on coordination and synchrony of the sensorineural pathways.

Recovery takes time and commitment to therapy, but most patients are able to manage some oral intake. Some patients may require short-term nutritional support via a nasogastric tube. This is a bedside procedure to insert a small tube into the nostril, passing down through the pharynx, into the stomach. Patients with significant dysphagia or nutrition issues may require long-term enteral feeding. This is the intake of food via the gastrointestinal (GI) tract via a tube (gastrostomy) that goes directly to the stomach or small intestine. A short surgical procedure is required to insert a gastrostomy, and there are a variety of different gastrostomy types. Requirement for gastrostomy should be considered before treatment commences (NICE 2004) and removal considered once oral intake is sufficient to maintain nutrition and hydration needs.

Trismus

Reduced jaw opening is referred to as trismus (Figure 14.2). Trismus in head and neck cancer can be caused by the location of a tumour, surgery, or radiotherapy. Trismus can cause serious functional problems including speech and chewing difficulties and access for oral hygiene (Cardoso et al. 2021). SLTs can advise on specialist cutlery or strategies for patients who have difficulty fitting standard cutlery in their mouth. Some patients may have such significant trismus that they are unable to use standard toothbrushes. SLTs work with dental colleagues to advise appropriate tools for oral hygiene.

Trismus assessment involves assessment of jaw opening and movements alongside patient-reported symptoms of tightness and pain. Trismus rehabilitation requires intensive therapy and can be a lifelong commitment to manage. Therapy can involve active exercises, such as functional chewing, and passive resistance exercises to rehabilitate the muscles of the jaw (van der Geer et al. 2020). The SLT team educate patients about the risk of trismus prior to their treatment. If trismus occurs, SLTs then manage and train patients to manage these difficulties independently. For some patients, trismus will resolve completely with treatment, but for others, the goal of therapy is maintenance of their current jaw opening.

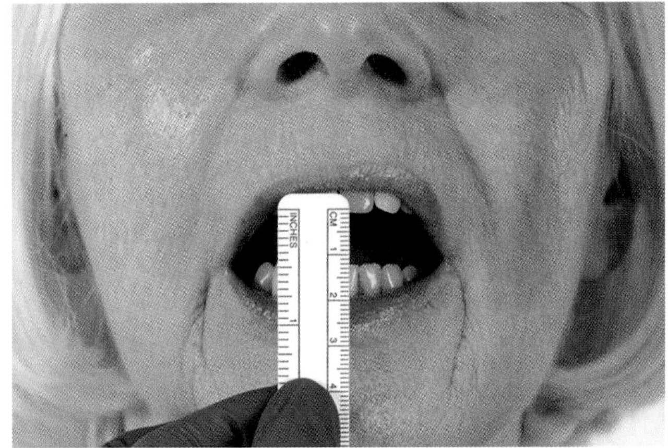

Figure 14.2 Trismus after head and neck cancer.

Altered Airways

SLTs have highly specialist skills to support and manage patients who have undergone voice box removal (laryngectomy) (Clarke et al. 2016). They provide education and training to patients and their carers before surgery and are involved with these patients for the rest of their lives. Following laryngectomy, patients breathe through a permanent stoma (hole) in their neck. As they cannot breathe through their mouth and nose, these patients are unable to heat or filter the air before it reaches their lungs. SLTs assess the need for different products to support respiratory rehabilitation (RCSLT 2020a). SLTs also assess and manage communication after laryngectomy that may be nonverbal, use of an electrolarynx (electronic device that mimics the voice box externally) or oesophageal speech (the patient learns to inject air into the oesophagus for speech). Most patients choose a voice prosthesis where a one-way valve is inserted into the wall between the trachea and the oesophagus. SLTs support patients in learning how to look after their voice prosthesis and troubleshoot any difficulties (Evans et al. 2010). Most laryngectomy patients are able to eat and drink by mouth, but some patients do have difficulties swallowing. SLTs can support diagnosis and treatment of swallowing difficulties after laryngectomy.

Some people with head and neck cancer require a tube in their neck to help them breathe (tracheostomy). Tracheostomies can be temporary or permanent. Some patients have a planned tracheostomy; for example, if upper airway swelling is expected postoperatively or there is a known risk of airway occlusion. Other patients may require an emergency tracheostomy due to acute airway obstruction or breathing difficulties. Tracheostomy can impact communication and swallowing (RCSLT 2021). SLTs provide assessment, education, and management of any difficulties. Communication may be verbal or nonverbal. SLTs manage swallowing difficulties with tracheostomy as these patients are often at a higher risk of aspiration and may require advice on managing secretions. Following tracheostomy the upper airway can become desensitised and sensory rehabilitation may be required (Wallace and McGrath 2021). SLTs are part of the multidisciplinary team who assess safety for tracheostomy removal.

Dietitians

SLTs work closely with dietitians throughout the patient pathway. SLTs assess swallowing physiology and function. Dietitians are experts in assessing nutritional status and intake, calculating nutritional requirements, and providing nutrition recommendations (BAHNO 2021b). Adequate and well-managed nutrition is essential for wound healing and recovery from treatment (Villegas 2018). Dietetic advice may include fortification of foods, support for managing appetite and taste changes, supporting oral nutrition with supplements, or alternative routes for nutrition and hydration including nasogastric feeding, gastrostomies, and, in rare cases, total parenteral nutrition. The team work together to support patients to maintain sufficient and safe nutrition and hydration during their head and neck cancer journey.

Training

A degree in speech and language therapy is required to become an SLT. Undergraduate degrees are either a three-year degree or up to six years part time. There is a range of undergraduate and postgraduate courses in the UK. Training involves a theoretical grounding in a wide range of core subjects including anatomy and physiology, linguistics, and neurology. Clinical placements are a core area in speech and language therapy degrees and allow students to gain a range of adult and paediatric experience. Further postgraduate training is required for specialist areas such as dysphagia, altered airway management (tracheostomy and laryngectomy), and instrumental assessments of swallowing and voice (videofluoroscopy, FEES, and EEL).

References

British Association of Head & Neck Oncologists (2021a, 26 May). Speech & Language Therapists https://bahno.org.uk/speech_language_therapist.aspx

British Association of Head & Neck Oncologists (2021b, 25 August). AHPs – dietitians https://bahno.org.uk/ahps-dietitians.aspx

Brady, G.C., Goodrich, J., and Roe, J.W.G. (2020). Using experience-based co-design to improve the pre-treatment care pathway for people diagnosed with head and neck cancer. *Support Care Cancer* 28: 739–745. https://doi.org/10.1007/s00520-019-04877-z.

Carding PN, Jones S, Morton V, Robinson F, Slade S and Wells C (2008). Speech and language therapy endoscopy for voice disordered patients. Royal College of Speech and Language Therapists position paper 2008.

Cardoso, R.C., Kamal, M., Zaveri, J. et al. (2021). Self-reported trismus: prevalence, severity and impact on quality of life in oropharyngeal cancer survivorship: a cross-sectional survey report from a comprehensive cancer center. *Support Care Cancer* 29: 1825–1835. https://doi.org/10.1007/s00520-020-05630-7.

Clarke, P., Radford, K., Coffey, M., and Stewart, M. (2016). Speech and swallow rehabilitation in head and neck cancer: United Kingdom national multidisciplinary guidelines. *J. Laryngol. Otol. 130* (S2): S176–S180. https://doi.org/10.1017/S0022215116000608.

Elaldi, R., Roussel, L.M., Gal, J. et al. (2021). Correlations between long-term quality of life and patient needs and concerns following head and neck cancer treatment and the impact of psychological distress. A multicentric cross-sectional study. *Eur. Arch. Otorhinolaryngol.* 278: 2437–2445. https://doi.org/10.1007/s00405-020-06326-8.

Evans E, Hurren A, Govender R, Radford K, Robinson H F, Batch A, Samuel P, Prosthetic surgical voice restoration (SVR): the role of the speech and language therapist. Royal College of Speech and Language Therapists policy statement 2010

Farneti, D., Turroni, V., and Genovese, E. (2018). Aspiration: diagnostic contributions from bedside swallowing evaluation and endoscopy. *Acta otorhinolaryngol. Ital. 38* (6): 511–516. https://doi.org/10.14639/0392-100X-1967.

National Institute for Health and Care Excellence. (2004). *Improving outcomes in head and neck cancers* [NICE cancer service guideline CSG6]. https://www.nice.org.uk/guidance/csg6

Patterson, J.M. (2019). Late effects of organ preservation treatment on swallowing and voice; presentation, assessment, and screening. *Front. Oncol. 9*: 401. https://doi.org/10.3389/fonc.2019.00401.

Pezdirec, M., Strojan, P., and Boltezar, I.H. (2019). Swallowing disorders after treatment for head and neck cancer. *Radiol. Oncol. 53* (2): 225–230. https://doi.org/10.2478/raon-2019-0028.

Royal College of Speech and Language Therapists (2020a, 26 May) RCSLT clinical guidance for the management of total laryngectomy in the context of COVID-19. https://www.rcslt.org/wp-content/uploads/2020/11/RCSLT-COVID-19-Laryngectomy-guidance-041120.pdf

Royal College of Speech and Language Therapists (2020b, 26 May) RCSLT guidance: speech and language therapist-led endoscopic procedures in the COVID-19 pandemic. https://www.rcslt.org/wp-content/uploads/media/docs/Covid/RCSLT-COVID-19-SLT-led-endoscopic-procedure-guidance_FINAL-(2).PDF?la=en%26hash=8101575091FE8F1ABA41B4B472387DAFB023A39D

Royal College of Speech and Language Therapists. Videofluoroscopic evaluation of oropharyngeal swallowing function (VFS): the role of speech and language therapists. RCSLT position paper 2013

Royal College of Speech and Language Therapists (2021) Dysphagia guidance: vulnerability and risk issues. https://www.rcslt.org/members/clinical-guidance/dysphagia/dysphagia-guidance/#section-6

van der Geer, S.J., Reintsema, H., Kamstra, J.I. et al. (2020). The use of stretching devices for treatment of trismus in head and neck cancer patients: a randomized controlled trial. *Support Care Cancer* 28: 9–11. https://doi.org/10.1007/s00520-019-05075-7.

Villegas, B.C. (2018). Clinical swallow evaluation in head and neck cancer. In: *Dysphagia Management in Head and Neck Cancers* (ed. K. Thankappan, S. Iyer and J. Menon). Singapore: Springer https://doi.org/10.1007/978-981-10-8282-5_4.

Wallace, S. and McGrath, B.A. (2021). Laryngeal complications after tracheal intubation and tracheostomy. *BJA Edu. 21* (7): 250–257.

Williams, A.M., Lindholm, J., Siddiqui, F. et al. (2017). Clinical assessment of cognitive function in patients with head and neck cancer: prevalence and correlates. *Otolaryngol. Head Neck Surg.* 157 (5): 808–815.

15

The Role of the Restorative Dentist in the Management of Head and Neck Cancer Patients

Michael Fenlon

King's College London, London, UK

Introduction

The primary aim of treatment of head and neck cancer patients with curative intent is to eliminate malignant disease. Treatment offered to patients depends on the size, location, and type of tumour being treated. With some exceptions, cancers of the mouth, sinuses, and salivary grands are treated with primary surgery alone for small tumours and surgery combined with postoperative radiotherapy alone or radiotherapy combined with chemotherapy for more extensive disease. For tumours of the larynx, pharynx, base of tongue, and tonsils, the treatment of choice is radiotherapy alone or radiotherapy combined with chemotherapy, with surgery reserved for persistent or recurrent disease after radiotherapy.

The secondary aim of treatment of head and neck cancer patients is to restore appearance and function as nearly as possible to pretreatment conditions. This is where the restorative dentistry contribution is so important. Many patients fear mutilation, loss of function, and isolation after treatment for head and neck cancers. Restoring appearance (Kansy et al. 2018) and function are critical to restoring self-confidence after cancer treatment and to quality of life.

Alterations to appearance are sometimes unavoidable for patients who have surgery for head and neck cancers. However, every effort to minimise these changes or to disguise them should be made. Restoring missing teeth and providing soft tissue support make important contributions to ameliorating appearance changes as a result of surgery.

Problems Related to Rehabilitation of Head and Neck Cancer Patients

In the classic surgical approach to head and neck cancer, the 3Rs apply. These are resection, reconstruction, and rehabilitation. Resection and reconstruction are often done in the one visit to the operating theatre. However, rehabilitation is a lifelong task for the dentist and burden for the patient. Most rehabilitation relates to the consequences of treatment rather than being directly attributable to the tumour. For many surgical cases, postoperative radiotherapy or chemotherapy is necessary if the staging of the tumour is advanced or if there is any evidence of regional spread.

In the classic approach to tumours requiring radiotherapy and chemotherapy, treatment is provided over a period of six weeks. The treatment of choice is intensity-modulated radiation therapy (IMRT), with patients receiving a dose of 2.2 grays (Gy) on five consecutive days every week for six weeks with a target dose for the tumour in the region of 66 Gy. Radiation causes permanent damage to soft tissues and specialised tissues (Watters et al. 2011). Saliva glands are severely damaged by doses over about 30 Gy. Serous saliva glands, particularly the parotid gland, are seriously affected by radiotherapy, with salivary flow reduced by as much as 95% and the quality of saliva severely affected (Arrifin et al. 2018). In contrast, mucous salivary glands tend to continue to produce diminished amounts of mucous saliva. The combination of mucous saliva and very little serous saliva results in sticky, thick, unpleasant saliva. Radiation damage results in saliva with very limited buffering capacity and reduced immunoglobulins. Reduced buffering capacity in combination with a reduced saliva flow increases the risk of dental caries (Arrifin et al. 2018). So-called radiation caries is a result of changes to saliva flow because of radiation therapy. Radiation caries tends to manifest itself as dental caries rapidly advancing in areas not usually associated with dental caries, particularly caries at the incisal edges and cusp tips and annular root caries of teeth where there has been some recession. Radiation caries, once it

Care of Head and Neck Cancer Patients for Dental Hygienists and Dental Therapists, First Edition. Edited by Jocelyn J. Harding.

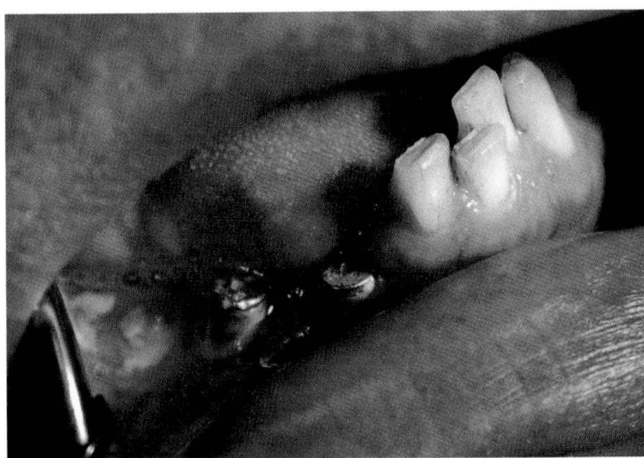

Figure 15.1 Osteoradionecrosis associated with dental implant placement.

becomes established, is difficult to control, and prevention is essential (Palmier et al. 2020). Careful oral hygiene combined with fluoride treatments are essential to prevent the onset of radiation caries. The wearing of removable partial dentures is undesirable. Removable partial dentures increase caries risk by up to five times in patients who have never had radiation therapy, and in patients who have had varied radiation therapy, the problem is even worse.

Radiation damages soft tissues, causing fibrosis in muscles and connective tissues, interfering with the mobility of joints, stretching muscles, causing limitation of opening of the mouth, reducing the ability of tissues to heal after trauma (Brook 2020), and increasing the risk of osteoradionecrosis. Osteoradionecrosis is the death of bone that has been in the radiation field. It is defined as bone exposed for three months or more in a radiation field. Osteoradionecrosis can occur spontaneously or can be the result of trauma currently as a result of extraction of a tooth (Nabil and Samman 2011). All patients who have tumours towards the back of the mouth in the larynx and pharynx tend to be treated primarily with radiotherapy. The dose to parotid glands, bone, muscles of mastication, and the temporomandibular joint tends to be very high, resulting in mandibular molars being included in highly irradiated fields in patients with limitation of opening. These factors make cleaning the teeth very difficult, and because of the risk of radiation, caries in combination with poor cleaning means the possibility of these teeth being lost is high. These teeth are particularly at risk of needing to be extracted, potentially causing osteoradionecrosis (Figure 15.1).

Restoring Function

Dentists tend to equate restoration of function in patients who are missing teeth with the ability to chew. However, posttreatment head and neck cancer survivors tend to be more concerned with the ability to speak comprehensibly; be understood when using the phone; and be able to eat and drink in company without food or fluids dripping out of the nose, causing gagging, prostheses dislodging, or any other of the multitude of embarrassing problems that can ruin social interactions for these patients (Melissant et al. 2021). These concerns represent social function rather than chewing function.

Chewing ability is not critical for nutrition, as food can be blended or delivered as supplements. However, this view ignores the very important role eating with friends and family plays in social well-being (Jovanovic et al. 2021). Effective chewing is important, not only from the positive experience of chewing foods of different textures but also being able to chew at a rate that is compatible with eating with others. A particular consideration for patients who have had radiotherapy and for those who have had surgery to the larynx and pharynx is the reduced ability to swallow food that has not been finely comminuted by chewing. Poorly chewed food can result in gagging, choking, and pain on swallowing.

The Head and Neck Cancer Multidisciplinary Meeting and the Contribution Made by the Restorative Dentistry Consultant

As a result of the reorganisation of head and neck cancer services after the millennium, the number of services offering head and neck cancer treatment was reduced dramatically. The aim was to have centres with a critical mass to provide comprehensive support for head and neck cancer patients, concentrate equipment in centres of expertise, and make sure that surgeons and oncologists were doing enough treatment to become experts in the field of head and neck cancer. As part of this arrangement is best practice according to the head and neck cancer manual published by the National Institute for Health and Care Excellence in 2004, multidisciplinary meetings (MDMs) for head and neck cancer patients became mandatory in each centre. These happen every week, and there is a specified list of attendees whose attendance is expected. These include oncologists, surgeons, cancer nurse specialists, restorative dentists, and representatives of the various therapies. Designated members from each of these specialties are required to attend at least 70% of meetings every year.

The Workings of the Head and Neck Cancer MDM

The main function of the MDM is to collate evidence in relation to diagnosis, to decide on appropriate treatment. Treatment may be curative intent or palliative where a cure cannot be achieved. The most appropriate treatment for some patients may be primary surgery, for others radiotherapy or chemoradiotherapy, or for a small group referral to other specialist MDMs, for example, lymphoma and myeloma MDMs. When initial treatment has been completed, the MDM considers evidence from pathology and radiology to decide on types of treatment that may subsequently be necessary to maximise the chance of cure. The role of the restorative dentist at the MDM includes the following:

- To identify patients who need pretreatment dental assessment (all patients with teeth).
- To establish if any devices or prostheses are required at the time of initial surgery, such as dressing plates, obturators, and cutting stents.
- To contribute to surgical planning and design. Where incisions are made and how resections are done may compromise a patient's rehabilitation is subsequently where small alterations may have made a major improvement in the patient's outcome in relation to rehabilitation.
- To arrange for extractions were necessary during cancer surgery in theatre.
- To contribute to planning of grafting and reconstruction to maximise the chance of optimal rehabilitation later.

The restorative dentist contributes to care of head and neck cancer patients at various stages of the treatment pathway:

- Participation in the head and neck cancer MDM to plan management of Head and neck cancer patients
- Pretreatment planning and preparation of patients
- For surgery patients, in theatre obturator placement and implant placement
- Prosthodontic rehabilitation after completion of treatment with curative intent
- Ongoing maintenance and surveillance.

The most important message related to head and neck cancer care is the collaborative nature of planning and treatment if the best survival rates are to be achieved and for patients to enjoy the best achievable quality of life under the circumstances.

Interventions Provided by the Restorative Dentist for Head and Neck Cancer Patients

In addition to contributing to planning at the MDM, the restorative dentist is responsible for precancer treatment dental assessment and planning for patients. Oral health of patients having radiotherapy or surgery should be as good as possible before cancer treatment. This may offer substantial benefits to healing after surgery or after radiotherapy, so vigorous initial interventions to reduce periodontal inflammation and infection burden should be delivered (Samim et al. 2016). Teeth with poor or hopeless prognosis that will be substantially involved in radiation fields should be extracted. Teeth that offer substantial risk of infection during radiotherapy, requiring cessation or pausing of radiotherapy, may cause reduced cure with radiotherapy and increased mortality rates (Fesinmeyer et al. 2010). Second and third molar teeth or teeth with deep periodontal pockets or poor root canal treatments within the high-dose radiation field should be considered for extraction.

Impressions for dressing plates may be necessary at this stage of initial assessment. Dressing plates are used in the palate and occasionally in the mandible to support soft tissue grafts where an area of soft tissue is being replaced.

Where patients will end up with a palatal defect after surgery, an immediate obturator may be necessary. These necessitate careful planning. Impressions are made at the earliest possible opportunity after diagnosis to ensure that the immediate obturator is available at the time of surgery.

At the time of surgery where a defect in the palate is anticipated, fitting of the immediate obturator is done by the restorative dentist in theatre at the time of the resection. When the palate has been resected, the obturator is fitted. The maxillary antrum and/or nasal spaces need to be packed and a seal achieved over the immediate obturator using a soft lining material such as Coe-Comfort. Two to three weeks after primary surgery, the restorative dentist returns to theatre to remove the immediate obturator, which has been left in place. At that visit the obturator is relined and a master impression made for a

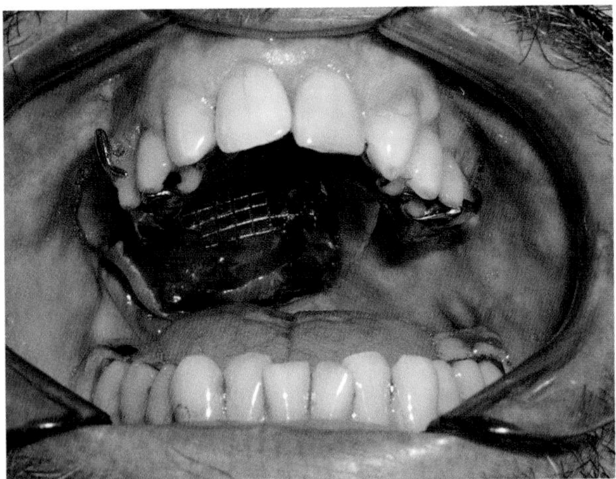

Figure 15.2 Obturator in a dentate patient.

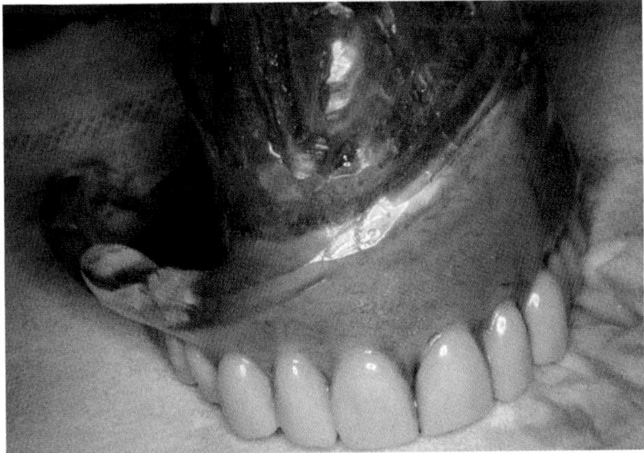

Figure 15.3 Obturator for an edentulous patient.

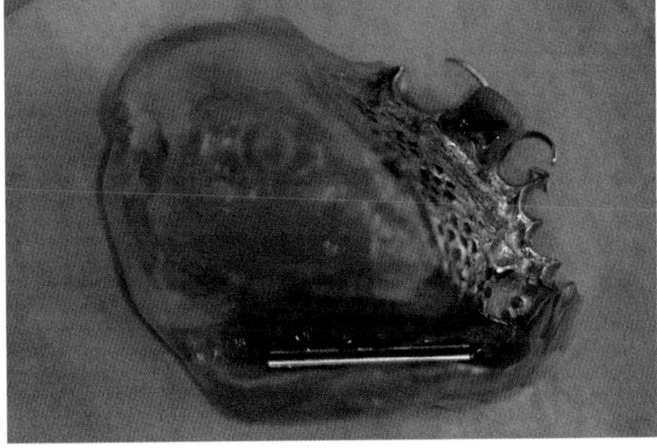

Figure 15.4 Implant-supported obturator.

replacement interim obturator. In the dental clinic the obturator is subsequently made. This obturator is an interim measure to provide the patient with some teeth and a seal between the mouth and the nose to allow speech and eating while healing is happening. Usually, six months and two years after the initial treatment new obturators are made and then approximately every five years thereafter (Figures 15.2–15.4).

Modern reconstruction methods allow closing of defects and in many cases placement of implants in the free tissue transfer graft. One of the benefits of modern grafting procedures is that surgeons can make large resections with the full knowledge that subsequently they will be able to reconstruct the defect (Barclay et al. 2018). This allows good margins around tumours without the mutilating effects of very large surgical defects. Typically, hard tissue grafts include fibula, iliac crest, radial forearm, and scapula bone. These grafts are free vascularised tissue transfer grafts where a graft of bone, soft tissue, and blood vessels is taken from a donor site, the bone is fixed in position to replace missing bone, soft tissues of the graft are arranged to replace missing soft tissues, and the blood vessels of the graft are connected to blood vessels in the head and neck area to keep this graft alive. More than 95% of grafts should survive (Ishimaru et al. 2016). Provided the graft survives in the area and is not subsequently heavily irradiated, dental implants may be possible, providing the patient with fixed or removable implant-supported prostheses where the function is predictable and the appearance is good (Curi et al. 2018) (Figures 15.5 and 15.6).

Until about 40 years ago, no treatment was provided for patients in the mandible where a discontinuity resulted from surgery. To avoid discontinuities in the mandible, surgery was kept small with adverse effects on survival. Where a discontinuity was created, there was nothing much that could be done because wearing conventional dentures under the circumstances was usually unsuccessful. In the era of successful vascularised grafting, CT scans of the mandible and donor sites including fibula and iliac crest allow rapid prototypes of the mandible and of graft sites to be made with careful planning of resection and reconstruction. Cutting stents can be made to ensure that shape and size of graft bone matches the amount and shape of the reselected bone in the mandible, resulting in optimisation of angulation of bone for implant placements and in good occlusion and good appearance after surgery.

Dental implant placement at the time of primary surgery should only be made in local rather than in grafted bone unless radiotherapy is planned. When grafts have become established two to three months after grafting, implants can be placed. Optimum implant placement requires careful planning and the use of implant-guidance stents or computer-aided navigation. Critical considerations for use of dental implants in head and neck cancer patients include general suitability for implants, interdependent diabetes, smoking, the amount of bone present, and radiation dose if any. Patients on intravenous bisphosphonates should not be provided with dental implants. Survival is reduced for implants placed in bone that has received a radiation dose of more than 50 Gy (Buddula et al. 2012).

A particular area of concern is the rehabilitation of edentulous patients treated for head and neck cancer. While wearing complete dentures always involves compromises, and many complete denture patients struggle to wear lower dentures, the situation for patients treated for head and neck cancer is markedly worse. Patients treated with surgery for oral cancer usually have deformities within the oral cavity that interfere with denture wearing and denture retention. Implant-supported overdentures work well in these patients. If in addition to surgery these patients have been treated with postoperative radiotherapy, placement of implants may be difficult or impossible because of radiation fields. In patients treated for cancers of the soft palate, base of tongue, tonsils, pharynx, and larynx, high doses of radiation are concentrated towards the back of the mouth, often affecting the posterior mandible as far forward as about the second premolar. In these patients, dry mouth can be a serious problem, and the effect of radiation on soft tissues tends to make soft tissues intolerant of mobile dentures because of their tendency to be traumatised and to heal poorly (Figure 15.7). In addition, their mobile complete dentures touching the mylohyoid ridges on the lingual side of the mandible posteriorly can induce osteoradionecrosis. The anterior mandible and most of the maxilla are usually spared substantial doses of radiotherapy, so implants can be placed in the mandible in the interforaminal area and in the maxilla if necessary. Implant treatment in the maxilla is necessary where the mouth is very dry or where patients are inclined to gag.

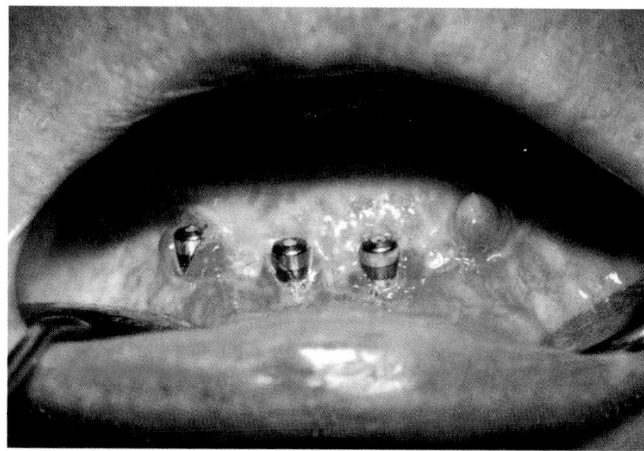

Figure 15.5 Implant bar and denture.

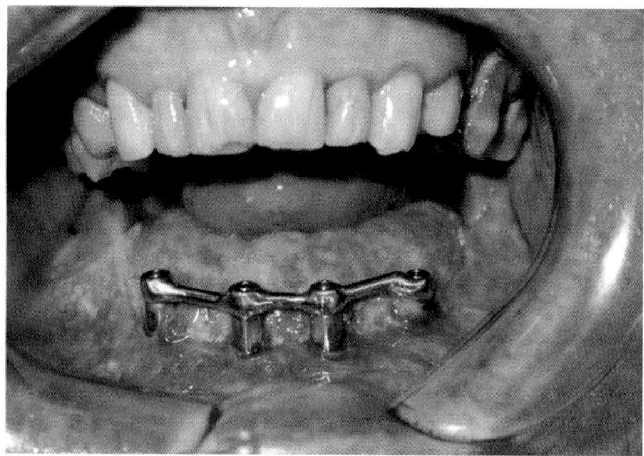

Figure 15.6 Implant bar and denture in situ.

Supporting Patients' Psychological Well-Being

While psychological well-being of patients is not the foremost consideration in dentistry, it is an important consideration, particularly in patients treated for head and neck cancer. Being diagnosed with life-threatening disease is a severe psychological blow for many patients. The treatment is arduous and in many cases results in changes to appearance and social function. Patients who have had radiotherapy often have bizarre changes in taste and smell and may have persistent pain that can be difficult to control in the long term. Many patients fear mutilation and social isolation as a result of surgery. While some of this concern is justified, modern approaches minimise these risks. It is important that patients be provided with up-to-date and correct information. There is good evidence that head and neck cancer patients' quality of life returns close to normal with the passing of time.

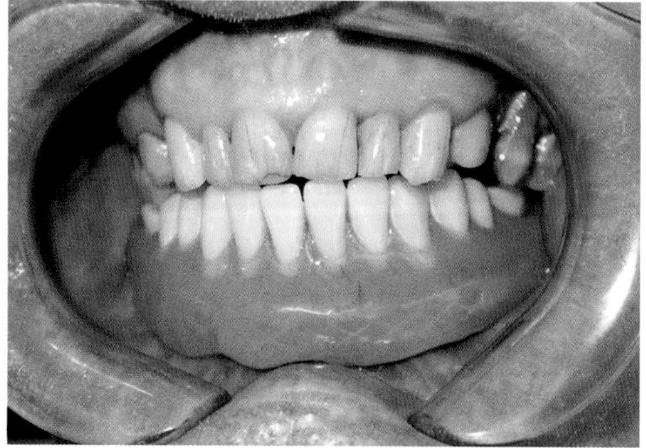

Figure 15.7 Hyperplasia around implants associated with poor oral hygiene. Note also incipient radiation caries.

About 2% of head and neck cancer patients commit suicide between time of diagnosis and end of primary treatment for cancer (Zeller 2006). Therefore, it is very important for every clinician to be aware of this possibility and to be on alert for any statements that might suggest suicidal ideation. Patients contemplating suicide usually mention their concerns to a health professional in the month before taking their own lives. While major resources are focused on saving lives by efficient and effective cancer treatment, appropriate referral of patients who mention the possibility of suicide is also a lifesaver (Klonsky et al. 2016).

Long-Term Prevention and Maintenance

The preservation of teeth where possible is highly desirable. In the case of patients who have had radiotherapy, keeping teeth in a healthy condition is challenging. Excellent oral hygiene, regular visits to the dentist and hygienist, and high fluoride and remineralising regimes become lifetime necessities if teeth are to be preserved in patients with radiation-related xerostomia.

After radiotherapy, substantial changes on oral flora take place, and these may influence survival of dental implants. Therefore, excellent hygiene of dental implants is an important consideration. Regular removal of implant-retained bridges to facilitate hygiene and to check implant stability, in addition to radiological surveillance, is important for maintaining osseointegration.

It is essential that dentures supported by implants as well as conventional dentures are replaced in a timely fashion before resorption causes uneven loading and tilting of dentures. If uneven loading happens in an area where radiotherapy dose has been delivered in substantial amounts, there is always a risk of osteoradionecrosis.

Ongoing Cancer Surveillance

There is a definite risk of recurrence of any cancer in the first two years, in particular for patients treated for head and neck cancer. The risk after five years becomes insignificant. Therefore, careful examination of the oral mucosa and original nodes is an important function for every clinician at every patient visit.

The risk unfortunately extends beyond that of recurrence. Patients who have had one head and neck cancer are at substantially elevated risk of having a new primary head and neck cancer (Priante et al. 2011). In particular, where patients have exposed themselves to the carcinogenic effects of alcohol and tobacco in large quantities over many years before being diagnosed with their first primary cancer, the soft tissues of the mouth, nose, paranasal sinuses, pharynx, and larynx are at increased risk of developing a new cancer. The risk may be as much as a hundred times above baseline; therefore, careful monitoring for life by dental health professionals is very important.

References

Arrifin, A., Heidari, E., Burke, M. et al. (2018). The effect of radiotherapy for treatment of head and neck cancer on oral flora and saliva. *Oral Health Prev. Dent.* 16 (5): 425–429.

Barclay, C.W., Foster, E.C., and Taylor, C.L. (2018). Restorative aspects of oral cancer reconstruction. *Br. Dent. J.* 225 (9): 848–854.

Brook, I. (2020). Late side effects of radiation treatment for head and neck cancer. *Radiat. Oncol. J.* 38: https://doi.org/10.3857/roj.2020.00213.

Buddula, A., Assad, D.A., Salinas, T.J. et al. (2012). Survival of dental implants in irradiated head and neck cancer patients: a retrospective analysis. *Clin. Implant. Dent. Relat. Res.* 14: 716–722. https://doi.org/10.1111/j.1708-8208.2010.00307.x.

Curi, M.M., Condezo, A.F., Ribeiro, K.D., and Cardoso, C.L. (2018). Long-term success of dental implants in patients with head and neck cancer after radiation therapy. *Int. J. Oral Maxillofac. Surg.* 47 (6): 783–788.

Fesinmeyer, M.D., Mehta, V., Blough, D. et al. (2010). Effect of radiotherapy interruptions on survival in Medicare enrollees with local and regional head-and-neck cancer. *Int. J. Radiat. Oncol. Biol. Phys.* 78 (3): 675–681.

Ishimaru, M., Ono, S., Suzuki, S. et al. (2016). Risk factors for free flap failure in 2,846 patients. *J. Oral Maxillofac. Surg.* 74 (6): 1265–1270.

Jovanovic, N., Dreyer, C., Hawkins, S. et al. (2021). The natural history of weight and swallowing outcomes in oropharyngeal cancer patients following radiation or concurrent chemoradiation therapy. *Support. Care Cancer* 29 (3): 1597–1607.

Kansy, K., Hoffmann, J., Alhalabi, O. et al. (2018). Subjective and objective appearance of head and neck cancer patients following microsurgical reconstruction and associated quality of life — a cross-sectional study. *J. Craniomaxillofac. Surg.* 46 (8): 1275–1284.

Klonsky, D.E., May, A.M., and Saffer, B.Y. (2016). Suicide, suicidal attempts and suicidal ideation. *Annu. Rev. Clin. Psychol.* 12: 307–330.

Melissant, H.C., Jansen, F., Eerenstein, S.E. et al. (2021). Body image distress in head and neck cancer patients: what are we looking at? *Support. Care Cancer* 29 (4): 2161–2169.

Nabil, S. and Samman, N. (2011). Incidence and prevention of osteoradionecrosis after dental extraction in irradiated patients: a systematic review. *Int. J. Oral Maxillofac. Surg.* 40 (3): 229–243.

National Institute for Health and Care Excellence. (2004). Improving outcomes in head and neck cancers [NICE cancer service guideline CSG6]. https://www.nice.org.uk/guidance/csg6

Palmier, N.R., Migliorati, C.A., Prado-Ribeiro, A.C. et al. (2020). Radiation-related caries: current diagnostic, prognostic, and management paradigms. *Oral Surg Oral Med Oral Pathol Oral Radiol* 130 (1): 52–62.

Priante, A.V.M., Castilho, E.C., and Kowalski, L.P. (2011). Second primary tumors in patients with head and neck cancer. *Curr. Oncol. Rep.* 13: 132–137.

Samim, F., Epstein, J.B., Zumsteg, Z.S. et al. (2016). Oral and dental health in head and neck cancer survivors. *Cancers Head and Neck* 1 14.

Watters, A.L., Epstein, J.B., and Agulnik, M. (2011). Oral complications of targeted cancer therapies: a narrative literature review. *Oral Oncol.* 47 (6): 441–448.

Zeller, J.L. (2006). High suicide risk found for patients with head and neck cancer. *JAMA* 296 (14): 1716–1717. https://doi.org/10.1001/jama.296.14.1716.

16

The Role of the Dental Nurse in an Oral and Maxillofacial Unit

Laura Holdway

East Kent Hospitals University Foundation Trust, Ashford, UK

The dental nurse role in an oral and maxillofacial unit is varied. Our fundamental dental nursing skills are always needed; however, we are additionally trained to assist with consultant-led clinics, biopsies, and skin cancer surgery lists. For those of us who are radiographically trained, we also undertake cone-beam CT (CBCT) imaging upon consultant request (see Figures 16.1–16.3).

Once patients are referred, they are given an appointment to attend a consultant-led clinic. We see an array of problems that all fall within head and neck. One patient may have an unresolving neck lump, the next may have suspected lichen planus on their tongue that needs investigating. After this appointment the patient will either be discharged or, if the consultant thinks more investigation is necessary, the nurse helps organise review appointments, biopsies, and any imaging that may be needed. Some of the imaging can be done within our unit; otherwise, the patient will be given an appointment to attend main x-ray for larger imaging such as magnetic resonance imaging (MRI).

Biopsies of any suspicious areas are taken during minor oral surgery clinics. As dental nurses we assist with these procedures and are used to dealing with various sets of instruments and also making sure the diathermy is ready to use. Postoperative instructions are also given at this time so that the patient can look after the area and heal as quickly as possible. These samples are then taken to histology, and we organise for the patient to return for results.

One of the hardest parts of the job is assisting a consultant who needs to break the bad news of a cancer diagnosis to a patient. This never gets easier, but the consultants are excellent at having a robust treatment plan ready to tackle the patient's individual needs. As dental nurses we can offer comfort and support if the patient and family members need it.

If patients are having radiotherapy to the head and neck, they are routinely assessed by our restorative consultants to see if any dental treatment needs to be undertaken. Irradiation immediately increases a patient's chances of treatment-related complications such as xerostomia, oral infections, and osteoradionecrosis of the jaw. Our dental nurses work closely with the consultants to get these patients treated in a timely manner before they begin treatment.

We assist with skin cancer lists, which routinely remove basal and squamous cell carcinomas. Sometimes these patients require a skin graft at the time of surgery, and it is fascinating to be able to assist with these procedures. The great thing about nursing in an oral and maxillofacial unit is being able to help patients get through a cancer diagnosis and then be a part of their dental rehabilitation in a restorative clinic. Our restorative consultants are able to give patients their smile

Care of Head and Neck Cancer Patients for Dental Hygienists and Dental Therapists, First Edition. Edited by Jocelyn J. Harding.

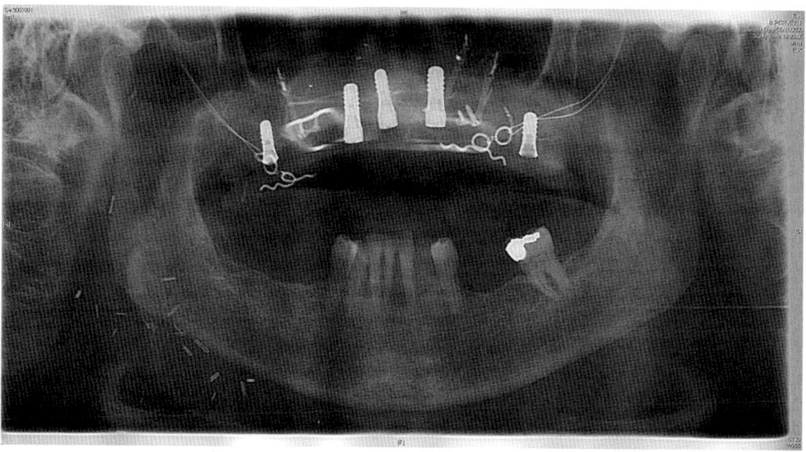

Figure 16.1 An orthopantomogram image that shows the final implants that support the implant-retained denture.

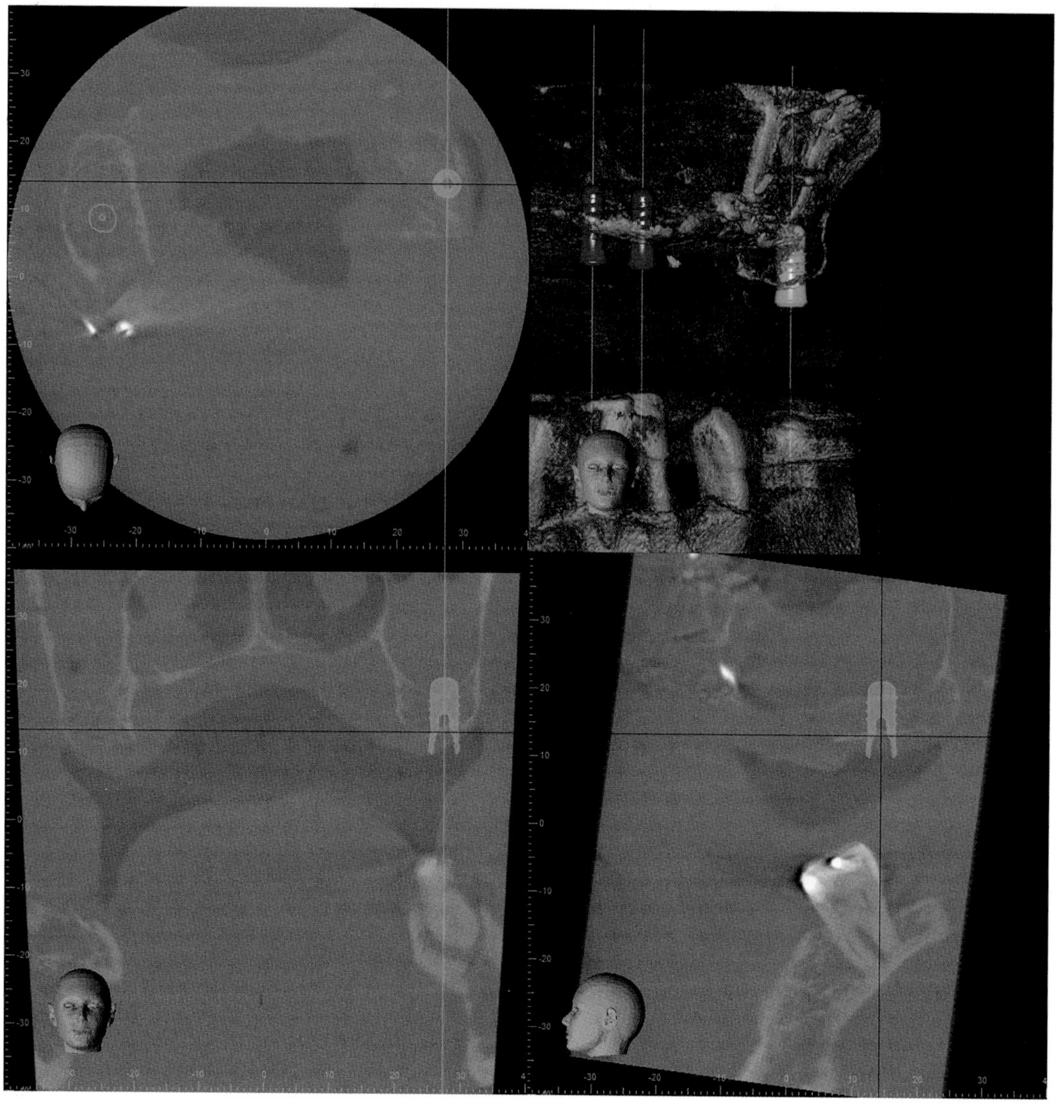

Figure 16.2 A snapshot of a surgeon's planning programme. The red and green highlighted areas represent proposed implants. Surgeons place the implants where they would ideally like them, and then the programme works out whether there is enough bone density to support the implants.

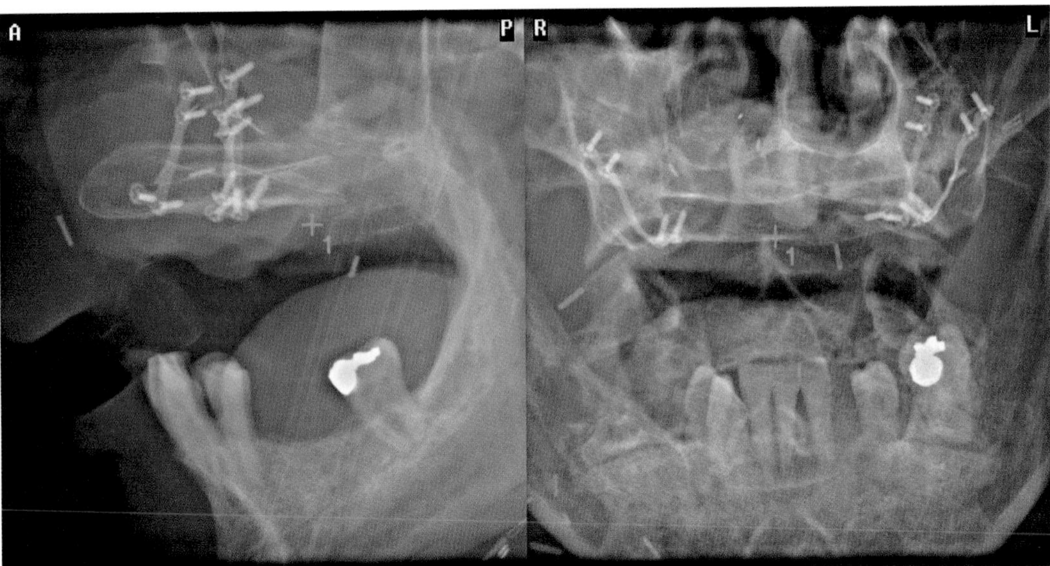

Figure 16.3 The actual image a dental radiographer sees while taking a CBCT image.

back and a functional bite, which is paramount for confidence and being able to eat properly and comfortably. We run nurse-led clinics in oral health, where we often come across these patients. Time is spent listening to them and going through brushing technique, which may have changed through limited opening and multiple surgeries, and how different oral hygiene aids may be beneficial.

Section 3

Types of Head and Neck Cancer Treatment

17

Chemotherapy: An Overview

Helen Davies

Cardiff and Vale University Health Board, Wales, UK

What Is Chemotherapy?

The Oxford Dictionary defines chemotherapy as 'the treatment of disease by the use of chemical substances, especially the treatment of cancer by cytotoxic and other drugs' (Lexico.com 2021).

How Does It Work?

The term 'cytotoxic' means 'toxic to living cells'. A tumor is caused by mutated cells dividing rapidly, so many chemotherapy drugs target cell division. Healthy, rapidly dividing cells, like the oral mucosa, will be affected but can repair and recover; most cancerous cells cannot. Unfortunately, this means there is an increased likelihood of patients experiencing dental problems during and after treatment, and the role of the dental team becomes paramount.

Chemotherapy is often used in four ways for head and neck cancer:

- Neoadjuvant chemotherapy (a high preloading dose prior to other treatments, most commonly radiotherapy)
- In conjunction with radiotherapy (concurrent)
- After surgery or radiotherapy (adjuvant)
- On its own (often for palliation).

Neoadjuvant Chemotherapy

Neoadjuvant chemotherapy is delivered prior to definitive treatment as a high preloading dose and is used to reduce the size of the tumor in cases where it is very large or there is extracapsular spread (nodal metastases that have spread beyond the lymph node capsule) (Myers et al. 2001). Local infiltration of a large tumor can make surgery problematic, hence the need to reduce the size of the primary tumor. In addition, the risk of distant metastases forming can be reduced by administering neoadjuvant chemotherapy.

Concurrent Chemotherapy

Most commonly, chemotherapy is given alongside a course of radiotherapy. Usually, radiotherapy is a six-week course of five-day treatment, with chemotherapy most commonly being administered every three weeks to allow for patient recovery. However, there are some clinical trials that administer chemotherapy in varying doses at different time intervals (Institute of Head and Neck Studies and Education 2021).

Care of Head and Neck Cancer Patients for Dental Hygienists and Dental Therapists, First Edition. Edited by Jocelyn J. Harding.

Adjuvant Chemotherapy

Adjuvant chemotherapy is administered after primary treatment (surgery or radiotherapy). The main purpose of this treatment is to reduce the likelihood of the cancer returning by 'mopping up' residual cancer cells in the bloodstream. These cells left untreated may lead to the formation of distant metastases in the future.

Palliative Chemotherapy

Palliative chemotherapy is used when the treatment intent isn't curative due to the advancement of the disease. The focus is to minimize symptoms and provide a more extended period before death while maintaining quality of life. It can also be used when other treatments cease to be effective, and the emphasis turns to minimizing the spread of the tumor. It is often administered at lower doses.

Types of Chemotherapy in Head and Neck Cancer

The following cytotoxic drugs are commonly used to treat head and neck tumors:

- Cisplatin/carboplatin
- Docetaxel
- Paclitaxel
- Fluorouracil (5FU)
- Gemcitabine.

The duration and time intervals of administration may vary depending on the type of chemotherapy given, part of a clinical trial, or the patient's specific needs.

Common Side Effects of Chemotherapy

Each drug has its own side effect profile, but the following symptoms are common to most:

- Fatigue (damage to healthy cells; the body needs to repair, using energy to do so)
- Mucositis (cells in the oral mucosa have a rapid turnover and so are more affected by chemotherapy)
- Metallic taste in the mouth
- Anaemia (patients typically present as feeling tired and breathless)
- Nausea and vomiting
- Hair loss
- Impaired immune response
- Bruising/bleeding, especially gingival
- Memory/concentration problems
- Neutropenia (see below).

How Is Chemotherapy Administered?

Chemotherapy can be administered intravenously (or less commonly, in tablet form orally). There are three main routes of administration for intravenous chemotherapy:

- Cannula (a needle inserted into a vein in the back of the patient's hand)
- PICC line (peripherally inserted central catheter, usually in the arm)
- Central line (inserted into the subclavian vein, internal or external jugular).

PICC lines remain in place for the duration of the treatment and must be monitored frequently to ensure there is no infection in the area.

A potential side effect of intravenous chemotherapy administration via cannula can be *extravasation*, where the chemotherapy agent leaks into the surrounding tissues and causes anything from minor irritation to tissue necrosis. An extravasation kit containing hyaluronidase or dimethyl sulfoxide (DMSO) is used by the oncology team to reduce inflammation in the area.

Patients are supported during their cancer treatment by a multidisciplinary team, which will be covered in more detail in the specific chapter of this book. For their chemotherapy, they will have the support of their oncologist and a clinical nurse specialist and input from a restorative dentist and dental hygienist or dental therapist.

Neutropenia is a condition where the number of white blood cells (neutrophils) is abnormally low and can be a common side effect of chemotherapy. This is why dental treatment should be delayed, if at all possible, during chemotherapy, as the potential release of bacteria into the bloodstream from a dental procedure could cause sepsis. Neutropenic sepsis carries a mortality rate of between 30% and 58% in high-risk patients, so this is critical (Clarke et al. 2013; Suárez et al. 2016: Office for National Statistics 2018).

Considerations When Treating Patients Undergoing/Having Had Chemotherapy

Patients under the care of a multidisciplinary team during their cancer treatment tend to seek advice and treatment from them, and it is rare that they would come to their general dental practitioner at this stage but not unheard of in the case of an emergency. The following points should be considered in this instance:

- Check the patient's medical history. If possible, ask patients beforehand to bring a list of medications, details of their cancer treatment, and the name of their oncologist.
- Some patients may be having ongoing regular chemotherapy or immunotherapy; neutrophil and platelet count must be checked prior to treatment.
- All routine dental treatment should be delayed during cancer treatment, specifically chemotherapy, and for at least three weeks after the last administration.
- Once chemotherapy has been completed, it is vital that the patient's oncologist be consulted prior to the formulation of a treatment plan.
- If emergency dental treatment is required, it should be minimally invasive where possible; an example of this would be a patient presenting with a fractured tooth. A temporary restoration could be placed without causing trauma or damage to the surrounding tissues (no local anesthetic, no matrix, no subgingival preparation).

Considerations for Patients during Treatment

The following should be considered for patients during their treatment:

- Patients may have impaired swallowing as a result of their treatment; they should be treated in a position that they feel comfortable in. Generally, patients will struggle in the supine position; head slightly elevated is helpful.
- Some patients struggle with nausea for a while after chemotherapy; again, raising patients so they are not lying flat will aid in this. The use of a rubber dam (if patients will tolerate it) can allow them to have a degree of reassurance that their gag reflex will not be provoked.
- Mucositis may persist for several weeks after chemotherapy; it is wise to avoid treatment during the active phase of mucositis (unless it is for an emergency) as this will be uncomfortable for patients, and their immunity takes time to recover.
- Patients may have a dry mouth after treatment. The author has found that moistening the mirror with water from a 3 in 1 tip before retracting the soft tissues is helpful, and also the use of a gel for dry mouth relief such as Oralieve or Bioxtra so that instruments do not adhere to the oral mucosa (ensure the patient is not allergic prior to administration of any product).
- Book longer than you would expect for their appointments; they may struggle with fatigue, have more questions about their treatment, and updating their medical history will take longer. They may also need to take frequent pauses during treatment. In addition to this, they may require more complex dentistry, which will increase the amount of time required.

- Unfortunately, patients with head and neck cancer are potentially at risk of recurrence, so a thorough intraoral and extraoral check is of the utmost importance. It is important to be aware that most patients will have a degree of anxiety around this, so reassurance is key.
- Often, patients may have had extensive dental reconstruction (including dental implants, dentures, obturators, or other prostheses). They may need extra support to look after and maintain these (see later chapter).

Summary

Chemotherapy is a treatment that aims to kill cancer cells, but unfortunately, it comes with a myriad of side effects, some of which are temporary, some permanent. These can impact patients' dental treatment in terms of their toleration of treatment and the complexity of treatment. It is of the utmost importance that there be good communication between the dental team and the patient's oncology team to facilitate effective and timely treatment for the patient. It is recommended that the oncologist is always consulted prior to any dental treatment being carried out in the primary care setting. The effects of cancer treatment on the oral cavity and surrounding structures can be long lasting, and it is vital that a good relationship is forged between patient and clinician.

References

Clarke, R.T., Jenyon, T., van Hamel Parsons, V., and King, A.J. (2013). Neutropenic sepsis: management and complications. *Clin. Med. (Lond.)* 13 (2): 185–187. http://doi.org/10.7861/clinmedicine.13-2-185.

Institute of Head and Neck Studies and Education (2021). Improving patients' lives through research. https://www.inhanse.org/patient-research/compare.

Lexico.com (2021). s.v. 'Chemotherapy'. https://www.lexico.com/definition/chemotherapy.

Myers, J.N., Greenberg, J.S., Mo, V., and Roberts, D. (2001). Extracapsular spread. *Cancer* 92 (12): 3030–3036. https://doi.org/10.1002/1097-0142(20011215)92:12<3030::AID-CNCR10148>3.0.CO;2-P.

Office for National Statistics (2018). Number of deaths from neutropenic sepsis where cancer was the underlying cause of death, by specified cancer types, sex and age groups, England and Wales, 2011 to 2016. www.ons.gov.uk/peoplepopulationandcommunity/birthsdeathsandmarriages/deaths/adhocs/007956numberofdeathsfromneutropenicsepsiswherecancerwastheunderlyingcauseofdeathbyspecifiedcancertypessexandagegroupsenglandandwales2011to2016.

Suárez, I., Böll, B., Shimabukuro-Vornhagen, A. et al. (2016). Letalität hämatoonkologischer Patienten in Neutropenie auf der Intensivstation [mortality of hematology-oncology patients with neutropenia in intensivecare]. *Medizinische Klinik, Intensivmedizin und Notfallmedizin* 111 (2): 84–91. https://doi.org/10.1007/s00063-015-0039-6.

18

Radiotherapy in Head and Neck Cancer

Muneeb Qureshi, Brindley Hapuarachi, and Bernadette Foran

Weston Park Cancer Centre, Sheffield Teaching Hospitals NHS Foundation Trust, Sheffield, UK

Radiotherapy

Radiotherapy (RT) is the use of high-energy x-rays (ionising radiation) to treat cancers and is the mainstay of HNC treatment. These high-energy x-rays interact with the water molecules inside the area targeted. This creates oxygen free radicals, which cause damage to the DNA of cells. The DNA damage limits a cell's ability to undergo further division and growth and causes cell death and tumour shrinkage. This damage also occurs in surrounding normal tissues and is the reason why there are side effects associated with RT.

The use of radiation in cancer treatment is reported as early as the late nineteenth century, when it was found to shrink tumourous growths. It was not until the mid to late twentieth century that the modern techniques of delivering radiation to cancers were developed and mastered, which revolutionized the use of RT in oncology as we see it today (Gianfaldoni et al. 2017).

In this chapter, we will discuss how head and neck RT is delivered with specific reference to intensity-modulated RT (IMRT) and what particular considerations are needed prior to RT in HNC patients, as well as side effects of RT.

Radiotherapy Techniques

The aim of RT is to deliver high doses of radiation to the tumour that result in cell death, whilst limiting the dose to the surrounding normal tissues, to minimise the side effects of the treatment. This is known as the *therapeutic ratio* (Okawa et al. 1987). The evolution of modern RT techniques has improved the therapeutic ratio, which has enabled oncologists to aim for higher doses of radiation to the cancer whilst at the same time reducing dose to surrounding critical structures. The ability to deliver RT accurately increases the chances of tumour control; reduces the dose to the normal critical structures, also known as *organs at risk* (OARs), such as parotid glands; and decreases the risk of toxicities from the treatment.

In the past, the limitation of imaging modalities meant that the tumour could only be targeted in two dimensions, namely length and width, which delivered a significant dose of radiation to the adjacent normal structures, causing side effects. With advancements in imaging techniques, it became possible to visualize and target the tumour in three dimensions, which led to the advent of 3-D conformal RT.

Three-dimensional conformal RT utilizes the accurate tomographic information from planning CT scans, which is uploaded into a software that creates a personalised treatment plan. This plan is linked to the linear accelerator, the machine that delivers external-beam RT to the tumour from outside the body and enables delivery of high doses of radiation to a volume of tissue, which is highly conformed to the actual tumour volume (see Figure 18.1). This multidimensional conformity reduces the dose received by surrounding OARs and increases the patient tolerance of treatment, improving the side effect profile.

Care of Head and Neck Cancer Patients for Dental Hygienists and Dental Therapists, First Edition. Edited by Jocelyn J. Harding.

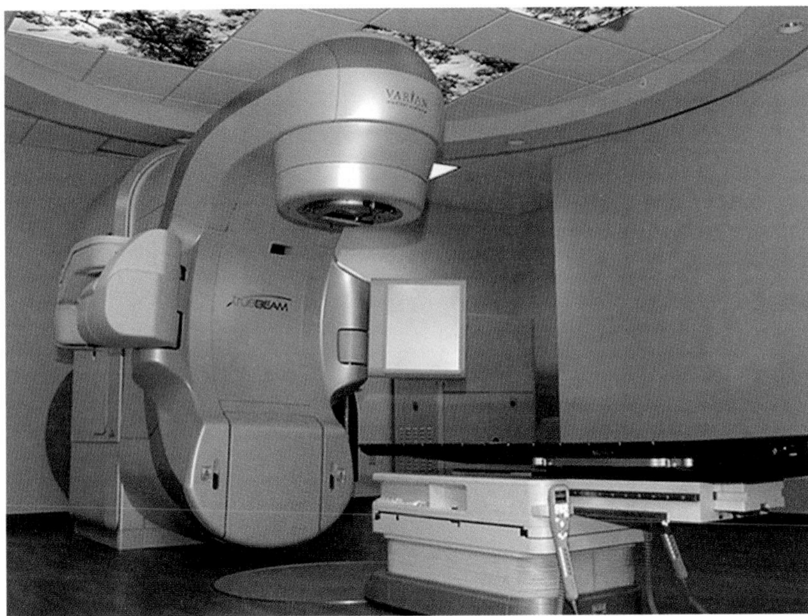

Figure 18.1 A VARIAN® linear accelerator. *Source:* Varian Medical Systems.

IMRT

IMRT is a step further in the evolution to deliver highly conformal RT to the cancer whilst minimising the dose to areas that do not require radiation. It uses the principles of 3-D conformal RT in precisely targeting the tumour whilst the radiation beam intensity can be controlled (modulated) at different time points during treatment delivery to ensure an accurate and homogenous dose distribution to the cancer and minimising dose to the OARs (see Figure 18.2). IMRT is now the standard of care in the radical RT for the cancers of the head and neck region as it reduces the side effect profile significantly whilst maintaining tumour control (Gupta et al. 2020; Wang and Eisbruch 2016).

Modern RT delivery systems also enable monitoring various parameters including patient and organ motion and any changes in shape of the patient anatomy and/or the tumour size. Image-guided RT (IGRT) enables correct patient positioning and accurate treatment delivery.

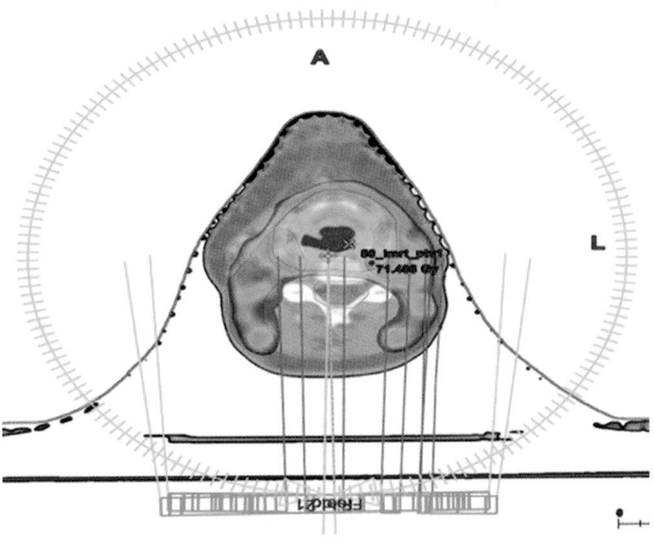

Figure 18.2 An IMRT treatment plan. The shaded areas represent the area of the body that will be targeted with radiation. The area coloured yellow is receiving the highest dose as it represents the site of cancer in the voice box (larynx), whilst the areas shaded blue receive a lower dose as they represent the areas of draining lymph nodes, which may contain microscopic deposits of cancer. The grey areas receive very little dose as they represent the normal tissues. The arc represents the path of the linear accelerator as it moves around the patient and delivers radiation in a very precise and controlled way.

Head and Neck Cancers

There are 12 200 new HNCs in the UK every year (Cancer Research UK 2022). Accounting for 3% of all new cancer cases. HNC is an 'umbrella' term that covers a diverse range of specific cancer subsites that can develop in the head and neck region (see Figures 18.3 and 18.4). This includes cancers of the oral cavity, oropharynx, hypopharynx, and larynx as well as less common sites such as the ear, salivary glands, nasal cavity, and sinuses. The majority of cancers that occur in the head and neck region are squamous cell carcinomas (HNSCCs). The percentages of cancer distribution stratified according to stage and estimated overall survival based on stage are shown in Table 18.1.

Prior to deciding on appropriate management for an individual cancer patient, it is essential to have knowledge of the following:

1) Site of cancer, for example, oral cavity
2) Stage of the cancer by TNM classification
3) Histological type of cancer
4) Patient fitness and performance status
5) Patient's wishes in respect to treatment.

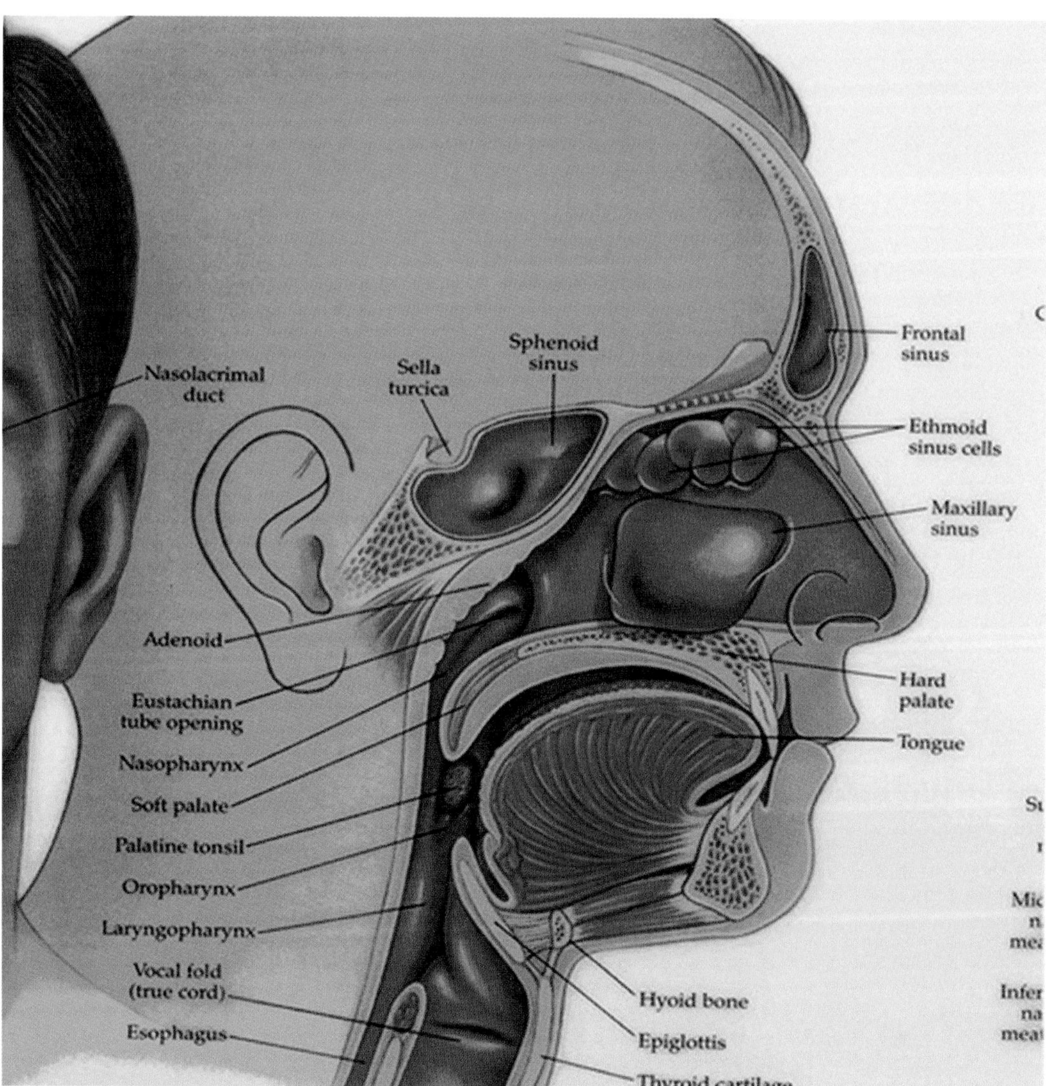

Figure 18.3 Head and neck anatomy; cancers can arise from different subsites.

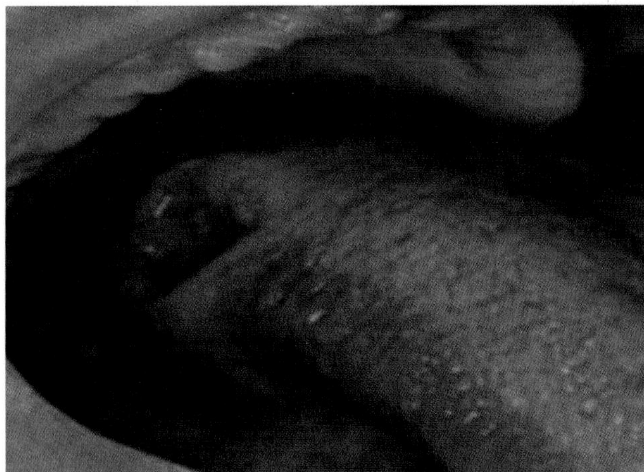

Figure 18.4 Cancer of the tongue.

Table 18.1 Cancer distribution according to stage and estimated overall survival based on stage.

	Presentation (%)	Five-year survival (%)
Stage 1	15%	90%
Stage 2	20%	70%
Stage 3	25%	55%
Stage 4	25%	40%
Inoperable/metastatic	15%	5–10%

As per Table 18.1, most patients present with local or locally advanced disease, and wherever possible radical (curative) treatment is offered. The mainstay of curative treatments in HNCs is surgery, RT, or a combination of the two. In some circumstances, due to the close proximity of critical normal structures, RT (with or without concomitant chemotherapy) may offer an attractive and effective treatment option for organ preservation.

RT is typically delivered in small daily doses known as *fractions*. This allows the normal tissues time to recover from the effects of radiation. In most cases the RT is delivered five days per week, Monday through Friday. Duration of treatment can vary from two to seven weeks of treatment (10–35 fractions) depending upon the site, stage, and intent of treatment. Early stage larynx cancers are usually treated with 15–20 fractions, whilst more advanced stage cancers are treated with 30–35 fractions. Palliative treatments can be given in 5–15 fractions depending upon the site and extent of disease and the patient's fitness.

Pre-RT Preparation and Planning

Patient selection is an important component of successful RT treatment. Due to the rigorous schedule and high-intensity treatments, it is essential to educate and counsel patients regarding the rationale, logistics, and usual side effects of treatment. Patients with a good performance status (PS), that is, normal levels of activity and fitness (PS 0, 1, and sometimes 2) are usually considered fit for radical RT treatments. Patients with poor baseline PS (PS 3, 4), that is, reduced activity and/or dependent on others for care, are usually considered inappropriate for intensive radical treatments but can still be considered for shorter palliative RT schedules.

Dental Assessment

Prior to planning, all patients undergoing radical head and neck RT should be counselled to maintain scrupulous oral and dental hygiene. Where appropriate, patients should also be counselled to stop smoking and reduce alcohol consumption.

Due to the potential consequences of RT on the mouth and dentition, patients are routinely referred for a pre-RT dental assessment. This is to try to reduce future dental complications. Teeth with a poor prognosis may need to be extracted before RT is planned. Any dental work that is required must be expedited to avoid any delays in starting RT treatment. Patients are often seen by a dental hygienist as well to discuss how to properly look after teeth, mouth, and gums during and after RT.

Following RT, the benefit of dental treatments must be carefully weighed against the risk of complications such as osteoradionecrosis.

Nutrition

All patients should also undergo formal dietetic assessments and reviews. In patients who are at risk of significant nutritional impairment and weight loss secondary to RT, a feeding tube called a gastrostomy may be placed. The most common type of feeding tube is a PEG tube. An alternate method of inserting a feeding tube is to site a RIG tube.

Despite placement of a feeding tube, all patients are encouraged to try to maintain oral intake as much as possible throughout the RT and during the period afterwards. The use of the muscles in and around the oral cavity and throat reduces the severity of RT-induced fibrosis and improves the functional outcomes, including long-term swallowing and speech function.

Patients are monitored regularly by dietitians during RT and in follow-up. Feeding tubes are removed as soon as oral caloric intake has improved back to acceptable levels. With the use of modern IMRT techniques, fewer than 5% of patients are feeding tube–dependent at the end of two years after RT completion.

SLT Assessment

Muscles that move the jaw and enable swallowing can become thickened and stiffened by RT. This can make mouth opening, speaking, and eating more difficult after RT treatment. Mouth and jaw exercises started before RT and continued long term can help reduce this complication. In most hospitals, patients due to undergo radical head and neck RT will be referred to the SLT team for instruction on exercises.

Immobilisation Device

The accurate delivery of RT to the target volume is achieved by minimising patient movement. This is achieved by use of a special thermoplastic head and shoulder shell, as illustrated in Figure 18.5. The manufacture of a personalised head and neck immobilisation shell is the first step in RT planning. Once the shell is made, the patient then undergoes a CT (planning) scan wearing the shell in the position that the RT will be given.

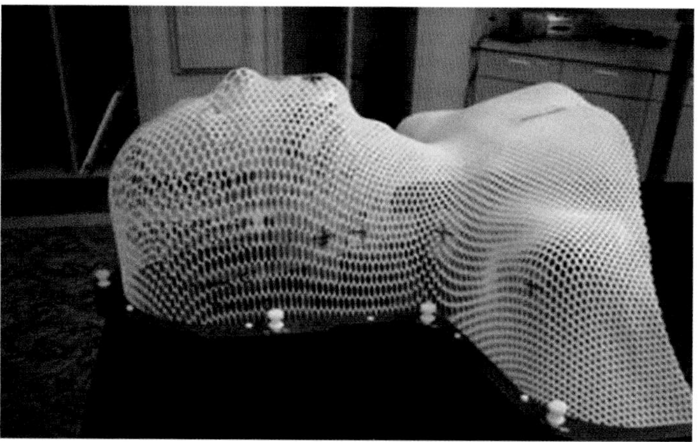

Figure 18.5 Head and neck immobilisation device (thermoplastic shell/mask).

RT Planning

Once the patient has undergone the CT planning scan, the oncologist is then responsible for contouring or delineating the area that requires the RT. This is known as the *target volume* and incorporates the area where there is known to be cancer but also areas that are at risk of harbouring microscopic disease, such as lymph nodes. The surrounding normal structure OARs such as spinal cord, brain stem, parotid glands, and larynx are also outlined. This contouring needs to be very precise and in some situations can take many hours to complete.

Once the oncologist has completed the contouring work, the RT planners then devise a 'recipe' (the RT plan) to deliver the treatment in the best possible way, that is, ensuring coverage of the target volume whilst minimising the dose as low as possible to the OARs.

Patients must provide written consent prior to commencing the RT.

Toxicities

The effects of head and neck radiation on normal tissues will result in significant side effects. These are divided into acute and late effects based on the timing of their onset in relation to the RT treatment schedule.

- Acute effects: side effects that start during RT and within 90 days of completing treatment. These are common and the majority are reversible.
- Late effects: side effects that start after 90 days. These are uncommon but likely to be irreversible when they occur.

The toxicity profile can be considered as a continuum of symptoms, which starts as an acute reaction to radiation and mostly settles in two to four months. Some symptoms can persist for a longer duration – for example, dry mouth – and may be permanent.The toxicities from treatments are graded using one of the validated grading systems such as common terminology criteria for adverse events (CTCAE), Radiation Therapy Oncology Group (RTOG), and WHO. The toxicities in CTCAE (National Cancer Institute 2017) are graded between grade 1 and 5:

- Grade 1 signifies mostly asymptomatic changes.
- Grade 2 signifies significant symptoms.
- Grades 3 and 4 are serious side effects that can sometimes require hospital admissions and consideration of treatment schedule changes/interruptions.
- Grade 5 is a loss of life because of an adverse effect.

Grade 3 and 4 toxicities in HNC treatments require an aggressive supportive approach towards toxicity management whilst aiming to continue the RT as planned. This is because, unlike other treatments, RT interruptions or delays can have a detrimental effect on the tumour control and cure rates.

Acute Effects

The acute effects of head and neck radiation include the following:

- Fatigue: Tiredness is multifactorial and results from a combination of RT effects, the intensive scheduling of treatment, and the reduction in caloric intake and dehydration.
- Skin reaction: Most patients experience a degree of skin inflammation, which can be very profound in some instances. Treatments include topical moisturisers for intact skin, anti-inflammatory topical steroid creams, and special topical preparations in case of skin breakdown (Figure 18.6).
- Mucositis: The oral mucosa becomes inflamed as a reaction to RT. The mainstay of treatment is the use of regular analgesia and mouthwashes. It is important to maintain good oral hygiene, use a soft toothbrush to avoid added injury to oral mucosa and gums, and detect and treat any superadded bacterial or fungal infections as and when they arise (Figure 18.7).

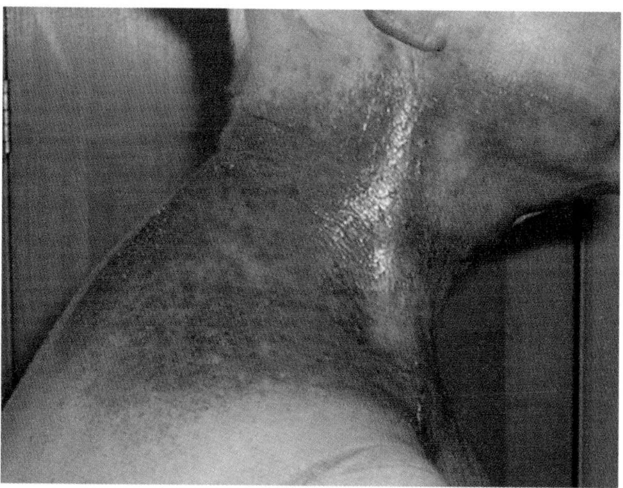

Figure 18.6 Skin toxicity from radiotherapy.

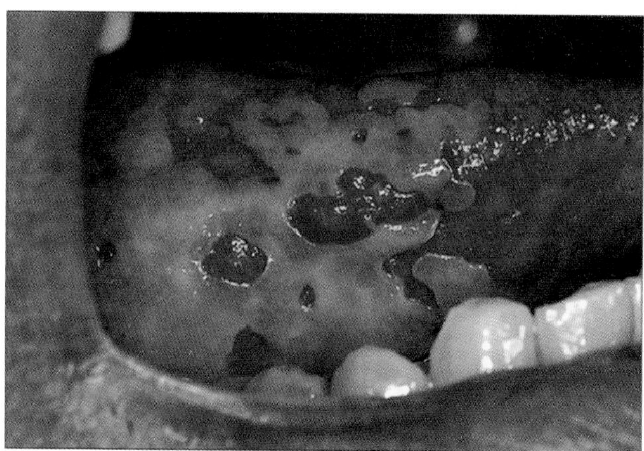

Figure 18.7 Mucositis.

- Swallowing, articulation, and speech impairment: The intense RT reaction also affects musculature of the head and neck region in addition to the mucosa and skin. The inflammation and pain affects function, and swallowing and speech becomes painful and difficult. SLT input and review may be required for instruction into mouth and jaw exercises as mentioned earlier but also for rehabilitation post-RT to maximise functional recovery.
- Pain: Pain is treated with a WHO analgesic ladder approach. The pain treatment should begin with a simple analgesic like paracetamol, then, if required, weak opioids and strong opioids can be added. It is important to monitor and treat the underlying topical causes of pain, for example, infection and inflammation of the oral cavity. Certain anaesthetic agents like lidocaine mouthwashes are best avoided as they may reduce the sensation in the area of concern and contribute to a worse functional outcome.
- Hearing loss: RT can cause inflammation and fluid build-up in the middle ear cavity, which can cause 'conductive' hearing loss. It usually settles slowly once the RT course is completed. Patients receiving concurrent chemotherapy with cisplatin along with radical RT are at risk of 'sensorineural' hearing loss, as the chemotherapy agents can damage the nerves involved in hearing. This kind of hearing loss can be permanent at times.
- Dry mouth/xerostomia: RT damages the major and minor salivary glands, in particular the parotid gland, which can cause significant dryness of the mouth. During the RT planning process, careful consideration is given to the radiation dose to each parotid gland, and the dosimetrists try to reduce the dose below a certain threshold to minimise the risk of toxicity where it is possible to do so. Patients are educated to keep the mouth well hydrated by using regular sips of water and by using artificial saliva in some cases. Dryness of the mouth can contribute to poor oral hygiene and dental problems.

- Weight loss: Weight loss is undesirable during RT treatments as it not only makes the patients unwell but also alters the local anatomy because of fat redistribution, and as a result the RT target volume position can change. Nutritional supplements and feeding tubes are used to prevent significant weight loss.
- Hair loss: RT can cause hair loss within the treatment field depending upon the dose received. HNC treatments mostly affect facial hair and hair around the upper neck and around the temple region. The hair loss is usually temporary, but the hair thickness and pigmentation changes in the hair can be longer term.
- Taste changes: Mucosal reaction secondary to radiation damages the taste buds and causes decrease, aversion, or complete loss of taste.

Late Toxicities

The late effects of head and neck radiation include the following:

- Skin tightening/fibrosis/trismus: Patients are encouraged to perform regular neck exercises to prevent significant tightening of the skin, muscles, and jaw in the head and neck region.
- Lymphoedema: Disruption of superficial lymphatics can cause accumulation of fluid in the subcutaneous tissues, known as *lymphoedema*. Patients are educated to carry out exercises and skin massage to help with the flow of fluid. In severe cases, patients can be referred to the specialist lymphoedema service.
- Osteoradionecrosis: Osteoradionecrosis is the term used when bone dies within the RT treatment field. It is thought to be due to damage to bone vasculature from the RT. It usually affects the lower jaw/mandible. Patients can present with a wide array of symptoms, including but not limited to pain, redness, infection, abscess formation, and bone erosion. Management requires specialist input from dental and maxillofacial teams, and recovery can follow a protracted course in some instances.
- Risk of second malignancy: RT causes a theoretical increase in the risk of a second malignancy within the treatment field. Usually the risk is very small, and the benefits of radical RT treatments will almost always outweigh this risk. The risk of radiation-induced malignancy is more relevant to younger subgroups of patients treated with radical intention who have high chances of long-term survival, for example, those with HPV-associated oropharyngeal cancers.
- Telangiectasias: Superficial skin veins can become dilated and tortuous and sometimes visible as 'spider veins' (Figure 18.8).
- Residual acute effects: Acute effects such as mucositis, speech difficulties, swallowing problems, taste changes, and dryness of mouth recover most significantly within the first 12 months after RT. After 12–24 months of treatment, patients reach a level of recovery that is usually established as their new functional baseline.

Follow-Up

During RT, patients are generally reviewed by the clinical team once a week to assess and manage toxicities associated with RT. After completion of treatment, the frequency of follow-up is quite often (usually every 4–12 weeks) for the first one to two years. This is to assess response to treatment but also to maximise rehabilitation and function. It is also recognised that the chances of recurrence are generally greatest in the first 24 months. Early detection may enable salvage treatment in some patients.

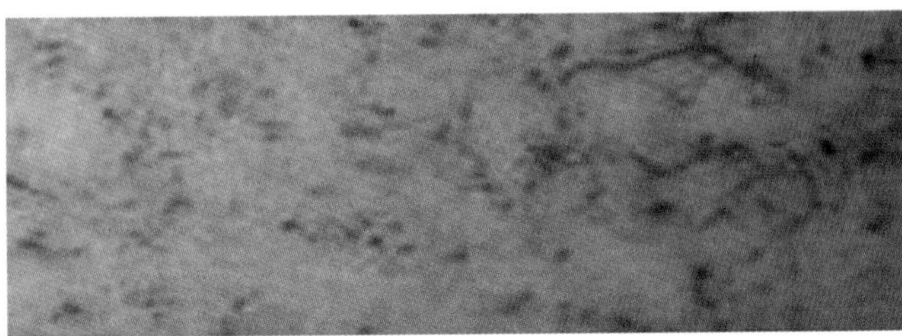

Figure 18.8 Telangiectasias of the skin.

The follow-up duration is increased progressively in year three to five (usually every three to six months). The follow-up includes assessment for late effects of RT, review of any new symptoms that may indicate disease recurrence, and thorough physical examination to rule out any local or regional recurrence. If any abnormalities are noted, then repeat imaging can be performed for further clarification of clinical findings.

References

Cancer Research UK (2022). Head and neck cancer statistics. https://www.cancerresearchuk.org/health-professional/cancer-statistics/statistics-by-cancer-type/head-and-neck-cancers (accessed 26 March 2021).

Gianfaldoni, S., Gianfaldoni, R., Wollina, U. et al. (2017). An overview on radiotherapy: from its history to its current applications in dermatology. *Open Access Maced. J. Med. Sci.* 5 (4): 521–525. https://doi.org/10.3889/oamjms.2017.122.

Gupta, T., Singha, S., Ghosh-Laskar, S. et al. (2020). Intensity-modulated radiation therapy versus three-dimensional conformal radiotherapy in head and neck squamous cell carcinoma: long-term and mature outcomes of a prospective randomized trial. *Radiat. Oncol.* 15: 218. https://doi.org/10.1186/s13014-020-01666-5.

National Cancer Institute (2017). Common terminology criteria for adverse events (CTCAE) v5.0. https://ctep.cancer.gov/protocoldevelopment/electronic_applications/docs/CTCAE_v5_Quick_Reference_5x7.pdf.

Okawa, T., Kita, M., and Goto, M. (1987). Therapeutic ratio in radiotherapy – clinical analysis and strategy. *Gan No Rinsho* 33 (13): 1527–1531. Japanese. PMID: 3694791.

Wang, X. and Eisbruch, A. (2016). IMRT for head and neck cancer: reducing xerostomia and dysphagia. *J. Radiat. Res.* 57 (Suppl 1): i69–i75. https://doi.org/10.1093/jrr/rrw047.

19

The Role of Immunotherapy in Head and Neck Cancer Management

Brindley Hapuarachi, Muneeb Qureshi, and Bernadette Foran

Weston Park Cancer Centre, Sheffield Teaching Hospitals NHS Foundation Trust, Sheffield, UK

Background

The majority of cancers originating in the head and neck region are HNSCCs. These can include cancers of the oral cavity, pharynx, and larynx (National Cancer Institute 2021). HNSCC is the seventh commonest cancer worldwide and has an annual incidence of 700 000 and a UK annual incidence of 12 200, accounting for 3% of all new UK cancer cases (Cancer Research UK 2022). Around 75% of HNSCCs are triggered by alcohol and tobacco use. HPV is also associated with HNSCC, especially that arising in the oropharynx region – tonsils, soft palate, and base of tongue. HPV-associated oropharyngeal cancer is associated with a better prognosis compared to HPV-negative HNSCC due to increased sensitivity to treatment (National Cancer Institute 2021).

In HNSCC, the main treatment modalities are surgery and radiotherapy either as single modality therapy in early stage disease or in combination for late-stage disease. Systemic anticancer therapies (SACTs) mainly in the form of chemotherapy are often utilised in specific patients where there is evidence that giving chemotherapy concomitantly (at the same time) with radiotherapy improves outcomes. This is called *chemoradiotherapy*. It is also used neoadjuvantly, prior to primary radiotherapy for patients where it is beneficial to try to reduce the bulk of the cancer before proceeding with radical radiotherapy or chemoradiotherapy. In the palliative setting, chemotherapy is used to try to improve a patient's symptoms where cure is not possible.

Although less than 5% of HNSCC patients have metastases at their initial diagnosis, around half of patients with locally advanced disease will develop a local recurrence and/or metastatic disease (Machiels et al. 2020). In the metastatic setting as well as in those with inoperable local recurrence curative treatment is not possible, but patients can be offered chemotherapy and/or immunotherapy in an attempt to control the cancer (Machiels et al. 2020).

In the palliative setting, traditional SACTs such as chemotherapy have varying and limited success in HNSCC patients. The introduction of immunotherapy within palliative treatment regimes in HNSCC has been a welcomed addition in recent years.

One of the key features of cancer cells is their ability to 'hide' from the body's immune system. Immunotherapy is a type of systemic anticancer treatment that works by utilising the body's own immune system to recognise and fight against cancer cells. This chapter will outline what immunotherapy is, how it works, when it is used in HNSCC and when it should not be used, and how it is administered as well as potential side effects and possible future use.

Immunotherapy interacts with different targets within the immune system, allowing recognition and removal of tumour cells. Immunotherapy has revolutionised treatments for many different cancer sites such as malignant melanoma, renal cell carcinoma, and certain lung cancers. In recent years the use in HNSCC has also started to be recognised. Ongoing research means it will continue to play a pivotal role in cancer management, including in HNSCC.

The concept of utilising the immune system in tumour control has been around since the nineteenth century, when a New York surgeon called William Coley looked into treating inoperable malignant tumours with killed cultures of bacteria with some evidence of success (Coley 1991). One of the first uses of immunotherapy in modern medicine was in 1976, when the attenuated tuberculosis vaccine bacillus Calmette-Guérin (BCG) was used in nonmuscle-invasive bladder cancer to reduce recurrence. This treatment is still used today (ScienceDirect 2022).

Care of Head and Neck Cancer Patients for Dental Hygienists and Dental Therapists, First Edition. Edited by Jocelyn J. Harding.

A major role of the immune system is to identify and eliminate abnormal cells in order to fight infection as well as to cease the early steps in malignant transformation, preventing cancer development (National Cancer Institute 2019). Inheritable and sporadic mutations (changes in the cell's DNA) can allow cells to develop ways to evade this process, making them to able proliferate into a tumour.

There are now several different types of immunotherapy in clinical practice that are classified by the mechanism of action. These include:

1) Immune checkpoint inhibitors
2) Monoclonal antibodies
3) Vaccines
4) Cell-based adaptive immunotherapies such as CAR T cells.

In this chapter we will focus only on immune checkpoint inhibitors, as this is the only type of immunotherapy currently licenced for use in head and neck cancers.

How Do Immune Checkpoint Inhibitors Work?

Immune checkpoint inhibitors follow this process:

1) A protein (immune checkpoint protein) called PD-1 on some immune cells binds with specific molecules on cancer cells. These molecules are called ligands.
2) When the PD-1 protein binds with the ligand, this has the effect of 'switching off' the immune system cell. This means it cannot protect the body by attacking the cancer cell.
3) Immune checkpoint inhibitors are drugs that bind with the PD-1 protein, which means it cannot bind with the ligand.
4) Blocking the ligand from binding with the PD-1 protein means the immune system is 'switched on' and can therefore do its work in attacking cancer cells.
5) This action gives us a therapeutic effect in some patients but can also be responsible for causing side effects.

Figure 19.1 illustrates how a cancer cell can hide from a T cell by using its PDL-1 cell surface receptor to bind to the PD-1 receptor on the T cell. This provides an inhibitory signal that tells the T cell to ignore the tumour cell, allowing a tumour mass to develop. Figure 19.2 illustrates how an anti-PD-1 agent blocks the inhibitory signal, allowing the interaction T cell to attack the cancer cell.

When Is Immunotherapy Used in HNSCC?

The immune checkpoint inhibitors currently available and licenced to be used in recurrent or metastatic HNSCC are the anti-PD-1 agents nivolumab (Opdivo®, Bristol Myers Squibb) and pembrolizumab (Keytruda®, Merck). There are several other anti-PDL-1 agents that are currently being investigated in HNSCC clinical trials. We do not currently have the

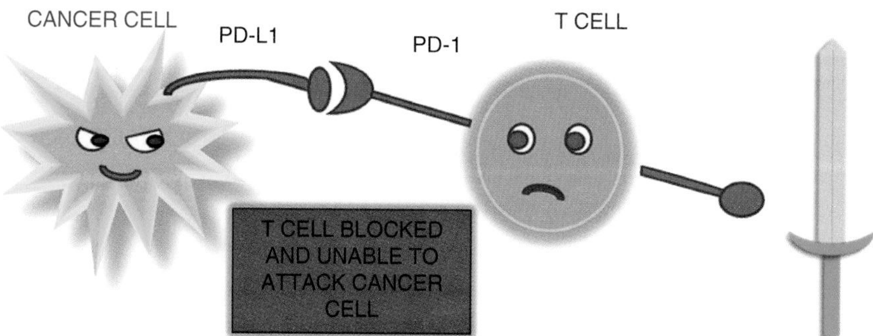

Figure 19.1 PD-1/PDL-1 inhibitory signalling pathway.

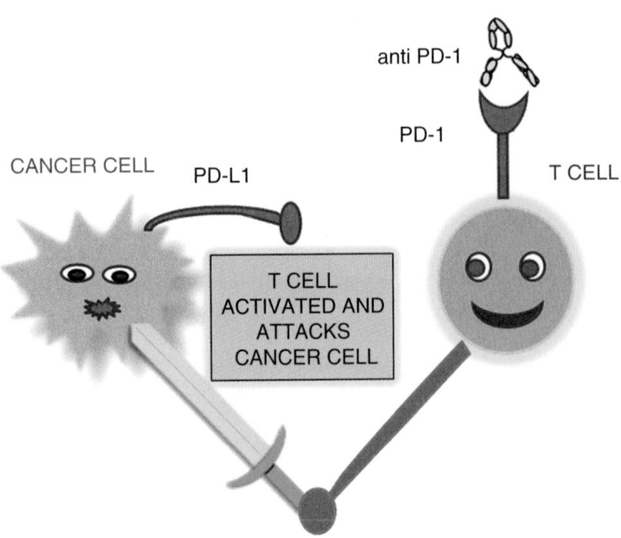

Figure 19.2 Anti-PD-1 mechanism of action.

evidence to support their use in other treatment indications; for example, in the curative setting. However, this is being looked at in a number of clinical trials that are currently in progress.

Pembrolizumab is indicated as a first-line treatment with palliative intent and can be used on its own or in combination with chemotherapy. Nivolumab can be used in patients whose cancer has progressed within six months of platinum-based chemotherapy treatment, that is, second-line treatment.

Patients with metastatic or inoperable recurrent HNSCC may have their tumour tested to see if PDL-1 (ligand) is expressed on their cancer cells. Those who have evidence of PDL-1 on their cancer cells can be considered for pembrolizumab monotherapy as first-line treatment through the high-cost Cancer Drugs Fund (CDF) within the NHS.

Benefits in HNSCC

Trials in HNSCC patients have shown that immunotherapy can improve life expectancy as a first and second line cancer treatment in the palliative setting in some patients. Compared to chemotherapy/targeted therapy, modest improvements of several months are seen on average (Machiels et al. 2020). The benefit from immunotherapy may often take some weeks/months to become apparent. In some patients, where rapid progression of the cancer may cause significant symptoms, such as difficulty swallowing or breathing, rapid shrinkage of the tumour is required. In these circumstances, studies have shown the combination of chemotherapy and immunotherapy is best utilised (Machiels et al. 2020).

Figures 19.3 and 19.4 show how an advanced recurrent tumour at the tongue base responded to immunotherapy, causing a complete response after 24 months of treatment, meaning that there was no measurable tumour following treatment. This particular patient went from being unable to safely swallow to now eating a relatively normal diet. The patient had undergone radical chemoradiation four years previously and had inoperable disease when the cancer recurred.

How Is Immunotherapy Administered?

Patients are seen and carefully assessed in the same way as they would be when receiving any other SACT such as chemotherapy. Prior to starting immunotherapy, the following blood tests are required due to risk of reactivation of these infections on immunotherapy:

- Viral hepatitis and HIV screen
- TB screen.

Prior to every treatment, the following blood tests are required for monitoring purposes with reasons explained in the side effects section:

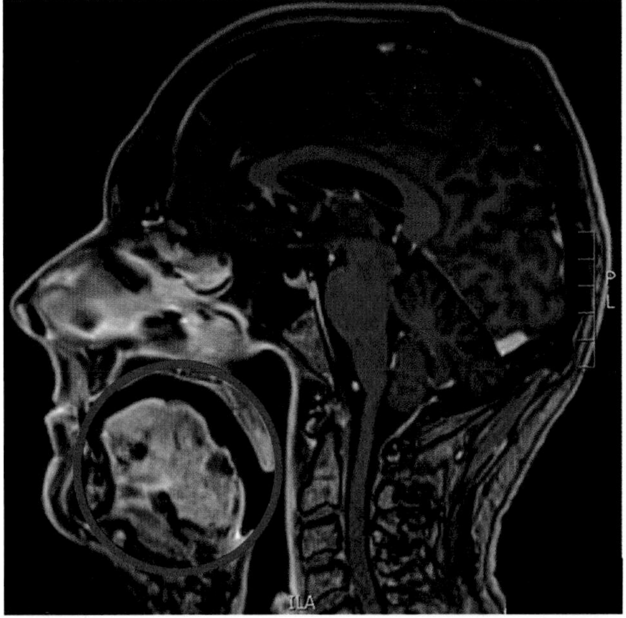

Figure 19.3 Magnetic resonance imaging (MRI) of the head showing an advanced recurrent base of tongue tumour immediately prior to commencing immunotherapy treatment. The entire tongue is affected by the cancer and is circled in red.

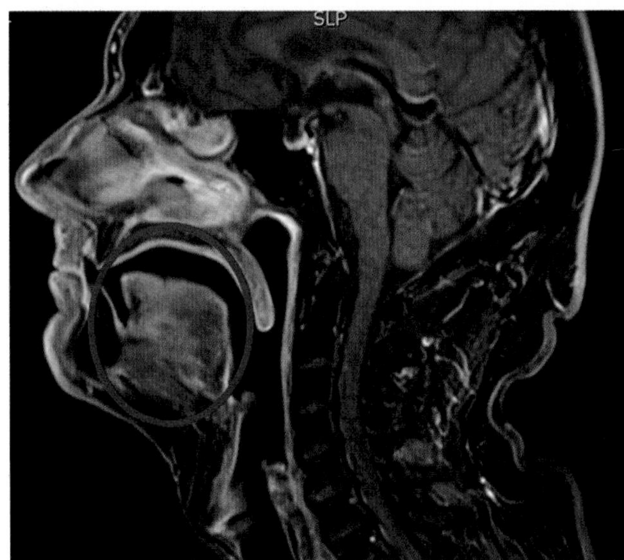

Figure 19.4 MRI of the head showing tumour response following three months of immunotherapy. The MRI demonstrates a marked reduction in the tumour bulk and the patient's symptoms of pain and difficulty eating had both markedly improved.

- Full blood count
- Kidney function
- Liver function
- Bone profile
- Glucose level
- Thyroid function
- Cortisol level.

When undergoing immunotherapy, it is very important that patients are not on significant steroid therapy. Steroids can cause immunosuppression, and this can negate any benefit from immunotherapy. Patients typically receive the drug through hospital outpatients or day case facilities within oncology units.

The drugs are administered intravenously at regular intervals (usually three to six weekly). The immunotherapy is continued as long as there is a response to the treatment and no significant side effects for up to a maximum of 24 months under the current CDF system. Whilst receiving the drug, patients are seen and assessed regularly by the clinical team to assess treatment response but also assessed for toxicity related to the treatment. This assessment includes clinical examination and blood tests as well as serial cross-sectional imaging (MRI, CT, or PET-CT).

Side Effects of Immunotherapy

The general principles of immunotherapy and the mechanism of action of inhibitors of the PD-1/PDL-1 pathway have been outlined above. They allow recognition and destruction of cancer cells that could otherwise evade the immune system. Unfortunately, by suppressing inhibitory pathways, they also allow the immune system to potentially attack normal and healthy cells, which can cause a wide range of toxic side effects.

In essence, immunotherapy works by 'switching on' different parts of the immune system. In patients with pre-existing autoimmune conditions, such as rheumatoid arthritis, this could lead to worsening of the condition; therefore, this is usually seen as a contraindication for its use.

The side effects profile with immunotherapy differs significantly from the side effects associated with chemotherapy agents (immunosuppression, nausea and vomiting, hair loss). Common nonspecific immunotherapy side effects include:

- Fatigue
- Fever
- Chills
- Muscle aches.

The range of immunotherapy side effects reflects the fact that overactivation of the immune system can lead to attack and inflammation of any cell system or organ within the body. Common and mild adverse effects can be seen in the skin, gut, and endocrine system (Puzanov et al. 2017). Table 19.1 shows some examples of how immunotherapy can affect different systems.

In Figure 19.5, the arrow is pointing to patchy white shadowing that can be seen covering both lungs. This shadowing is due to inflammation of the lung tissue that leads to symptoms of shortness of breath and cough that can potentially be life-threatening. There are many different types of adverse skin reactions to immunotherapy. Figure 19.6 shows an area of a patient's abdomen that was flat, red, and itchy along with other parts of the body (classed as grade 3), requiring steroids.

Table 19.1 Immunotherapy-related adverse events.

Organ system	Toxicity	Symptoms
Thyroid	Underactive (hypo-)/overactive (hyper-) thyroid	Lethargic, weight gain/loss, sweating, hair loss, tremor. *Note:* If patient becomes hypothyroid, treatment is with levothyroxine.
Lungs	Inflammation of lung tissue (pneumonitis) (see Figure 19.5.)	Shortness of breath, cough, chest pain, low oxygen levels, potentially life-threatening.
Liver	Inflammation of liver tissue (hepatitis)	Usually asymptomatic, diagnosis on blood tests, can lead to liver failure if untreated.
Kidneys	Inflammation of kidney tissue (nephritis)	Initially asymptomatic, diagnosis on blood tests, may lead to kidney failure if untreated with reduced urine output.
Bowel	Inflammation of bowel walls (colitis)	Diarrhoea with varying degree of severity, leading to bowel perforation if severe.
Skin	Skin inflammation (dermatitis) (see Figure 19.6)/ vitiligo (autoimmune skin depigmentation)/ psoriasis/more severe blistering skin conditions such as Steven-Johnsons syndrome/toxic epidermal necrolysis	Depends on diagnosis, commonly can cause red rash with varying degrees of severity up to potentially life-threatening.
Pancreas	Diabetes	High blood sugars, possible diabetic complications such as diabetic ketoacidosis.

Source: Based on Puzanov et al. (2017).

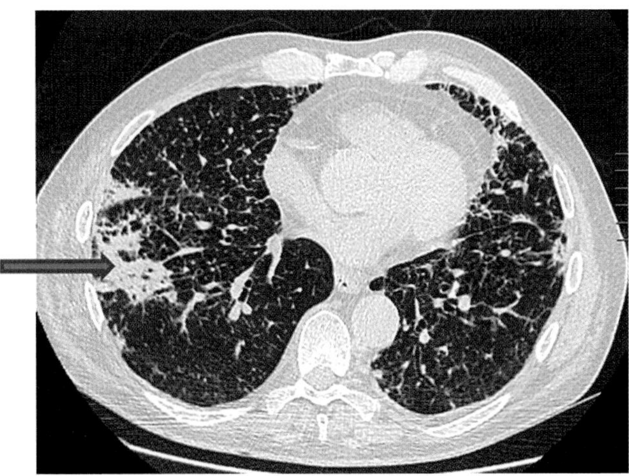

Figure 19.5 Computerised tomography (CT) scan of the lungs showing pneumonitis secondary to immunotherapy.

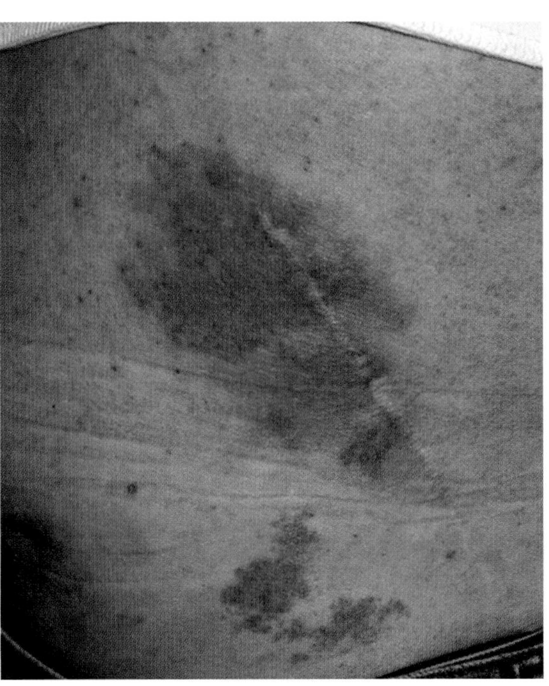

Figure 19.6 Skin rash secondary to immunotherapy.

Management of Immunotherapy-Related Adverse Events

Management of immunotherapy-related adverse events (IrAE) depends upon how severe they are. Oncologists will grade toxicities on a scale of 1–5 (asymptomatic/mild – life-threatening/death) using the CTCAE (National Cancer Institute 2017). Toxicities and approach for grades 1–4 are:

- Grade 1 can usually be monitored and immunotherapy can continue.
- Grade 2 usually requires a pause in treatment and use of oral steroids (prednisolone) to help treat the inflammatory response.
- Grade 3 can require oral/intravenous (IV) steroids (methylprednisolone) and may also lead to discontinuation of treatment.
- Grade 4 requires discontinuation of treatment, hospitalization, and IV steroids.

It is important to note that, although less common, there are potentially life-threatening side effects such as pneumonitis, severe colitis, and encephalitis. Clinical trials report death related to immunotherapy in up to 2% of patients (Puzanov et al. 2017). Prompt and correct treatment is essential to allow for better outcomes. For this reason, prior to starting treatment, patients and their carers are carefully counselled regarding the side effects, what to look for, and who to contact should side effects occur.

IrAE of any grade have been noted in up to 90% of patients on immunotherapy (Puzanov et al. 2017). A recent study looking into real-world data of immunotherapy toxicities showed around a third of patients developed clinically significant adverse related events (grade 2 or more), of which the majority required oral steroids and 11% required steroid-sparing immunosuppression such as infliximab (a biological agent targeting tumour necrosis factor alpha [TNFα], which is a key signalling protein within the immune system) (Puzanov et al. 2017).

It is important to note that compared to chemotherapy, immunotherapy side effects can have a delayed and prolonged course and have been reported to occur months to years after stopping treatment, which subsequently can lead to inappropriate management (Puzanov et al. 2017).

Future Use of Immunotherapy in HNSCC

Multiple trials are currently ongoing in HNSCC looking at whether immunotherapy could help to improve cancer control rates if given at the time a patient is first diagnosed with locally advanced cancer. The question is whether immunotherapy given alongside radiotherapy (with or without chemotherapy) and surgery might improve oncological outcomes and chances of cure in certain patients.

We hope that results of these trials will be available in the next couple of years.

References

Cancer Research UK (2022). Head and neck cancer statistics. https://www.cancerresearchuk.org/health-professional/cancer-statistics/statistics-by-cancer-type/head-and-neck-cancers (accessed 26 March 2021).

Coley, W.B. (1991). The treatment of malignant tumors by repeated inoculations of erysipelas: with a report of ten original cases. *Clin. Orthop. Relat. Res.* 262: 3–11. https://doi.org/10.1097/00000441-189305000-00001.

Machiels, J.P., Leemans, C.R., Golusinski, W. et al. (2020). Squamous cell carcinoma of the oral cavity, larynx, oropharynx and hypopharynx: EHNS–ESMO–ESTRO clinical practice guidelines for diagnosis, treatment and follow-up†. *Ann. Oncol.* 31 (11): 1462–1475. https://doi.org/10.1016/j.annonc.2020.07.011.

National Cancer Institute (2017). Common terminology criteria for adverse events (CTCAE) v5.0. https://www.meddra.org (accessed 26 March 2021).

National Cancer Institute (2019). Immunotheraphy to treat cancer. https://www.cancer.gov/about-cancer/treatment/types/immunotherapy (accessed 26 March 2021).

National Cancer Institute (2021). Head and neck cancers. https://www.cancer.gov/types/head-and-neck/head-neck-fact-sheet (accessed 26 March 2021).

Puzanov, I., Diab, A., Abdallah, K. et al. (2017). Managing toxicities associated with immune checkpoint inhibitors: consensus recommendations from the Society for Immunotherapy of Cancer (SITC) toxicity management working group equal contributors. *J. Immunother. Cancer* 5: 95. https://doi.org/10.1186/s40425-017-0300-z.

ScienceDirect (2022). Immunotherapy. https://www.sciencedirect.com/topics/immunology-and-microbiology/immunotherapy (accessed 26 March 2021).

20

Proton Therapy in the UK

Karol Sikora and John Pettingell

Rutherford Cancer Centres, UK

Introduction

Radiotherapy is currently used in 50% of cancer patients. Proton therapy (PT) allows the more precise delivery of radiotherapy and can reduce the long-term damage to normal tissues surrounding a cancer that results in unpleasant symptoms many years later. But it is expensive, costing 2–10 times more than traditional radiotherapy, depending on the system type. Meaningful, large-scale, randomised trials with protons versus photons are unlikely for all clinical indications. Instead, the pretreatment comparison of PT versus state-of-the-art IMRT in individual patients using preset metrics of plan quality will be used for deciding whether PT has significant advantages. This assessment can be made objectively by treatment planning software systems. Payers, government and insurers, will use set criteria to assess the value of PT in an individual using a comparative equation incorporating tumour control, early and late toxicity, and overall lifetime costs of care. Such analyses will determine logically the level of the therapeutic plateau in the relationship of cost to gain in clinical outcome. The range of published estimates for the optimal use of protons in radical radiotherapy ranges from 1% (UK, NHS) to 20% in the US. Recent policy studies from several European countries indicate a 10–15% conversion to protons in patients treated with radiotherapy with radical intent. That would require 15–20 treatment rooms across Britain. We were one of the last European countries to have an operational PT service and now need to catch up.

The Evolution of Precision Radiotherapy

The advent of more precise imaging methods and dramatic advances in information technology has led to the much more accurate delivery of radiation dose to tumours. A greater understanding of the distribution of critically sensitive organs at risk – each with their different toxicities – has reduced both the early and, most significantly, the late toxicity of radical treatments. Figure 20.1 shows the timeline of advance over the last 60 years.

The transition from radioactive cobalt to the linear accelerator (LINAC) took place mainly in the 1970s. This was the forerunner of computer-controlled collimators placed in the beam line to individualise the shape of each treatment field in real time. Millimetre accuracy was established by 1990 when conformal therapy emerged – creating a specific and often irregular shape to the delivered radiation that exactly followed the shape of the cancer being treated.

Further developments in beam shaping with IMRT and real-time checking using image guidance heralded an era of even greater precision. Currently, we are seeing further developments with stereotactic, ablative radiotherapy and real -time magnetic resonance imaging allowing changes to field dimensions as the tumour shrinks – four-dimensional or adaptive radiotherapy. It is likely that digital fusion images from multiple sources will create a continuous monitoring of tumour shrinkage during treatment, so again reducing toxicity to surrounding normal tissues. The considerable technical challenge of using magnetic resonance imaging concurrently with beam delivery has been solved, and two commercial systems are now available.

Care of Head and Neck Cancer Patients for Dental Hygienists and Dental Therapists, First Edition. Edited by Jocelyn J. Harding.

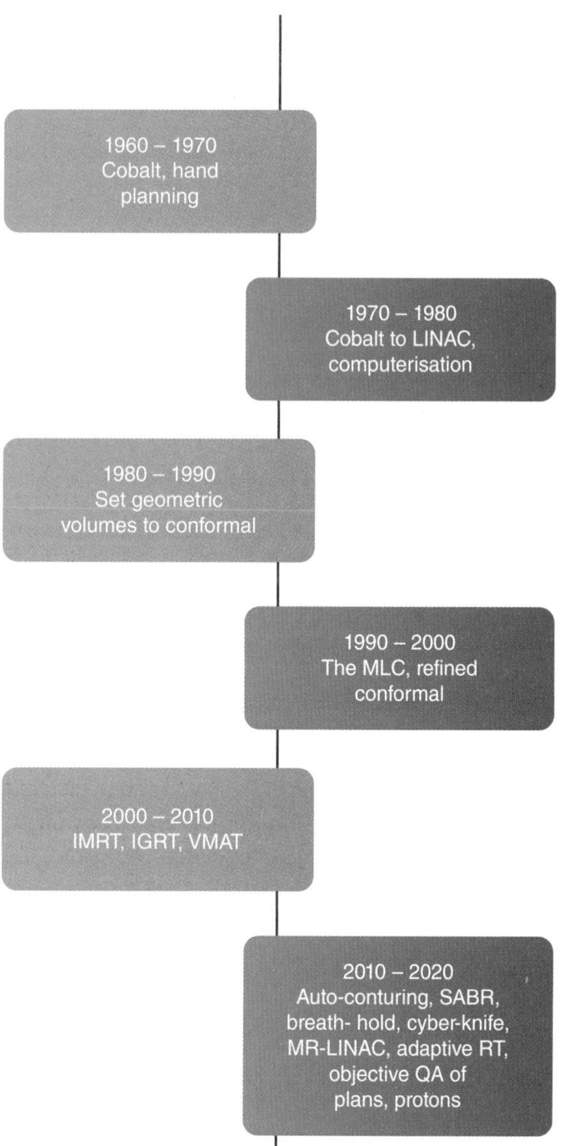

Figure 20.1 The evolution of precision radiotherapy. IGRT, image-guided radiotherapy; IMRT, intensity-modulated radiotherapy; LINAC, linear accelerator; MLC, multileaf collimator; MR-LINAC, magnetic resonance linear accelerator; QA, quality assurance; SABR, stereotactic ablative radiotherapy; VMAT, volumetric modulated arc therapy.

Why Protons?

The discovery of x-rays and gamma rays in the late nineteenth century led to a revolution in the diagnosis and treatment of cancer. In 1903, William Bragg, a British physicist, discovered the very surprising behaviour of particle radiation. But it was Ernest Rutherford in 1917 who first identified the proton as the key positively charged nuclear particle whilst working in Manchester. Protons are subatomic positively charged particles now produced by a circular accelerator called a cyclotron. The advantage of protons lies in something called the Bragg peak – they stop at a defined point and release all of their energy (Figure 20.2). This is the key to understanding why protons may be better for some patients by sparing critical radio-sensitive tissue adjacent to the cancer (Dvorak et al. 2013).

Before they reach the cancer, both proton and conventional radiation have to make their way through the patient's skin and surrounding tissues. X-ray photons have no mass or charge, and so x-ray beams are highly penetrating and deliver dose throughout any volume of tissue irradiated. However, most of the radiation is delivered only half a centimetre from the patient's skin, depending on the energy it was initially given. It then gradually loses this energy until it reaches the target. As tumours are almost always deeply located in the body, the photon actively interacts with outer healthy cells and drops only a small remaining dose of ionizing radiation on the deeper diseased cells. Moreover, as photons are not all stopped by human tissue, they leave the patient's body and continue to emit radiation as they do so. This is called the exit dose.

Protons, on the other hand, exhibit Bragg peak behaviour (Figure 20.2), and the depth of the peak depends on the energy given to the protons by the accelerator system. Therefore, by choosing the appropriate energy, a proton beam can be tuned to deliver maximum dose to the tumour with less dose to healthy tissue in front of the tumour and no dose at all to healthy tissue behind the tumour.

The aim of radiotherapy is to deliver as high a dose as possible to the cancer but to spare critically sensitive normal tissues around it as much as possible (Price and Sikora 2014). Certain organs are particularly sensitive – the spinal cord, base of brain, eye, intestine, liver, and kidneys. The Bragg peak allows a more precise delivery of radiation dose to the cancer yet sparing any tissues downstream of the beam.

In most patients, the extra spread-out dose from x-ray beams is clinically acceptable – where no significant side effects are likely, and patients are older so the possibility of secondary cancers is not an issue. In those circumstances, x-ray treatments may be preferred as they are less sensitive to possible errors in patient setup or position than proton beams. They offer more convenience as treatment is available locally. But in a small minority of patients, the extra targeting achieved with proton beams and the reduction in dose to surrounding tissues are vitally important.

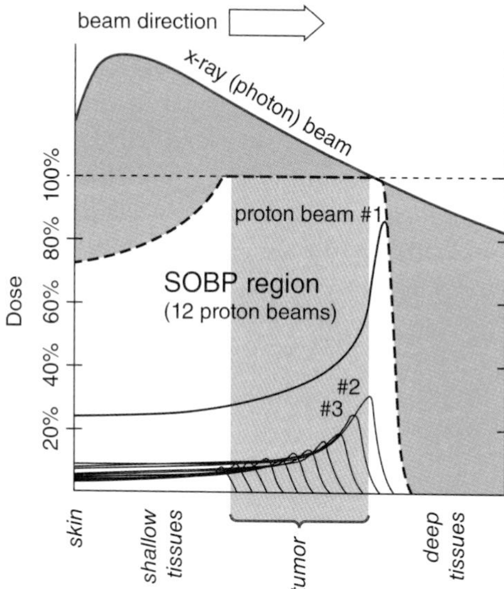

Figure 20.2 The different energy distribution of protons versus photons. SOBP, spread-out Bragg peak.

The Cost of PT

The problem is cost. Protons are 1835 times as big as electrons and require far more energy to get them moving, so a cyclotron is used to accelerate them round and round in circles getting faster and faster. These are large and expensive, costing up to £80 m with another £25 m for the building to house them (Table 20.1). Recently, costs have fallen and a compact model costs £15 m. This still compares unfavourably with £1.5 m for a conventional radiotherapy machine. The staffing requirements are also much higher for protons – often by four times compared to a LINAC. This all means that the total cost per fraction of radiotherapy delivered is inevitably considerably more.

However produced, PT is currently significantly more expensive than conventional LINAC-based radiotherapy. With legacy systems, the cost ratio of protons/conventional radiotherapy is nearly 10-fold. Such Varian systems are being installed at two sites by NHS England. With compact systems such as those installed by Rutherford Cancer Centres (RCC), this falls to below two. As the price differential diminishes, it is likely that there will be increasing demand for protons where the planned target volume can be achieved with greater critical normal tissue sparing than by using photons. There has been rapid global growth in the cumulative number of operational proton beam therapy (PBT) centres and the number of patients being treated in them. This is rising exponentially as more facilities become operational.

Table 20.1 Cost of delivering a single proton fraction (base cost LINAC photon fraction with state-of-the-art IMRT and IGRT £500).

Manufacturer	Vaults	Total pts	Cost	Staff	Cost/fraction
Varian	4	750	£110 m	80	5 K
IBA	1	500	£20 m	20	1 K
Mevion	1	500	£25 m	20	1 K
Hitachi	4	700	£35 m	40	2 K
AVO	2	750	£30 m	25	1.5 K
LINAC	1	500	£2.5 m	8	0.5 K

Clinical Trials of PT

There are 140 observational (mainly phase 2) studies across a range of tumour types (Verma et al. 2016). There are also 11 randomised control (phase 3) studies in a range of tumours including prostate, lung, breast, and brain. It is now unlikely that there will ever be further large-scale randomised clinical trials but rather a pretreatment comparison of proton versus conventional radiotherapy in individual patients using predetermined metrics of plan quality. This assessment would be made objectively by treatment planning software systems. Payers, both governments (including the British NHS) and insurers, will use these criteria to assess the value of PT to an individual patient using the equation

$$\text{VALUE} = \frac{\text{POTENTIAL SIDE EFFECT REDUCTION}}{\text{COST}}.$$

Current Indications for PT

1) *Absolute indications:* Mainly children and young adults with spinal cord and base of brain tumours. A recent 2018 Freedom of Information request revealed that during 2018, 216 patients were sent abroad from the UK for PBT at a total treatment cost of £24.19 m. There are estimated to be at least 750 of such patients a year who would benefit from PT in the UK.
2) *Cancer types where a significant proportion of patients are likely to benefit:* Lung, left breast, head and neck, and oesophageal through reduced long-term side effects (Mishra et al. 2017).
3) *Patients where the anatomy of the tumour and critical normal tissues favour a dose distribution with protons:* This could be of any cancer type or site where radical radiotherapy is being proposed. That means the radiation is being given with the aim of eradicating the cancer, so curing the patient. To determine whether protons will be indicated, it will be necessary to construct the proton and photon plans and conduct a comparative analysis of the dose volume histogram carried out manually or by computer scoring. This will require the development of normal tissue complication probability (NTCP) models, which are applied to each patient to calculate their individual change in NTCP (ΔNTCP). This represents the difference between proton and photon treatments to different organs at risk. Purchasers of care can set the threshold for PT based on a percentage of ΔNTCP above which protons are preferred for different organs at risk (Langendijk et al. 2013).

It is likely that the European consensus of 10–15% of radical radiotherapy delivered by protons will emerge as the most realistic future scenario, and this is now the basis of health department strategic planning in Holland, Germany, France, Italy, and Scandinavia. This is at considerable variance with current NHS plans as outlined in NHS England's strategy document, *A Vision for Radiotherapy 2014–2024*, which calls for only the two facilities now under construction by the NHS (Samuel and Boon 2014). The pooled European strategy data suggests a need for 10–20 PBT facilities in the UK. NHS England is planning for only 1% of radical radiotherapy to be delivered by protons. This compares unfavourably against other European countries' plans. Indeed, Dr. Adrian Crellin, NHS England Clinical Lead on Proton Therapy, wrote in December 2014 (Crellin and Burnet 2014):

> *Full business case approval is anticipated in early 2015 and the first patients are due to be treated in 2018. These centres will have a capacity to treat up to 1500 patients per annum with a secure revenue stream through NHS England. This represents just 1% of radiotherapy in England. For continental Europe, facilities are already in place in Italy, Germany, France, the Czech Republic and Switzerland. The confirmed strategy for PT in Sweden, Denmark and Holland is for proton capacity to deliver 14, 15 and 10% of radiotherapy workload, respectively.*

Since this was written, the dynamic has changed (Crellin 2018). There have been delays in the construction of the two NHS PT systems. Three independent sector facilities are now fully operational, with two more under construction and two at the planning stage.

Challenges for PT in the UK

1) *Total PT capacity requirement:* For the last 10 years, the NHS has sent increasing numbers of patients abroad for PBT as stated above, mainly to Jacksonville in Florida. Other patients have been treated in Switzerland and Germany. From 2019, this was no longer necessary. Two NHS facilities were planned, the first at Christie Hospital, Manchester, started treating in December 2018. The second, at University College Hospital, London, is now delayed until at least 2022. Seven private sector units are also being created. But even when all are operational there will be a predictable lack of capacity. We are the last sizable European country to have an operational proton service. Unless there is an urgent policy change, the overall quality of British radiotherapy will again fail to keep up with that of neighbouring countries. We need to evaluate the actual need for PT in the UK in order to build up realistic capacity. Comparative estimates from other European countries suggest that between 15 and 20 PT facilities working at full capacity will be required by 2022. This would ensure that 10% of patients currently receiving radical radiotherapy would receive protons. This will require a major policy change in the organisation of radiotherapy services and their IT networks.
2) *Speed of rollout:* Figure 20.3 shows the rollout of PT facilities in the UK over the last five years. Once complete, this would still only provide for a 5% radical radiotherapy capability even when at full capacity with double shifts and weekend working. Further investment, either public or private, is necessary at this stage in view of the time taken to construct and commission PT facilities.
3) *NHS Wales:* The Welsh government's Department for Health and Social Services approved an initial collaboration between Rutherford Health and NHS Wales to explore the delivery of a range of cancer services. The specialist commissioners, Welsh Health Specialised Services Committee, produced a commissioning document for PT, which, once all the quality and safety criteria were met, saw Welsh patients treated at the Rutherford Cancer Centre, South Wales. This clinic was successfully registered with Healthcare Inspectorate Wales in 2018, the equivalent of the English Care Quality Commission, and is treating patients. All radiotherapy plans are peer reviewed by the proton team at the University of Pennsylvania Hospital, Philadelphia prior to delivery.

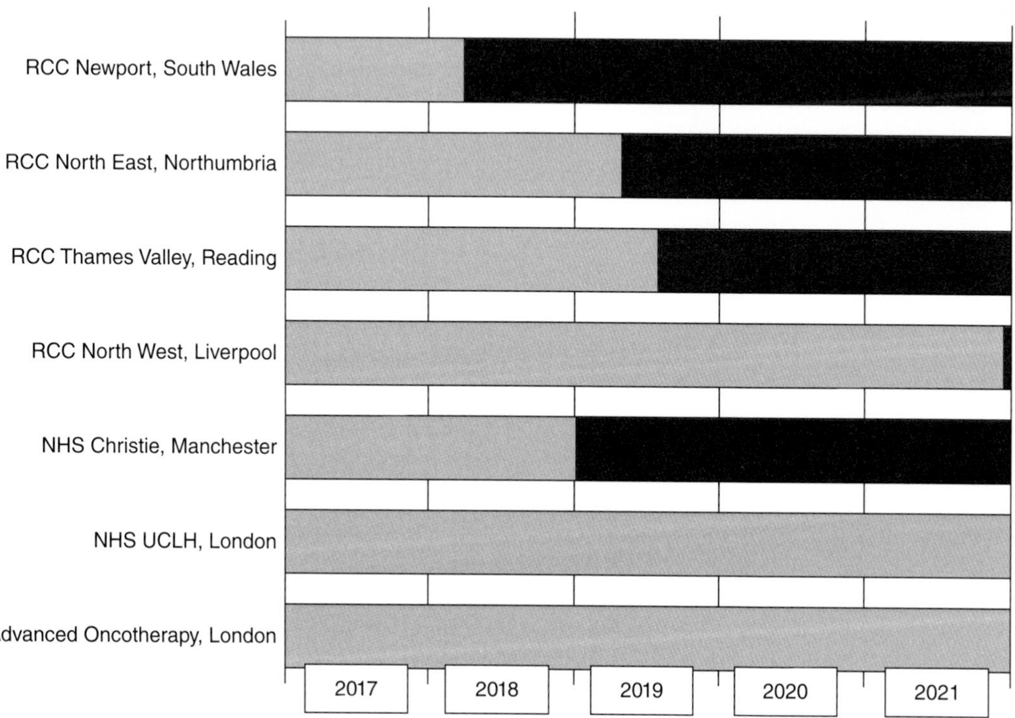

Figure 20.3 Timeline of operational proton facilities in the UK. *Source:* Adapted from Hall et al. (2017), but please note – no high-energy working prototype of this technology is as yet available.

Conclusion

Unless there is an urgent policy change, the quality of UK radiotherapy will again fail to keep up with that of neighbouring countries. There will be a repeat of the 10-year time lag to introduce previous new radiotherapy technology – IMRT and IGRT – into timely routine clinical practice. This has now been at least partially corrected by the direct intervention of the Prime Minister's Radiotherapy Fund. A leading US observer has commented that a network of small proton centres interconnected by a high-performance computer network in a public-private partnership is a rational way forward (Zietman 2018). In view of the time required to construct the necessary facilities, we need to encourage such innovative collaborations if we are to ensure that all cancer patients get the best care possible.

References

Crellin, A. (2018). The road map for National Health Service proton beam therapy. *Clin. Oncol.* 30 (5): 277–279. https://doi.org/10.1016/j.clon.2018.02.032.

Crellin, A.M. and Burnet, N.G. (2014). Proton beam therapy: the context, future direction and challenges become clearer. *Clin. Oncol.* 26 (12): 736–738. https://doi.org/10.1016/j.clon.2014.10.009.

Dvorak, T., Fitzek, M.M., and Wazer, D.E. (2013). Utilization of proton therapy: evidence-based, market-driven, or something in-between? *Am. J. Clin. Oncol.: Cancer Clin. Trials* 36 (2): 192–196. https://doi.org/10.1097/COC.0b013e3182438d92.

Hall, M., Hill, D. and Pave, G. (2017). Advanced oncotherapy delivery of LIGHT. http://www.directorstalkinterviews.com/wp-content/uploads/2017/03/15.03.17-delivery-of-light.pdf.

Langendijk, J.A., Lambin, P., De Ruysscher, D. et al. (2013). Selection of patients for radiotherapy with protons aiming at reduction of side effects: the model-based approach. *Radiother. Oncol.* 107 (3): 267–273. https://doi.org/10.1016/j.radonc.2013.05.007.

Mishra, M.V., Aggarwal, S., Bentzen, S.M. et al. (2017). Establishing evidence-based indications for proton therapy: an overview of current clinical trials. *Int. J. Rad. Oncol. Biol. Phys.* 97 (2): 228–235. https://doi.org/10.1016/j.ijrobp.2016.10.045.

Price, P. and Sikora, K. (ed.) (2014). *Treatment of Cancer*, 6e. CRC Press. Available at: https://doi.org/10.1201/b17751.

Samuel, E. and Boon, J. (2014). Vision for radiotherapy 2014-2024. https://www.cancerresearchuk.org/sites/default/files/policy_feb2014_radiotherapy_vision2014-2024_final.pdf.

Verma, V., Mishra, M.V., and Mehta, M.P. (2016). *A systematic review of the cost and cost-effectiveness studies of proton radiotherapy. Cancer* https://doi.org/10.1002/cncr.29882.

Zietman, A.L. (2018). Too big to fail? The current status of proton therapy in the USA. *Clin. Oncol.* 30 (5): 271–273. https://doi.org/10.1016/j.clon.2017.11.002.

21

Transoral Robotic Surgery

Naseem Ghazali

Royal Blackburn Teaching Hospital, Blackburn, UK

Introduction

Surgeons have traditionally relied on open surgery because this method provides good access for adequate visualisation of the pathologies, which is a basic prerequisite in accomplishing the aim of surgical treatment. Lying within the neck, the upper aerodigestive tract is essentially a tubular structure with a confined luminal space. With this anatomical configuration, pathologies of the upper aerodigestive tract are difficult to visualise and would require surgeons to make large incisions on skin/mucosa and into the underlying tissues (i.e. lip-splitting incision, pharyngotomy), including drilling and cutting through jaw bone (i.e. mandibulotomy), to directly approach the target area. This procedure is highly invasive, as normal tissues are injured and damaged during the process.

Minimally invasive surgery (MIS) includes surgical procedures that are usually accessed through natural anatomical openings, where additional incisions are avoided or significantly minimised, thereby causing the smallest collateral damage possible to normal structures. When compared with traditional open surgery, MIS results in less pain, lowered risk of infection, shorter hospital stay, quick recovery time, and reduced blood loss.

The mouth provides a natural opening for surgical access to the upper aerodigestive tract, that is, transoral access. Transoral MIS is usually endoscopic-based procedures because it is the only way that visualization and instrumentation can coexist in a confined space once accessed through the mouth. Transoral robotic surgery (TORS) is emerging as a minimally invasive alternative to open surgery, or conventional transoral MIS, that is, transoral laser surgery, for the treatment of some head and neck pathologies.

The TORS approach was first introduced by Weinstein et al. (2005), and the US Food and Drug Administration (FDA) approval for TORS head and neck surgery was subsequently obtained in 2009. The main improvements of the TORS approach over traditional transoral MIS are the advantage of 3-D high-definition (HD) endoscopic visualisation of the laryngopharyngeal structures and the high precision and dexterity afforded by the wristed robotic instrumentation (Weinstein et al. 2009). Technically challenging tasks, such as endoscopic suturing in confined spaces, may be performed with relative ease robotically.

The introduction of TORS has resulted in an increase in the use of surgery to the upper aerodigestive tract. The main anatomical areas where TORS has been applied are the oropharyngeal subsites, the skull base (i.e. parapharyngeal), larynx, and hypopharynx. The role of TORS is particularly significant in the management of oropharyngeal cancers. This coincides with the rising incidence of HPV-driven oropharyngeal cancers, which present with small primary tumours that are highly amenable to surgical resection. Application of the TORS technique has also expanded into the management of sleep apnoea and other benign conditions of the salivary glands.

This chapter will briefly discuss the da Vinci robotic surgical system, the TORS setup, the indications and contraindications, postoperative care, and complications related to TORS when it is used for head and neck cancers. A final section will also discuss the surgical training required for TORS and the challenges of this approach.

Care of Head and Neck Cancer Patients for Dental Hygienists and Dental Therapists, First Edition. Edited by Jocelyn J. Harding.

Robotic Surgical System

The main robotic system currently used in head and neck surgery worldwide is the da Vinci robotic surgical platform (Intuitive Surgery). This system is based on the 'master-slave' relationship, whereby the movement of the robot is fully 'master' controlled by the surgeon. This system consists of three components: the surgeon's console, the patient-side cart, and the vision cart (Figure 21.1).

Patient-Side Cart

The patient-side cart is the operative 'slave' unit of the robotic system and is positioned closest to the patient during surgery. The patient-side cart incorporates the camera arm and the instrument arms (Figure 21.2).

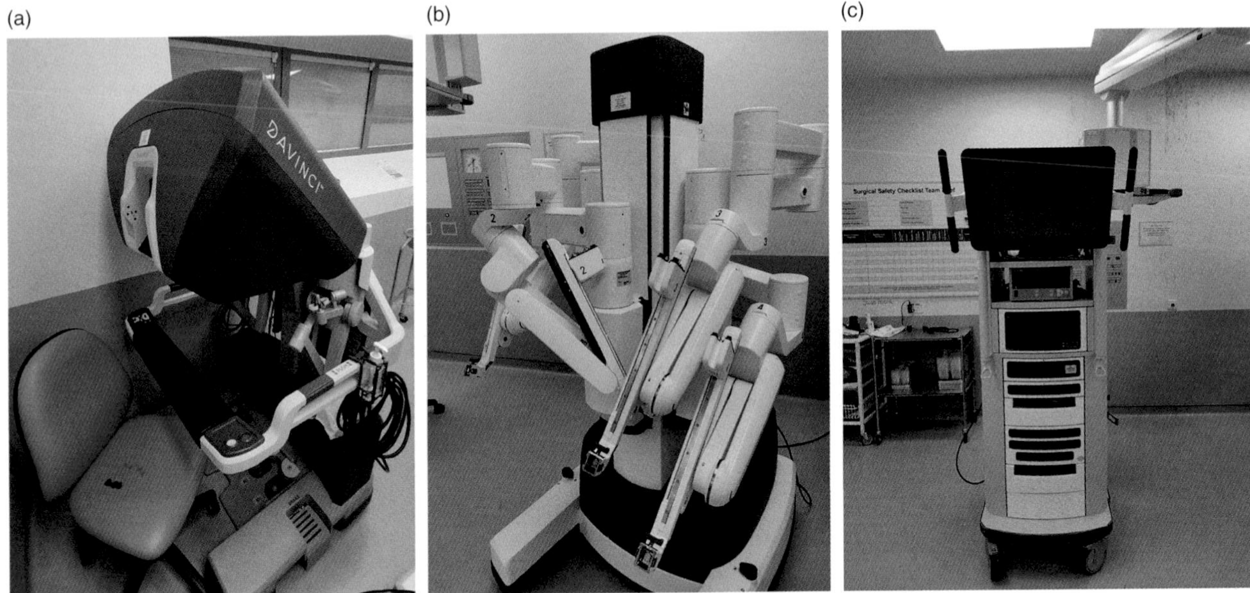

Figure 21.1 The three components of the da Vinci robotic surgical platform: (a) the surgeon's console, (b) the patient-side cart, and (c) the vision cart.

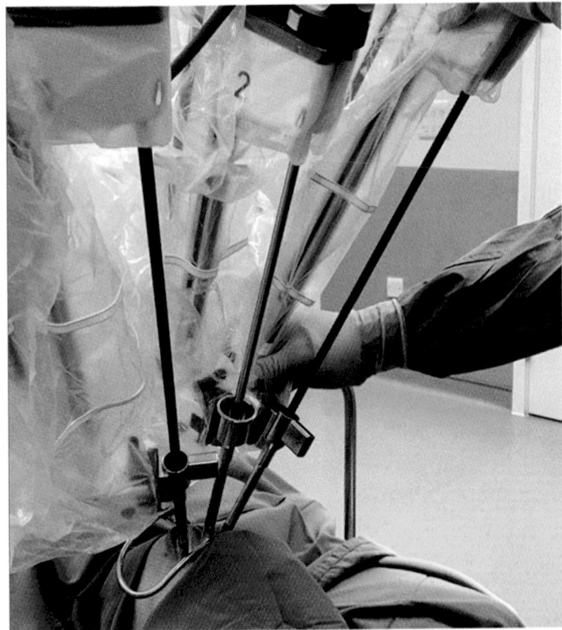

Figure 21.2 The patient-side cart incorporates the camera arm and the instrument arms.

The instrument arms provide the interface for the EndoWrist instruments, which are small (diameter 8 mm and 5 mm) wristed instruments that enable the surgical actions in the surgical field, for example, cutting, tissue grasping, and needle driving (Figure 21.3a).

The robotic camera is a rigid, 3-D HD stereoscopic endoscope, which is flat (0°) or angled (30°) and available in 8 mm or 12 mm diameter (Figure 21.3b).

A robotic assistant surgeon is usually positioned near the patient-side cart and operates it, mainly exchanging instruments and endoscopes at the robotic arms, and performs other surgical assisting activities, for example, suctioning, application of vascular clips, and cutting sutures.

(a)

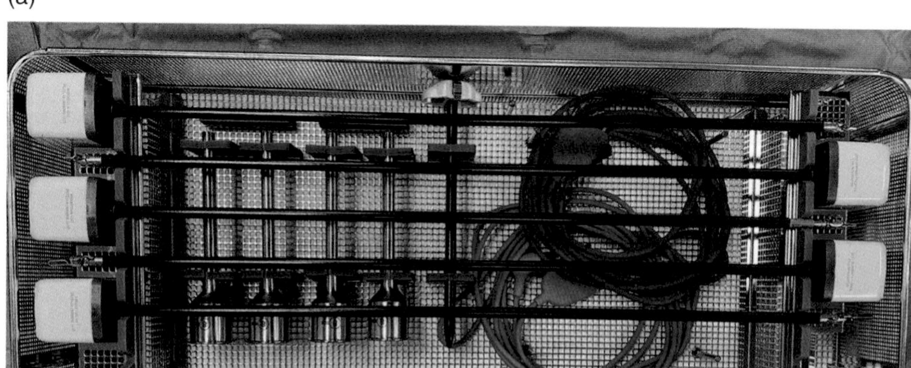

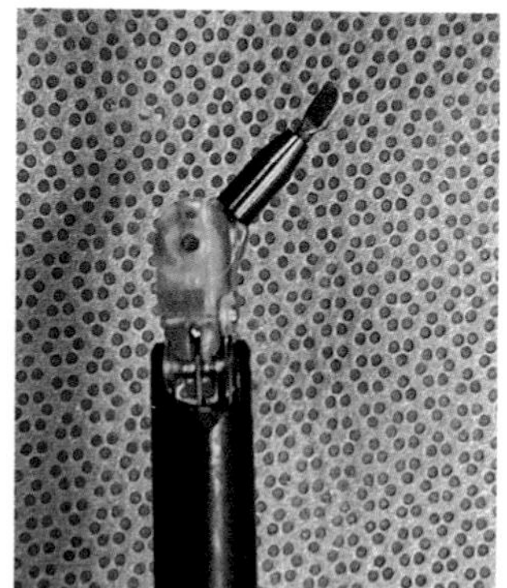

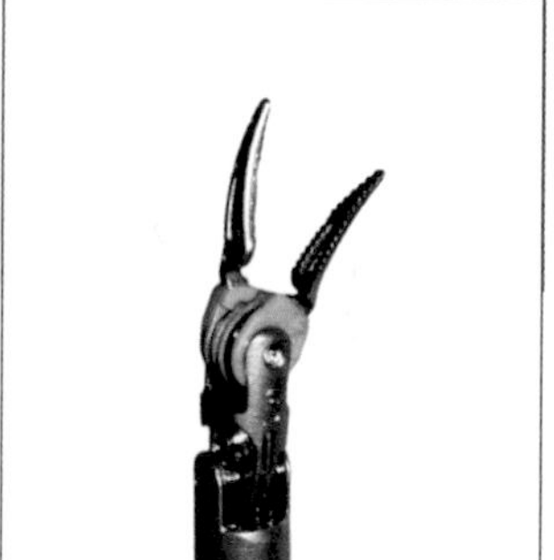

(b)

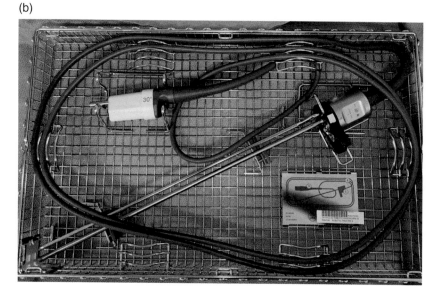

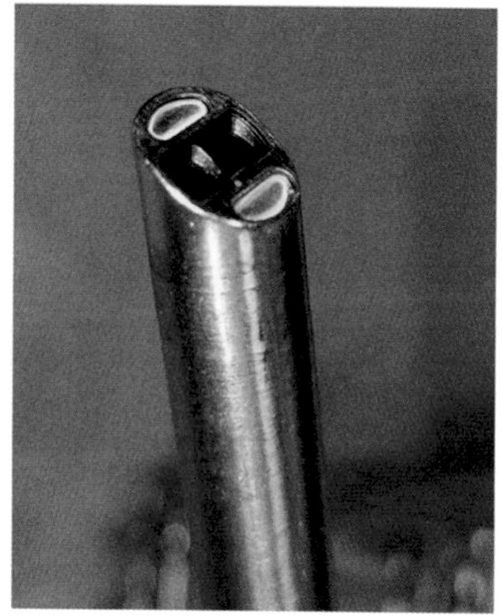

Figure 21.3 (a) Left, EndoWrist instruments with the cannulas in the surgical tray. Right, closeups of the ends of the EndoWrist instrument examples: the electrocautery spatula (top right) and the Maryland forceps (bottom right). (b) Left, the 3-D HD endoscopic camera; and right, closeup of the 30° endoscopic camera.

Surgeon's Console

The surgeon's console is where the surgeon sits and operates remotely during surgery (Figure 21.4a). The console is the 'master' unit of the robotic system. The EndoWrist instruments at the surgical field are fully controlled by the surgeon's hand movements through the 'master arms' at the surgeons console. The 'master arms' are formed by a pair of articulated arms with a finger clutch (i.e. where the surgeons place their finger and thumb) (Figure 21.4a) and a master controller. Using haptic technology, the 'master controller' senses the surgeon's hand movements and converts them electronically into real-time, scaled-down micromovements (i.e. motion scaling) to manipulate the smaller EndoWrists instruments in the surgical field. Natural hand tremor is also filtered out. Tremor reduction and motion scaling allow for high-precision work to be done.

The display system allows the surgeon to view the surgical field through the console binoculars (Figure 21.4a).

The view provided by the 3-D HD stereoscopic camera is highly magnified with true depth perception, allowing visualisation of tissue planes clearly and identification of structures, and this enables the surgeon to remain oriented in the anatomy. The EndoWrist instrument tips appear to align with the surgeon's hands during movement, simulating the natural eye, hand, and instrument alignment of open surgery (Figure 21.4b). Thus, the robotic platform enables the surgeon to be as dexterous as in open surgery while operating in a minimally invasive environment (Mishra n.d.).

The footswitch pedals enable the surgeon to manipulate the camera and control the energy instruments during surgery (Figure 21.4b).

The integrated control touch pad gives the surgeon control of video, audio, and system settings for the console surgeon. These include the options between 2-D and 3-D display, multi-image display (TilePro technology), fine-tuning of motion scaling, camera perspectives including Firefly fluorescence imaging, and personalising ergonomic settings.

Vision Cart

The vision cart accommodates the image-processing equipment of the robotic system. It has a 2-D vision touch screen that allows the robotic assistant to view the surgery in real time and ancillary staff to modify camera and energy instrument settings (Figure 21.5).

(a)

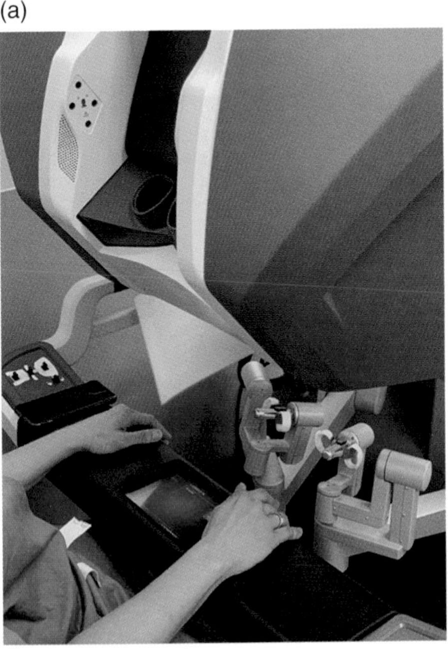

(b)

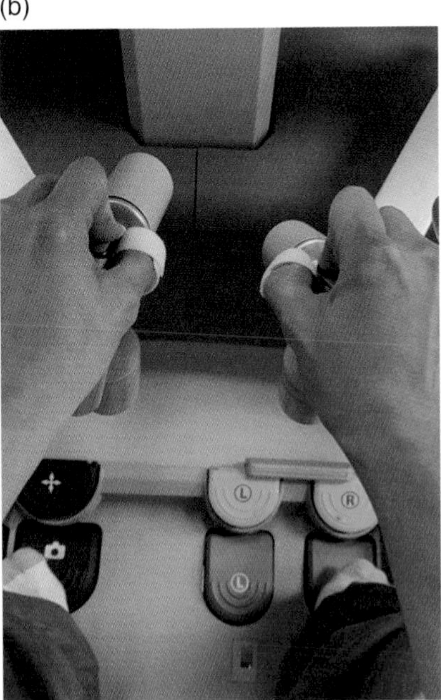

Figure 21.4 (a) A surgeon sits at the console during surgery and manipulates the 'master arms' with the finger clutch to control the EndoWrist instruments. (b) The human–robot interface with the surgeon's fingers at the finger clutch and feet at the foot pedals, which allow full control of the camera (via the left foot) and the energy of the EndoWrist instruments.

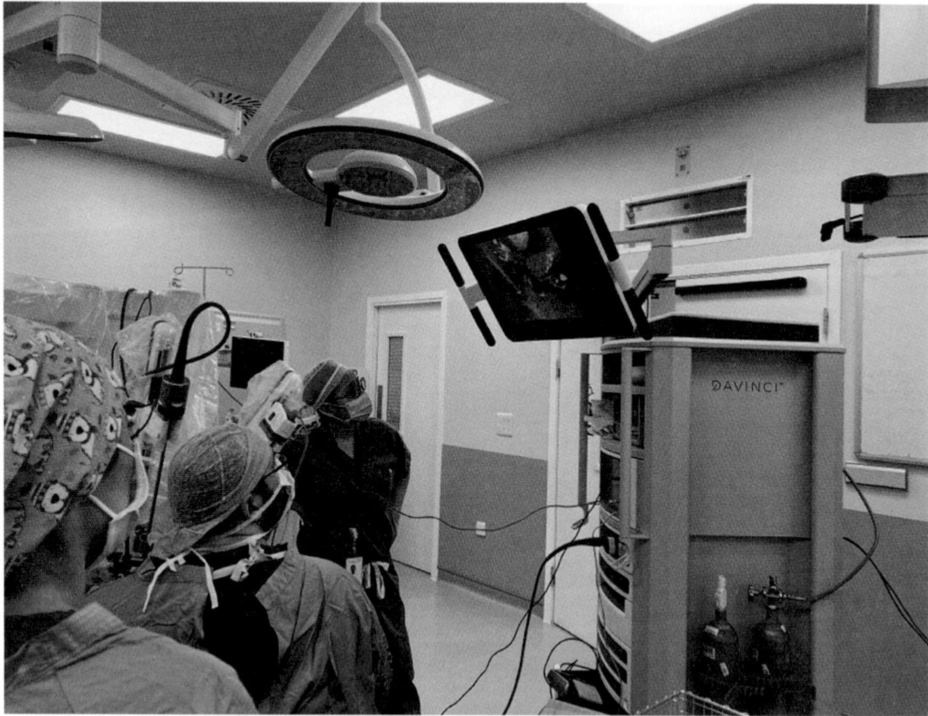

Figure 21.5 The vision cart accommodates the image-processing equipment for the robotic system. It provides 2-D HD vision for the robot surgical assistant and houses the electrocautery mechanism.

TORS Surgical Setup

The setting up of the team and the operating room (OR) environment for TORS includes the following:

1) Theatre preparation: It is critical to the success of TORS when the OR team and the environment are primed for the procedure. A team brief is held before the start of surgery where details relating to the patient, the procedure, the equipment, and availability of pathology support are discussed. The immediate steps to be taken during any intraoperative emergency, for example, fire in the airway, are also reviewed. As potential airway swelling and bleeding are a concern postoperatively, access to critical care or high-dependency bed postsurgery is considered at this stage.
2) Equipment: The robotic system is checked for any equipment malfunction. The robotic patient-side cart is draped. The headlight, robotic, and nonrobotic surgical instruments and medicaments, for example, adrenaline, are prepared.
3) Patient positioning and preparation: The recommended OR configuration is shown in Figure 21.6. The anaesthetised patient is laid supine, with the neck extended. The eyes and teeth are protected with eye shields and bite guards, respectively (Figure 21.7). The surgeon examines for adequate transoral visualisation of the tumour and evaluates if it is still feasible to undertake a TORS resection due to rapid tumour growth in some instances.
4) Placement of appropriate retractor to maintain mouth opening: The retractors are used to ensure a stable, transoral access throughout the procedure. The choice of retractor is down to surgeon preference and site of primary cancer (Figure 21.8).
5) Robot docking and positioning of the robotic arms and EndoWrist instruments: The patient-side cart is driven at a 30° angle into the ideal bedside position; that is, where the position of the foot of the patient cart relative to the base of operating table is shown in Figure 21.9. The robotic camera is positioned where optimal visualisation can be achieved and where it will not clash with the instrument arms during manipulation. The instrument arms are positioned where the arms can move about with minimal stress on the perioral tissues and the mouth gag during manipulations.

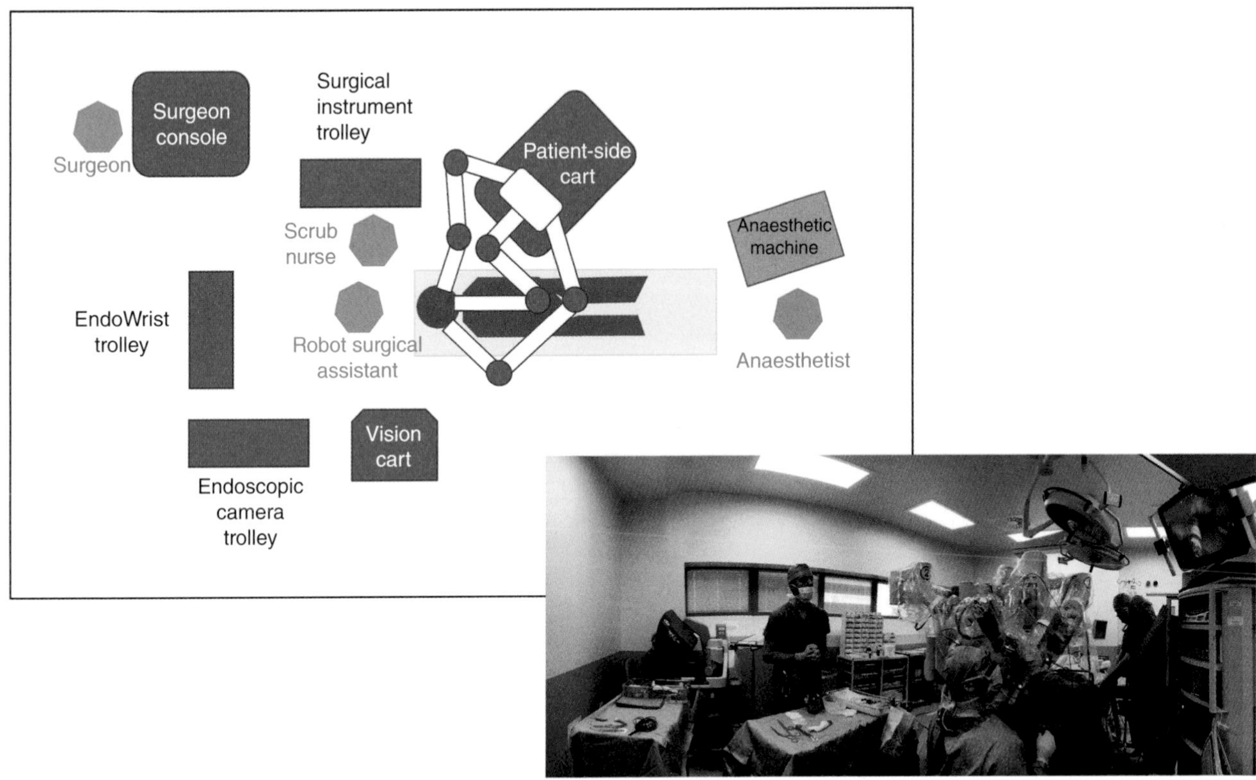

Figure 21.6 Operating room configuration for transoral robotic surgery.

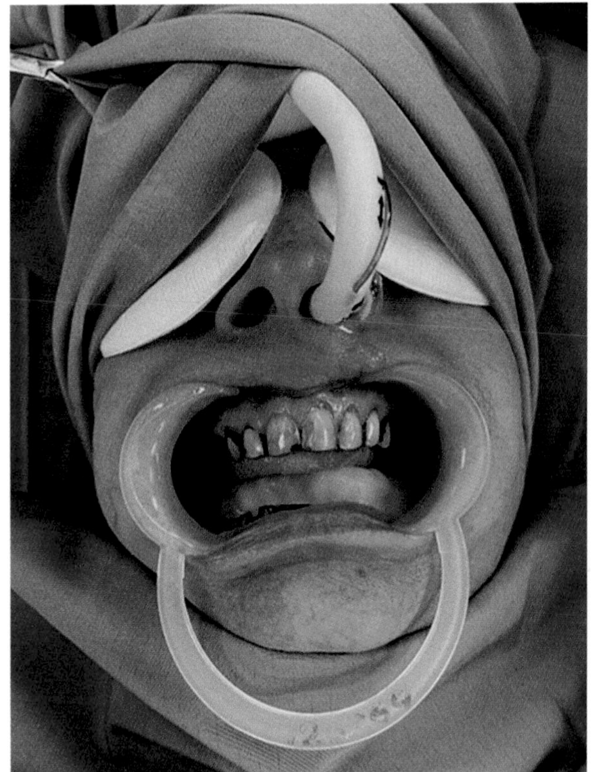

Figure 21.7 The eyes and teeth are protected with eye shields and bite guards.

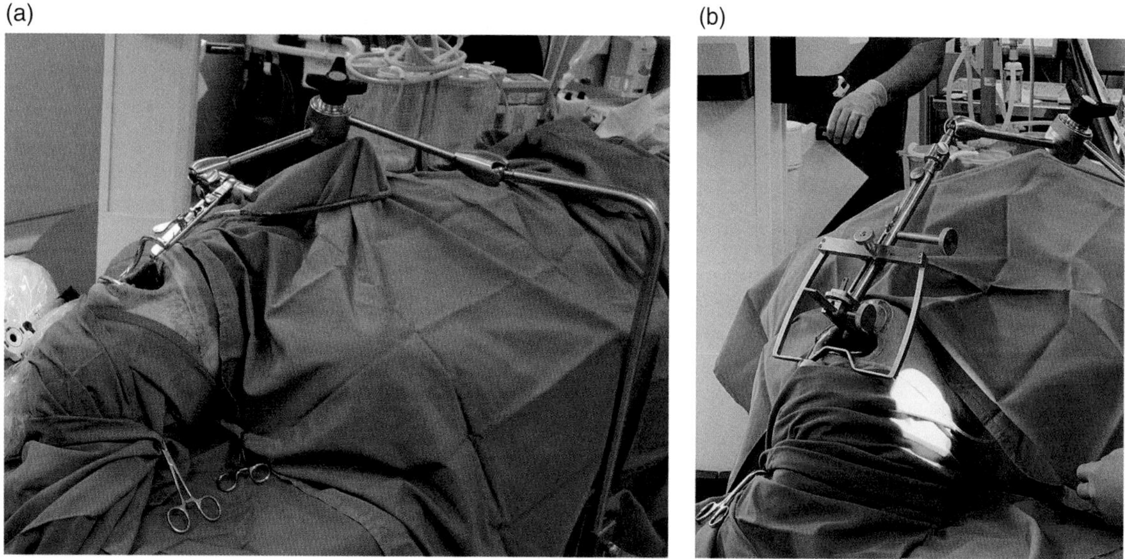

Figure 21.8 Two different retractors commonly used for transoral robotic surgery: (a) the Boyle Davis tonsil retractor and (b) the FK retractor.

Figure 21.9 Patient-side cart docked relative to patient position. The instruments and camera arms are positioned to allow optimal movement and visualization during surgery.

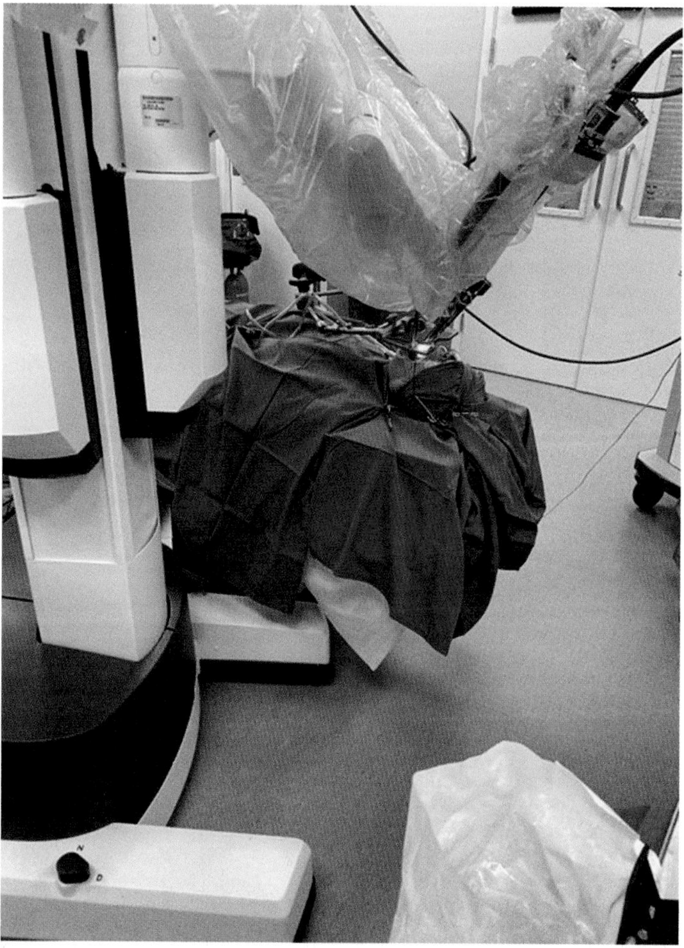

The Clinical Indications and Contraindications

Which Patients are Suitable for TORS?

To determine if TORS is a suitable treatment option, there are patient-related and tumour-related factors that must be considered. Patient-related factors may broadly fall into two categories: (i) patient comorbidity affecting fitness for surgery and anaesthesia and (ii) factors that can limit endoscopic access. Potential TORS candidates must be able to bear these possible risks and be expected to recover and heal from the procedure (Baskin et al. 2018). In general, the wounds created with TORS are often left open and to heal by secondary intention. Thus, the postoperative course may involve bleeding, airway compromise, dehydration, and malnutrition. Table 21.1 lists the strong relative and absolute contraindications for TORS.

Getting maximum transoral access is critical to TORS success. Patient-related factors that require consideration are the so-called the '8Ts' of endoscopic access, that is, teeth, trismus, transverse mandibular dimensions, tori, tongue, tilt, treatment (prior radiation), and tumour. The main contraindications to TORS are factors that can prevent robotic access, that is, limited mouth opening, limited neck extension, morbid obesity, micrognathia, microstomia, and craniofacial abnormalities. Relative contraindications are prominent teeth, large tongue, and body mass index (BMI) of >40.

What Characteristics of a Tumour Make It Amenable to TORS?

It is absolutely important to review the characteristics of each tumour when evaluating its suitability for TORS (Baskin et al. 2018). Careful consideration is given to the exact tumour location and its involvement with the adjacent structures, while deducing the extent of resection required to obtain a negative margin. TORS is suitable for early oropharyngeal, hypopharyngeal, and laryngeal carcinomas, that is, T1–T2 (up to 4 cm), usually with low-volume neck involvement. Table 21.2 lists the contraindications for TORS (Weinstein et al. 2015).

The TORS Procedure

In general, the following steps are undertaken. Once the robot and instrument arms are docked and good visualisation of the tumour is achieved, the surgeon begins the operation. The aim of the procedure is to remove the tumour en bloc – that is, one single piece rather than piecemeal – with adequate negative margins. Blood vessels encountered during the procedure are either cauterised or clipped to maintain haemostasis. Once the tumour is completely removed, it is sent for histopathological examination.

The wound is inspected; in particular, for any possible communication between the oropharynx and the neck, which can sometimes occur when the neck dissection is done at the same time as the TORS. In this situation, the communication may need to be repaired either directly with the surrounding tissues or with the use of a flap. Otherwise, TORS wounds are usually left open to heal by secondary intention, that is, granulation. Ligation of branches of the carotid artery is routinely done during neck dissection to stop significant postoperative bleeding, which can occur when the open wounds become secondarily infected.

Nasogastric feeding tubes are placed electively to provide nutritional support if oral intake is inadequate in the early postoperative stages. In some instances, a tracheostomy is placed at the surgeon's prerogative, usually when significant

Table 21.1 Strong relative and absolute contraindications for TORS.

Immunosuppression
Congestive heart failure
Chronic obstructive lung disease (COPD)
Connective tissue or rheumatologic disease
Conditions that prevent holding anticoagulation
Poorly controlled diabetes
Malnutrition

Table 21.2 Contraindications for TORS.

Vascular contraindications
Tonsillar malignancy with a retropharyngeal carotid artery
Tumour at the midline of the tongue base or vallecula
Tumour adjacent to the carotid bulb or internal carotid artery
Encasement of the carotid artery by tumour or metastatic neck nodes
Functional contraindications
Tumour resection requiring ≥50% of the deep tongue base musculature or posterior pharyngeal wall
Resection of the tongue base and entire epiglottis
Oncologic contraindications
T4b cancers
Unresectable neck disease
Multiple distant metastasis
Neoplastic-related trismus
Involvement of the prevertebral fascia
Involvement of the mandible or hyoid
Tumour extension into the soft tissues of the lateral neck
Eustachian tube involvement

Source: Based on Weinstein et al. (2015).

airway swelling is anticipated postoperatively. The majority of elective tracheostomies are often decannulated within a few days of surgery, and there is a trend towards decreasing tracheostomy placement rates over time as surgeons' experience increases (Yeh et al. 2015).

Postoperative Care and Complications

In the postoperative period, all TORS patients will experience a degree of pain, swelling, and dysphagia. If these are not managed adequately, normal sequelae can lead to complications that can be serious and life-threatening, such as poor pain control leading to prolonged dysphagia, weight loss/dehydration due to dysphagia, aspiration pneumonia, and secondary wound infection leading to catastrophic bleeding (Lubek and Ghazali 2022).

Thus, the expected TORS sequelae are usually managed pre-emptively by the multidisciplinary head and neck team (HN-MDT) via a combination of patient engagement through information, the use of multimodality analgesia featuring opioid-sparing regimens (i.e. paracetamol, nonsteroidal anti-inflammatory drugs, anticonvulsants, and steroids), and by early swallowing assessment and rehabilitation in anticipation of a quick return to normal safe oral swallowing. These elements are incorporated in a specific Enhanced Recovery After Surgery protocol for TORS patients (Ganti et al. 2020).

Most TORS patients will require a short in-hospital stay to manage the initial postoperative pain and altered swallowing. Most patients will be discharged once their overall condition is stable and when there is absence of active bleeding and infection. Occasionally, some patients are discharged with a temporary nasogastric feeding tube in place. Permanent feeding tubes (i.e. PEG) have been reported for patients who have required postoperative radio(chemo)therapy after TORS, but rarely is it required post-TORS alone. Table 21.3 lists the potential complications of TORS.

Outcomes of TORS

Surgical Margins and Cancer Outcomes

A systematic review of studies reporting transoral MIS in oropharyngeal cancers (Gorphe and Simon 2019) indicates that the rate of positive (involved) margins with TORS was 8.1%, which is slightly higher than the overall rate of all transoral

Table 21.3 Potential complications of TORS.

Sequelae and complications	
Pain	
Dysphagia	
Airway oedema	
Bleeding	
Iatrogenic orocutaneous communication and pharyngocutaneous fistula formation	
Aspiration pneumonia	
Nerve injury, including taste disturbance	
Other	
	Trismus and other musculoskeletal issues
	Iatrogenic injury, for example, dental injury; soft tissue laceration, burns
	Cervical spondylodiscitis

Source: Lubek and Ghazali (2022).

surgery for oropharyngeal cancers (7.8%). Overall, the positive margin status in transoral surgery for oropharyngeal cancers is related to a reduction in local control.

Functional Outcomes

When compared with the open approach, TORS cases have reduced operative time, less blood loss, fewer critical care admissions, less postoperative pain, shorter hospitalisation, fewer complications, and better cosmetic results as TORS obviates the need for external facial incisions (Kelly et al. 2014). Most patients who underwent TORS with or without adjuvant therapy report a return to baseline quality of life and swallow function by 6–12 months posttreatment (Castellano and Sharma 2019). It is possible that chemoradiotherapy may be avoided in about one-third of patients who undergo TORS, and in this group, the adverse side effects of CRT are avoided completely (de Almeida et al. 2014).

Training for TORS and Challenges

Surgeons who embark on TORS training (Richmon et al. 2011) typically enrol in an online course on the theoretical aspects of the energy instrumentation, the components of the robotic system, and the control of the surgeon's console. Time is spent on the robotic simulator doing exercises that help the surgeon grasp the depth of vision afforded by the robotic camera and obtain good control of the robotic arms and instrumentation at the console. Surgeons proceed to improve on their dexterity by undertaking tasks on models, including suturing. These exercises also enable the surgeon to continue developing the use of sight alone when undertaking robotic surgery, as all natural tactile feedback during open surgery is eliminated because the surgeon no longer manipulates the instrument directly.

Surgeons may attend live demonstrations of TORS and participate in cadaveric and/or animal TORS experience. Dry runs may be undertaken to mock the procedure, usually done prior to undertaking the first TORS case and also in situations when a new TORS procedure is to be introduced. Once these are completed satisfactorily, the novice robotic surgeon undertakes TORS with the supervision and support of an experienced TORS surgeon. This can be facilitated by dual console operating and via live video link mentoring.

There is a learning curve for all robotic surgeons. The TORS surgeon must master specific anatomy to ensure the ability to undertake the so-called 'inside-out' approach in TORS as opposed to the traditional open approach, where the incision begins from outside and works towards the inside of the body. The 'inside-out' approach requires knowledge and familiarity of the changing anatomy and landmarks inherent with this approach (Gorphe and Simon 2019). It is suggested that 20 is the number of cases needed to reach the peak of a learning curve for TORS.

However, the speed at which the learning curve reaches a plateau is not solely down to the surgeon but multifactorial. This includes the volume of suitable TORS cases, regular access to the robot, and close team working, that is, in the OR and with the HN-MDT. It is important to ensure that a defined, trained assistant robotic surgeon is available in all TORS cases. Maintenance of a core robotic OR team consisting of scrub nurses and theatre support workers is key in reducing overall OR time during TORS and ensures patient safety, particularly as the team will be familiar with the established emergency plans in case of uncontrolled bleeding, airway compromise, or robot malfunction. Discerning of suitable cases for TORS requires engagement and continued education of the HN-MDT.

Wider adoption of TORS in head and neck cancer remains a challenge. The robotic system is not widely available as its purchase may be cost-prohibitive for most hospitals. Individual hospitals that have acquired the robot may not necessarily have TORS service as a business strategy. There may be scepticism of a new technology among some on the HN-MDT, along with lingering concerns that adequate cancer surgery in the laryngopharyngeal region cannot be achieved by TORS and poor functional outcomes may follow TORS.

The scepticism of TORS as a surgical tool may be lessened as more surgeons become exposed and trained in TORS. Even though there has been a decade of post-TORS outcomes published in the medical literature, acceptance of TORS as a standard of care will only be established with the evidence obtained from randomised controlled trials that are currently ongoing.

Conclusion

TORS is a viable minimally invasive alternative to open surgery for the treatment of some head and neck pathologies, particularly oropharyngeal carcinoma. It is increasingly used based on evidence of good oncological outcomes and the prospect of better long-term functional and quality of life outcomes by the avoidance of chemoradiation or adjuvant radiotherapy.

Acknowledgement

The author thanks Mr Gioele Attardo, certified robot assistant, advanced surgical practitioner and adult learning lecturer, University of Central Lancashire, for his assistance with the video recordings and photography used in this chapter.

References

Baskin, R.M., Boyce, B.J., Amdur, R. et al. (2018). Transoral robotic surgery for oropharyngeal cancer: patient selection and special considerations. *Cancer Manag. Res.* 10: 839–846.

Castellano, A. and Sharma, A. (2019). Systematic review of validated quality of life and swallow outcomes after transoral robotic surgery. *Otolaryngol. Head Neck Surg.* 161 (4): 561–567.

de Almeida, J.R., Byrd, J.K., Wu, R. et al. (2014). A systematic review of transoral robotic surgery and radiotherapy for early oropharynx cancer: a systematic review. *Laryngoscope* 124 (9): 2096–2102.

Ganti, A., Eggerstedt, M., Grudzinski, K. et al. (2020). Enhanced recovery protocol for transoral robotic surgery demonstrates improved analgesia and narcotic use reduction. *Am. J. Otolaryngol.* 41 (6): 102649.

Gorphe P, Simon C. A systematic review and meta-analysis of margins in transoral surgery for oropharyngeal carcinoma. *Oral Oncol.* 2019; 98:69–77. doi: https://doi.org/10.1016/j.oraloncology.2019.09.017.

Kelly, K., Johnson-Obaseki, S., Lumingu, J., and Corsten, M. (2014). Oncologic, functional and surgical outcomes of primary transoral robotic surgery for early squamous cell cancer of the oropharynx: a systematic review. *Oral Oncol.* 50 (8): 696–703.

Lubek JE, Ghazali N. (2022) Transoral Robotic Surgery In Management of Complications in Oral and Maxillofacial Surgery 2nd edition, Miloro M, Kolokythas A (eds.), Wiley Blackwell Publishing 2022, Chapter 21 pp 465–480. [ISBN-13: 978-1119710691]

Mishra RK (n.d.). System components. Robotic Surgery. https://www.laparoscopyhospital.com/Book/Ch-03.pdf.

Richmon, J.D., Agrawal, N., and Pattani, K.M. (2011). Implementation of a TORS program in an academic medical center. *Laryngoscope* 121 (11): 2344–2348.

Weinstein, G.S., O'Malley, B.W., and Hockstein, N.G. (2005). Transoral robotic surgery: supraglottic laryngectomy in a canine model. *Laryngoscope* 115 (7): 1315–1319.

Weinstein, G.S., O'Malley, B.W. Jr., Desai, S.C., and Quon, H. (2009). Transoral robotic surgery: does the ends justify the means? *Curr. Opin. Otolaryngol. Head Neck Surg.* 17 (2): 126–131.

Weinstein, G.S., O'Malley, B.W., Rinaldo, A. et al. (2015). Understanding contraindications for transoral robotic surgery (TORS) for oropharyngeal cancer. *Eur. Arch. Otorhinolaryngol.* 272 (7): 1551–1552.

Yeh, D.H., Tam, S., Fung, K. et al. (2015). Transoral robotic surgery vs. radiotherapy for management of oropharyngeal squamous cell carcinoma – a systematic review of the literature. *Eur. J. Surg. Oncol.* 41 (12): 1603–1613.

22

Photobiomodulation Therapy for Management of Oral Complications Induced by Head and Neck Cancer Treatments

Reem Hanna

Department of Oral Surgery, King's College Hospital NHS Foundation Trust, London, UK
Department of Surgical Sciences and Integrated Diagnostics, University of Genoa, Genoa, Italy

Introduction

Oral complications induced by head and neck cancer (HNC) therapies are associated with a negative impact on patients' quality of life (QoL) (Epstein et al. 2012; Elting et al. 2008; Cooperstein et al. 2012; Hunter et al. 2013; Verdonck-de Leeuw et al. 2014). A multidisciplinary team to care for patients living with HNC is crucial for a patient's journey from diagnosis to treatment and continuing aftercare. In this context, nurses and therapists play an important role that can have an influence on patients with HNC by focusing on management of symptoms developed as a result of their treatments (Kagan 2009). Dental hygienists and therapists (DHTs) have become an essential part of HNC patients' care and aftercare (Chang et al. 2019).

The Multinational Association of Supportive Care in Cancer and the International Society for Oral Oncology (MASCC/ISOO) have addressed these complications, from an initial diagnosis of HNC throughout the treatment and survival. However, many interventions have limitations and are primarily palliative in nature (Zecha et al. 2016). Hence, noninvasive effective therapy has emerged to overcome these limitations. Photobiomodulation (PBM) therapy is one such therapy. Much evidence-based science and practice have demonstrated the efficacy of this therapy and its effectiveness to eliminate or reduce the symptoms of oral complications induced by HNC treatments (Zecha et al. 2016; Lalla et al. 2014). PBM has extensive benefits in improving patients' functionality, allowing HNC therapies without interruption, and ultimately enhancing HNC patients' QoL (de Pauli Paglioni et al. 2020; Yifru et al. 2021; Gautam et al. 2013).

MASCC/ISOO has approved the use of PBM therapy in the management of oral mucositis (OM) induced by chemotherapy (CT) and radiotherapy (RT) in HNC patients (Lalla et al. 2014; Elad and Zadik 2016). This has also been supported by the National Institute for Health and Care Excellence (NICE) in the UK (NICE 2018).

This chapter covers PBM mechanism of action, benefits, and clinical applications. It also addresses the current clinical PBM protocols in the management of various oral complications induced by CT and RT, in terms of therapeutic and preventive approaches. Moreover, it emphasises the vital role of DHTs in the management of oral complications within a multidisciplinary team in secondary care as well as in primary care setups. Finally, it discusses the future of DHTs training in the field of laser in dentistry in general with a focus on PBM therapy.

Photobiomodulation

What Is Photobiomodulation and Does It Work (Mechanism of Action)?

PBM is the current term that has replaced various other terms used prior to 2014, such as low-level laser therapy or soft laser (Anders et al. 2015). The word *photobiomodulation* is made up of the following: *photo* for light, *bio* for life, and *modulation* for manipulation of the cellular activities to generate desirable outcomes.

Red light and near-infrared (NIR) light are able to induce significant physiological changes inside the tissue. The PBM mechanism of action remains evolving, but the current presumed mechanism is related to the absorption of the light

Care of Head and Neck Cancer Patients for Dental Hygienists and Dental Therapists, First Edition. Edited by Jocelyn J. Harding.

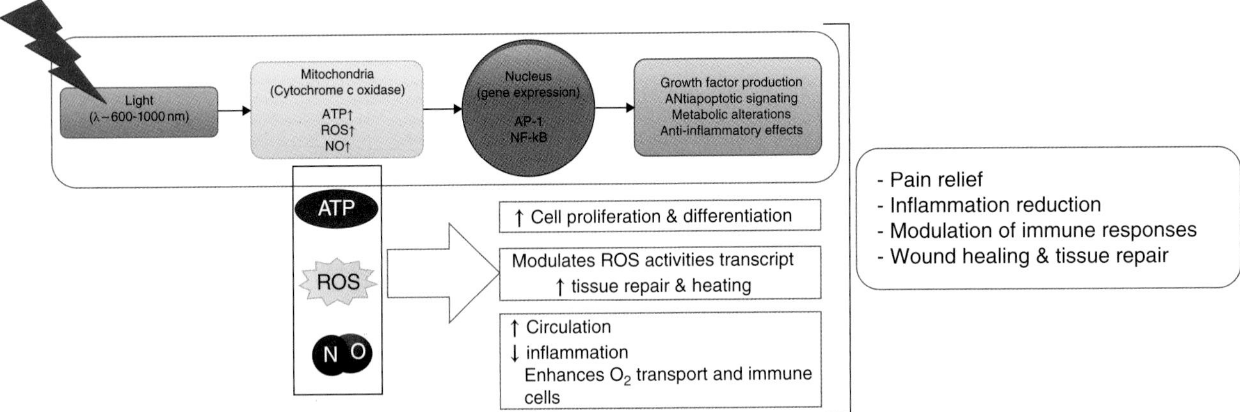

Figure 22.1 The current PBM mechanism of action. ATP, adenosine triphosphate; NO, nitric oxide; ROS, reactive oxygen species. *Source:* Based on Prindeze et al. (2012).

source by the mitochondrial enzyme called *cytochrome c oxidase* (a photoacceptor), resulting in an improvement in the mitochondrial respiration and oxygen consumption (de Freitas and Hamblin 2016; Wang et al. 2017), where a cascade of the following cellular and molecular activities occurs: an increase in adenosine triphosphate, modulation of reactive oxygen species (ROS), and an increase in nitric oxide. This shift in cellular metabolism leads to gene expressions and growth factor production (Figure 22.1) (Prindeze et al. 2012). Ultimately, this would have a great impact on such clinical outcomes as pain relief, reduction in inflammation, modulation of immune responses, and acceleration of tissue healing (Hanna et al. 2019, 2020, 2021; Amaroli et al. 2017, 2018). PBM can be utilised in forms such as laser and light-emitting diodes of red (630, 633, 655, 670 nm) and NIR (780, 808, 810, 880, 904, 940, 1064, 1072 nm) wavelengths.

How Do Photons Interact with Biological Tissue (Laser–Tissue Interaction)?

There are five phenomena related to light–matter interaction, as follows (Wieneke and Gerhard 2018, 3-1–3-42) (Figure 22.2):

Refraction: Laser light tends to bend when it travels through matter.

Transmission: Laser light passes through the medium and emerges as a light without interaction with the matter.

Reflection: Laser light bounces off an object (smooth surfaces), and this can occur at an angle, that is, if the beam is divergent, then the reflected beam will diverge.

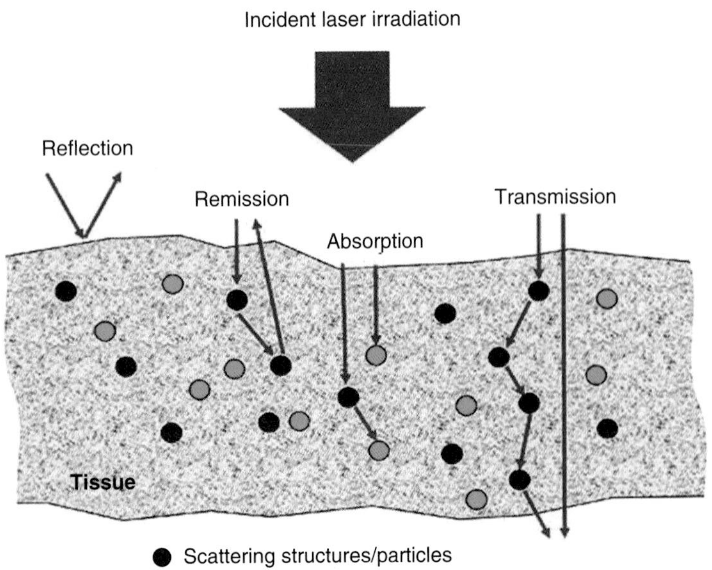

Figure 22.2 The laser–tissue interaction phenomena. *Source:* Adapted from Wieneke and Gerhard (2018).

Absorption: Absorption occurs when the photonic energy of the light wave is absorbed by the predominant chromophore of that matter. Each wavelength of an electromagnetic spectrum has an affinity to a certain chromophore, in order to achieve a desirable outcome.

Scattering: Scattering is a process where the laser light rays divert from a straight path or the matter particles are deflected.

The most important phenomena of laser–tissue interaction are absorption and scattering, for the following reasons:

1) Light penetration inside the biological tissues depends on the laser parameters, where wavelength and the optical properties of the tissue are most important (Ansari et al. 2009, 746–750).
2) The optical properties of the tissue determine the energy scattering (Jacques 2013).
3) The attenuation of light refers to the reduction in its intensity as it travels through a medium due to absorption or scattering of photons (Jacques 2013).

Essential Laser Terminology

Table 22.1 (Huang et al. 2009) and Figure 22.3 (Benedicenti and Benedicenti 2016) show the most fundamental laser parameters that require full understanding, as they are essential when laser treatment protocol is formulated.

What are PBM Effects on Clinical Outcomes?

The potential therapeutic benefits of PBM therapy include that it enhances microcirculation, improves lymphatic drainage, induces analgesia, increases proliferation and differentiation of epithelial cells, and increases fibroblast production and activity, resulting in accelerating collagen synthesis (Chung et al. 2012; Abramoff et al. 2008; Maegawa et al. 2000; Andrade et al. 2014; Bjordal et al. 2006). Table 22.2 shows a summary of PBM influences and PBM clinical benefits.

Table 22.1 An overview of PBM parameters.

Irradiation parameter	Unit of measurement	Comment
Wavelength	Nanometre (nm)	Wavelength is measured in nanometres (nm)
Irradiance	Watt/cm^2 (W/cm^2)	Power (W)/area (cm^2)
Pulse structure	Power (W), pulse frequency (Hz), pulse width (sec), duty cycle (%)	Average power (W) = peak power (W) × pulse width (s) × pulse frequency (Hz)
Energy	Joules (J)	Energy (J) = power (W) × time (seconds)
Energy density	J/cm^2	Refers to 'dose'
Irradiation time	Seconds	Referred to as an irradiation exposure time per spot
Time interval	Hour(s), days, weeks	Time interval between each irradiation session
Duration of treatment	Days, weeks	Total number of sessions over a period of time

Source: Adapted from Huang et al. (2009).

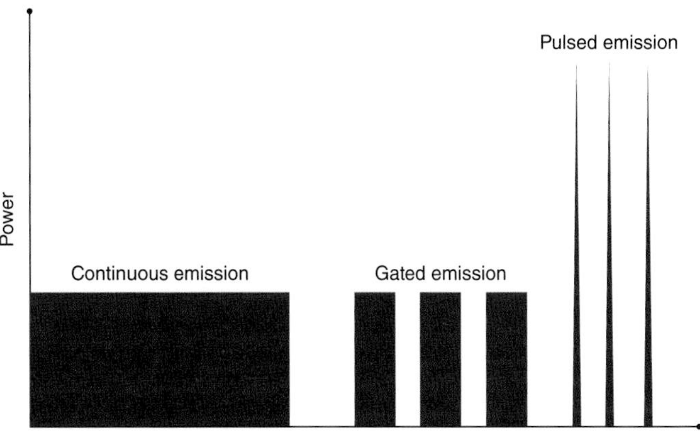

Figure 22.3 Types of emission mode. Pulsed mode represents pulse width (duration) in seconds as well the pulse interval; pulse frequency represents the number of pulses per second (Hz); gated emission represents the percentage of the duty cycle (%); and continuous emission (CW) represents a continuous duty cycle of 100%. *Source:* Adapted from Benedicenti and Benedicenti (2016).

Table 22.2 The influence of PBM effects on oral clinical effects. Based on

Results of PBM	Clinical outcomes
1) Stimulation of β endorphin 2) Reduction in the conduction of c-fibres	Reduction of pain
Reduction in the release of histamine, bradykinins, and acetylcholine	Reduction of pain association with an inflammation
An increase in neutrophil and macrophage migration and proliferation	Reduction in the inflammation and enhance tissue repair and healing
An increase in the lymphatic flow and increase vascularisation	Decrease the oedema (swelling)
Stimulation of cell proliferation and differentiation, such as fibroblasts, osteoblasts, chondroblasts, odontoblasts	Regenerative effects in wound healing, bone, extracellular matrix of cartilage, dentine, respectively

What are the Oral and Dental Complications Induced by CT and RT in Patients with HNC?

The following are complications induced by CT and RT (Sroussi et al. 2017; Zecha et al. 2016):

- Oral mucositis
- Hyposalivation (reduction in salvia) or xerostomia (dry mouth)
- Dysphagia (difficulty in swallowing)
- Trismus (limitation in mouth opening)
- Medication-related osteonecrosis of the jaws (MRONJ)
- Radiation dental caries
- Periodontal diseases
- Halitosis (bad breath)
- Aphthous ulceration
- Candida fungal infection
- Nutritional deficiency
- Voice/speech alteration.

What Is the Role of PBM Therapy in Management of Complications?

Oral Mucositis

CT- or RT-induced OM is a complex multifactorial tissue destruction linked to patient and treatment risk factors (Sonis et al. 2004b; Cawley and Benson 2005) (Figure 22.4). The pathophysiological process resulting in OM can be described in five phases (Lalla et al. 2008; Sonis 2004a) :

1) *Initiation of tissue injury:* induces cellular damage, generating ROS (free radicals)
2) *Upregulation of inflammation via messenger signals generation:* leads to stimulation of the pro-inflammatory cytokines
3) *Signaling and amplification:* significant inflammatory cells and further upregulation of inflammatory cytokines
4) *Ulceration phase:* the mucosal ulceration stage
5) *Healing phase:* involves proliferation and differentiation of cellular activities, leading to tissue restoration.

What are the Potential Benefits of PBM Therapy in OM?

Understanding OM pathophysiology is essential in order to plan a suitable therapy. On this note, PBM therapy has shown to reverse the oral tissue destruction caused by CT or RT. The exact mechanism remains unclear; however, the current understanding of PBM effects in this indication is as follows (see also Figure 22.5) (Hanna et al. 2020; Karu 2003; Hansen and Thorøe 1990; Walker 1983):

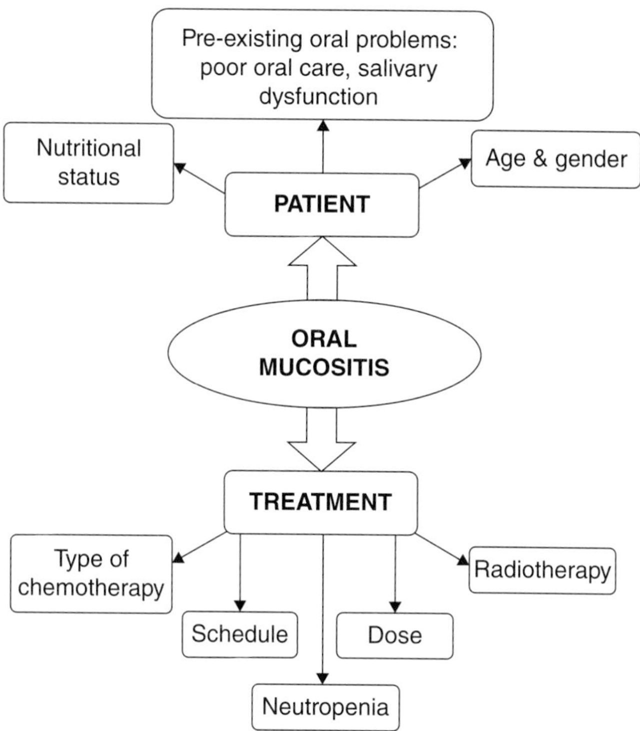

Figure 22.4 The patient and treatment contributing factors in OM severity. *Source:* Based on Sonis (2004b) and Cawley and Benson (2005).

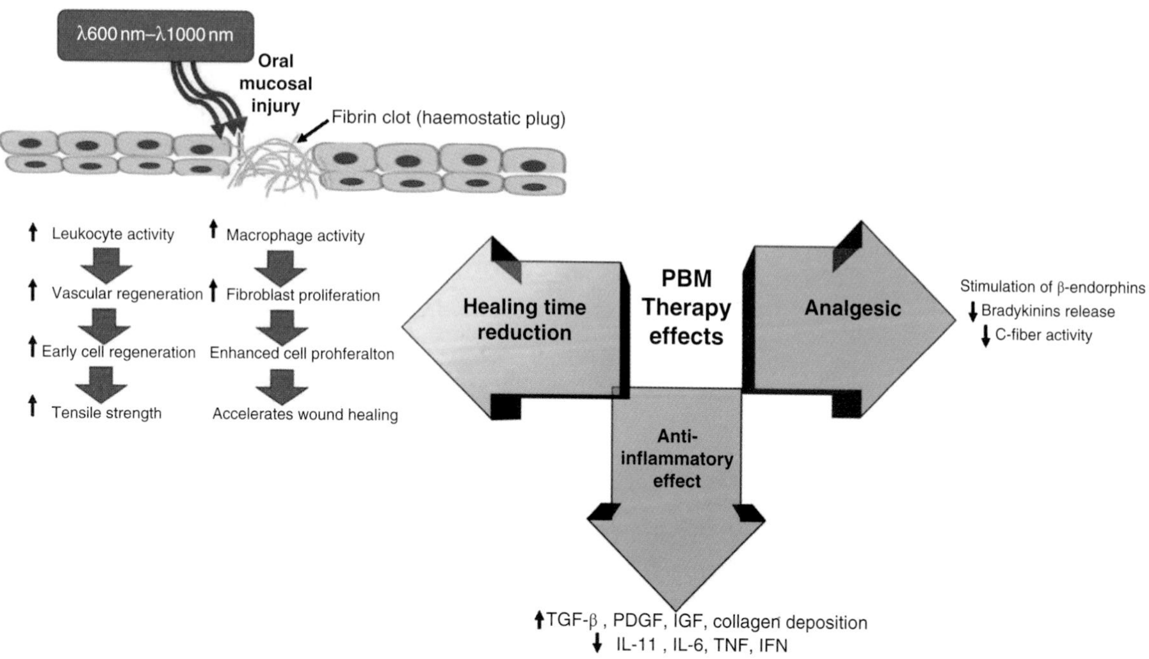

Figure 22.5 The cellular and molecular effects of PBM therapy of red and infrared light sources in OM, in terms of analgesic, anti-inflammatory, and healing. IFN, interferon; IL, interleukin; PBM, photobiomodulation; PDGF, platelet-derived growth factor; TGF-β, transforming growth factor beta; TNF, transforming necrotic factor; ↑, an increase; ↓, a decrease. Based on Chung et al. (2012); Karu (2003); Hansen and Thorøe (1990); and Walker (1983).

1) *Anti-inflammatory effect*: PBM therapy inhibits the production of prostaglandins and interleukin (IL)-1 and IL-6. This would induce ROS, leading to the following events: upregulating the expression of growth factors (transforming growth factor beta [TGF-β] and platelet-derived growth factor [PDGF]), encouraging collagen synthesis, and increasing formation of blood vessels (angiogenesis).
2) *Analgesic effects:* These effects are due to following events: stimulation of β-endorphins, a reduction in the release of bradykinins, and a decrease in C-fiber activity, which ultimately alters pain threshold.
3) *Regenerative and repair effects:* Regenerative and repair effects are related to an increase in leucocytes and fibroblast proliferation activities as well an increase in the vascular regeneration process, which ultimately leads to acceleration of wound healing and an increase in the tensile strength.

What Is the Evidence-Based Practice of PBM Therapy in OM Management?

OM is one of the most common complications of HNC treatments presented, as an inflammatory oral mucosa that has been graded on a severity scale from grade I to grade IV according to WHO, as shown in Figure 22.6 (World Health Organization 1979).

Preventive (Prophylactic) and Therapeutic Approaches of PBM Therapy

Several randomised controlled trials (RCTs) and prospective observational studies have demonstrated the effectiveness of PBM as a therapeutic (Antunes et al. 2017; Legouté et al. 2019) or preventive (prophylaxis) approach (Zanin et al. 2010; He et al. 2018) in reducing OM severity of grade II or III, which can result in pain reduction. This ultimately improves the functional limitation associated with diet/swallowing (Soto et al. 2015) and eventually can enhance patients' QoL (Silva et al. 2015; Bezinelli et al. 2016). These results are beneficial for both adult and paediatric patients with HNC (Hodgson et al. 2012; Legouté et al. 2019; Whelan et al. 2002).

A systematic review conducted by He et al. (2018) has reported that prophylaxis PBM therapy can significantly reduce the OM severity or reduce its prevalence in children and young adults with HNC. Further RCT studies with large data are warranted. On the other hand, a recent systematic review conducted by Zadik et al. established PBM recommendation protocols for OM prevention in patients who underwent one of the following treatments: hematopoietic stem-cell transplantation (HSCT), head and neck (HN) RT, and HN RT-CT. Two clinically effective PBM therapy protocols emerged; one for red light (633–685 nm) and another one for NIR (780–830 nm) (Zadik et al. 2019). In this regard, a pilot study by Soto et al. (2015) showed the effectiveness of combined intra- and extraoral approaches of PBM therapy in preventing OM in paediatric patients who underwent HSCT (Soto et al. 2015). The noninvasive and convenient approach of PBM therapy has been well-received by patients. Additionally, the positive achieved results have made this therapy feasible for OM prevention and treatment among young patients (Abramoff et al. 2008; Legouté et al. 2019). Tables 22.3–22.5 show the recommended suggested protocols (Zecha et al. 2016) for PBM red and infrared lasers and light-emitting diodes (LEDs) in the management of OM and other various complications induced by HNC treatments linked to an evidence-based literature and expert opinions and explained in this chapter.

Impact of PBM on Cost-Effectiveness and Economic Status

Several studies have examined the benefits of PBM therapy from an economic and cost-effectiveness standpoint. The results have shown that PBM therapy has reduced patients' hospital stay and has prevented HNC treatment interruption (Kwong et al. 1997; Sonis et al. 2001; Campos et al. 2020).

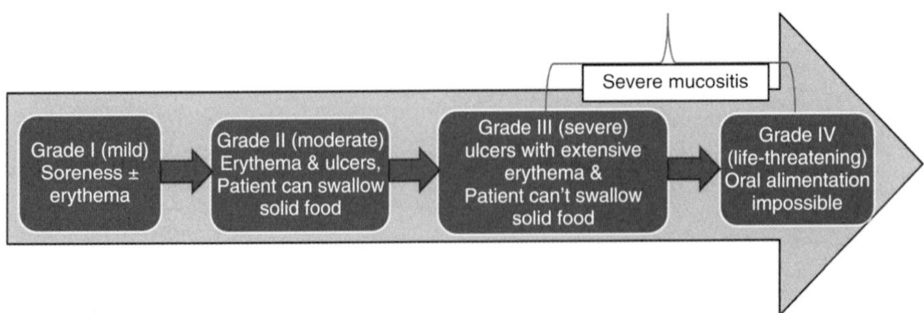

Figure 22.6 WHO oral mucositis severity scale. *Source:* Based on World Health Organization (1979).

Table 22.3 PBM therapy protocols for oral mucositis, radiation dermatitis, and dysphagia.

Complication	Treatment protocol**	Treatment area	PBM device characteristics and application	Therapeutic PBM dose	Optional target tissues
Oral mucositis	*Prophylactic:* *Chemotherapy:* Protocols vary. Start PBM treatment at first day of CT or prior to therapy and continue during all courses of chemotherapy. *Radiotherapy:* Start PBM treatment the first day of RT or prior to RT and continue during all days of RT (no requirement regarding the timing of PBM sessions, before or after RT session). *Therapeutic:* Continue treatment at least three times a week until symptoms improve. Daily treatment is recommended in case of severe mucositis.		*Extraoral:* IR LED cluster or mixed red and IR LED cluster 20–80 mW/cm² *Intraoral:* 630–830 nm 20–80 mW	*Extraoral:* 3 J/cm² IR LED cluster *Intraoral:* *Prophylactic:* 2 J per point *Therapeutic:* 4 J per point until the whole area involved is covered (2J for prophylactic use)	*Extraoral:* Lips, cutaneous surface corresponding to the buccal mucosae, bilateral cervical lymphatic chain.* *Intraoral:* *Prophylactic:* Treat each of the at-risk mucosal surfaces.* *Therapeutic:* Sites vary, depending upon the site of mucositis.
Dysphagia	*Prophylactic:* *Radiotherapy:* Start treatment the first day of radiotherapy and continue all days of radiation (no requirement regarding the timing of laser sessions, before or after radiation session). *Therapeutic:* Continue treatment at least three times a week until symptoms improve.	*Extraoral:* Lateral and ventral pharynx and larynx *Intraoral:* Soft palate, oropharynx	*Extraoral:* IR laser diodes or LED cluster 750–830 nm 20–80 mW/cm² *Intraoral:* 630–680 nm 20–150 mW	*Extraoral:* *Prophylactic:* 3 J/cm² laser diodes or LED cluster *Intraoral:* *Prophylactic:* 3 J per point	*Extraoral:* Midline neck and lateral neck anterior to sternocleidomastoid muscle. *Intraoral:* Bilaterally, 4 points to soft palate and onto oropharynx.

Note: These PBM therapy protocols for oral mucositis, radiation dermatitis, and dysphagia are based on evidence derived from literature and expert opinion and are intended only to provide clinical guidance and to serve as a starting point for research ** and * Zecha et al (2016) (courtesy of Prof. R.J. Bensadoun). LED cluster probe dose has been expressed in J/cm², and single-point laser dose has been expressed in joules per point. For LED cluster probes, treatment time (s) = dose (J/cm²) / power density (W/cm²).
Abbreviations: Light emitted diode (LED) cluster probe dose has been expressed in J/cm², and single point laser dose has been expressed in joules per point. For LED cluster probes, treatment time (s) = dose (J/cm²) / power density (W/cm²).

Table 22.4 PBM therapy protocols for hyposalivation/xerostomia, dysgeusia, and trismus.

Complication	Treatment protocol**	Treatment area	PBM device characteristics and application	Therapeutic PBM dose	Optional target tissues
Hyposalivation and xerostomia	*Prophylactic:* *Radiotherapy:* Start PBM treatment the first day of RT and continue daily with radiation (no requirement regarding the timing of PBM sessions, before or after RT session).		*Extraoral:* IR laser diodes or LED cluster 750–830 nm 20–80 mW/cm² *Intraoral:* 630–680 nm 20–150 mW	*Extraoral:* *Prophylactic:* 3 J/cm² laser diodes or LED cluster *Intraoral:* *Prophylactic:* 3 J/cm² per point	*Extraoral:* Major salivary glands, bilaterally (parotid, sublingual, and submandibular).* *Intraoral:* Total of 6 points (3 each side) targeting major salivary glands and minor salivary glands (on vestibular side, in the rear of salivary ducts).

(*Continued*)

Table 22.4 (Continued)

Complication	Treatment protocol**	Treatment area	PBM device characteristics and application	Therapeutic PBM dose	Optional target tissues
Dysgeusia	*Therapeutic:* Continue treatment from the day the patient complains of taste alterations, at least two or three times a week until symptoms improve.		*Intraoral:* 630–680 nm 20–150 mW	*Intraoral:* Dorsal and lateral tongue at 3 J/cm^2	*Intraoral:* A total of 10 points on the dorsum of the tongue.
Trismus	*Prophylactic:* *Radiotherapy:* Apply PBM on pterygoid/temporomandibular joint, at least three times a week, when high-dose RT is given in that region (oropharyngeal and nasopharyngeal carcinoma, e.g.) *Therapeutic:* Continue treatment from the day of diagnosis at least two or three times a week.		*Extraoral:* IR laser diodes or LED cluster 750–830 nm 20–80 mW/cm^2 *Intraoral:* 630–680 nm 20–200 mW	*Extraoral:* 3–6 J/cm^2 laser diodes or LED cluster *Intraoral:* 3 J per point	*Extraoral:* Bilaterally over the temporalis muscle, temporomandibular joint, masseter muscle, buccinator muscle.* *Intraoral:* Bilaterally over the region of pterygoids/pterygomandibular raphae (may be difficult clinically) and other muscles of mastication.*

Note: These PBM therapy protocols for hyposalivation/xerostomia, dysgeusia, and trismus are based on evidence derived from literature and expert opinion and are intended only to provide clinical guidance and to serve as a starting point for research ** and * Zecha et al (2016) (courtesy of Prof. R.J. Bensadoun).

Table 22.5 PBM therapy protocol for osteonecrosis.

Complication	Treatment protocol**	Treatment area	PBM device characteristics and application	Therapeutic PBM dose	Optional target tissues
Osteonecrosis	*Therapeutic:* Continue treatment at least two or three times a week until symptoms improve. Daily treatment is recommended. Combination with other medical/surgical treatment approaches may be needed.		*Extraoral:* IR laser diodes or LED cluster 750–830 nm 20–80 mW/cm^2 *Intraoral:* 630–680 nm 20–200 mW	*Extraoral:* 6 J/cm^2 laser diodes or LED cluster *Intraoral:* 6 J per point	*Intraoral:*5 or more points (1 cm apart) along lingual and buccal aspects of maxilla and/or mandible depending on site and size of region affected.*

Note: This PBM therapy protocol for osteonecrosis is based on evidence derived from literature and expert opinion and is intended only to provide clinical guidance and to serve as a starting point for research ** and * Zecha et al (2016) (courtesy of Prof. R.J. Bensadoun).

Hyposalivation (Reduction in Saliva) or Xerostomia (Dry Mouth)

Hyposalivation (a decrease of saliva) is one of the most significant long-term adverse effects of RT to salivary gland (Jensen et al. 2008). This has an impact on taste and speech, resulting in difficulty in chewing and swallowing (Porter et al. 2010). Also, it can increase the risk of developing candidiasis, gingivitis, and caries (Porter et al. 2010; Basu et al. 2012).

Understanding PBM mechanism of action in terms of stimulating saliva remains unclear; however, studies have shown that PBM therapy significantly enhances the salivary secretion and improves antimicrobial features of secreted saliva by increasing the level of secretory immunoglobulin A (sIgA). It also improves regeneration of salivary duct epithelial cells (Lončar et al. 2011). In this context, a study conducted by Simoes et al. reported that the use of PBM can increase salivary flow rate and amylase activity in rat parotid glands (Simoes et al. 2008). The authors of the latter also conducted a study on patients with HNC and reported that PBM given concurrently with RT could prevent hyposalivation and xerostomia and has had an impact on the composition of saliva (Simoes et al. 2010), thereby leading to an improvement in patients' QoL (Palma et al. 2017). A recent systematic review conducted by Louzeiro et al. highlighted that PBM therapy minimises radiation-induced hyposalivation (Louzeiro et al. 2020). Table 22.4 shows PBM laser and LED parameters and treatment trigger points for hyposalivation management (Zecha et al. 2016).

Radiation Dental Caries

Patients who receive RT can be at risk of the following: radiation dental caries (RDC), RT-induced hyposalivation, a rapid demineralisation of the tooth structure causing possible alterations to the tooth enamel, dietary changes, insufficient fluoride exposure, and poor oral hygiene (Basu et al. 2012; Palmier et al. 2018).

The therapeutic and preventive approaches of PBM therapy in dental caries management include the following:

- PBM therapy can possibly induce modification of the enamel organic matrix content, which may then lead to an increase in the resistance against demineralisation (Vlacic et al. 2007). A prospective randomised study conducted by Nemeth et al. concluded that PBM therapy of major salivary glands in high-caries-risk patients can reduce the cariogenic bacteria in the saliva and improve some salivary parameters, thus reducing caries risk (Nemeth et al. 2020).
- PBM therapy plays a vital role as a therapeutic or preventive tool in management of RDC, aiding in remineralisation and fluoridation, respectively. Many studies have shown the effectiveness of PBM laser-activated fluoride with various wavelengths (830 nm, 488 nm), providing protection to dental enamel (Vlacic et al. 2007; Seefeldt et al. 2020). In terms of PBM therapeutic approach in this indication, clinical studies have shown that PBM therapy is effective in pulpotomy procedures, enhancing pulp healing in primary molars, which was based on clinical and radiographic evaluations over 6- and 12-month follow-up time points (Golpayegani et al. 2010; Joshi 2017).
- PBM therapy prior to cavity preparation reduces pain perception in paediatric dental patients (Joshi 2017).

Periodontal Diseases

Many studies have demonstrated the effects of PBM as an adjunctive therapy to scaling and root planing as follows:

1) The anti-inflammatory effect of PBM therapy can slow down or reduce the deterioration of periodontal tissues by reducing the volume of the periopathogens.
2) The regenerative effect is advantageous in enhancing bone regeneration and accelerating wound healing.

Ultimately, the aforementioned effects can lead to restoring the following clinical periodontal parameters: bleeding on probing, pocket depth, and clinical attachment level (Kumaresan et al. 2016; Mastrangelo et al. 2018; Angiero et al. 2020). Hence, adjunctive PBM therapy to standard care treatment can be a useful noninvasive tool in managing periodontal diseases, especially in HNC patients who have undergone RT or CT.

Dysphagia (Difficulty in Swallowing)

As highlighted in the 'Hyposalivation (Reduction in Salvia) or Xerostomia (Dry Mouth)' section, dysphagia is one of the side effects of hyposalivation. Hence, management of the latter can help in improving swallowing. Decreasing the severity of OM can also assist in improving swallowing and subsequently enhancing patients' nutrition. A study conducted by Yifru et al. concluded that it is important to integrate swallowing function evaluation in cancer therapy protocols to relieve the effect of dysphagia and improve QoL (Yifru et al. 2021). Table 22.3 shows a proposed recommended laser and LED parameter protocol for dysphagia management (Zecha et al. 2016).

Dysgeusia (Alteration in Taste)

The mechanisms of dysgeusia during HNC treatment are not well understood; however, it is believed that CT or RT can cause dysgeusia by destroying and rapidly dividing the taste bud cells and olfactory receptor cells (Zecha et al. 2016). Hence, a pilot study conducted by Romeo et al. reported that PBM irradiation on the taste buds may ameliorate psychogenic/neurological burning mouth symptoms including taste alterations (Romeo et al. 2010). Nevertheless, to our knowledge, there are no published studies on PBM for the management of taste problems in cancer patients. Table 22.4 shows proposed parameters that can be used for future studies (Zecha et al. 2016).

Candida (Fungal Infection)

Oropharyngeal candida is the most common and frequent infection that occurs in patients with HNC who receive RT (Bensadoun et al. 2011). A study conducted by Simunović-Soskić et al. showed the effectiveness of PBM therapy in decreasing the levels of the proinflammatory cytokines (TNF-alpha and IL-6) significantly ($p < 0.001$) compared to the control/sham. The authors concluded that PBM may be an efficacious choice of therapy in management of denture stomatitis (Simunović-Soskić et al. 2010).

Medication-Related Osteonecrosis of the Jaws

Osteoradionecrosis is an area of exposed bone that fails to heal due to lack of vascularisation resulting from RT (Epstein et al. 1987). PBM therapy is beneficial in MRONJ because of the following clinical effects:

1) Accelerating alveolar mucosa healing and reducing postoperative pain and consequently minimal usage of analgesics have been demonstrated by a double-blind randomised pilot study conducted by da Silva et al. when the following protocol was used; λ 808 nm, 40 mW, 100 J/cm^2, 70 seconds, 2.8 J/point, 14 J/session, and area of 0.028 cm^2 (da Silva et al. 2021). Further randomised clinical trials with large data are warranted to confirmed these findings.
2) For stimulating bone regeneration, several studies have suggested that the therapeutic approach of PBM has beneficial effects in management of MRONJ in patients who have received or are having bisphosphonate medication (Scoletta et al. 2010; Romeo et al. 2011; da Guarda et al. 2012). A study conducted by Vescovi et al. proposed a PBM prophylactic protocol for reducing MRONJ incidence following tooth extraction (Vescovi et al. 2015). To date, no clinical study has utilised PBM therapy in HNC patients. However, evidence-based science and practice have confirmed the effects of PBM in stimulating osteoblasts in terms of proliferation and differentiation of the cells and increasing tissue vascularisation (Hanna et al. 2019, 2021; Amaroli et al. 2018). Dental screening and treatment prior to CT or RT are important to minimise any oral complications post-CT and RT, and an atraumatic extraction is required (Mainali et al. 2011; Chang et al. 2007).

Trismus

To our knowledge, no studies to date have reported the effect of PBM in preventing or reducing the severity of RT-induced trismus in HNC patients. However, the effect of PBM therapy in reducing trismus after surgical removal of the mandibular third molar has been reported with positive outcomes (Tenis et al. 2018). Hence, the potential clinical benefit of PBM therapy in reducing fibrosis and promoting muscular repair justifies further studies, for which Table 22.4 provides a proposed laser protocol for trismus.

Safety and Cautions for Consideration

With regard to HNC, a balance between reasonable safety and potential benefit needs to be taken into account. One must be cautious when considering the possibility of residual tumour cells within the site and direction of the PBM beam. Although the results of *in vitro* studies of PBM on malignant cells vary, and clinical reports showed little or no indication of adverse events, there is a lack of robust data regarding potential protection and promotion of tumours (Nair and Bensadoun 2016). Hence, the use of PBM is effective with a safety profile (Legouté et al. 2019).

How Can DHTs Contribute in Management of RT- or CT-Induced Oral Complications?

DHTs play a crucial role in the management of oral complications induced by HCN treatments. These can be divided into:

- *Before cancer treatment*, the goal is screening all patients prior to commencing cancer treatment by treating the existing oral problems and educating the patients about the benefits of basic oral care.
- *During cancer treatment,* the goals are managing the oral complications induced by HNC treatments by reducing the severity and restoring any associated oral functions as well as improving QoL.
- *After cancer treatment*, the goals are to maintain a good aftercare and manage any long-term side effects of cancer and its treatment.

So far, PBM therapy is not within the DHT scope of practice at the UK General Dental Council, whereas in some European countries and the US, dental therapists, after extensive training in PBM, are licensed to use this type of therapy for various clinical applications based on a clinician's prescription.

The involvement of DHTs within multidisciplinary roles is vital. It is critically important to emphasise the importance of structured training, which is an integral part of building a successful PBM therapy protocol to manage complications induced by HNC therapies. It requires knowledge, skills, and expertise in practising this therapy safely and effectively for the best interests of patients; therefore, an approach to integrate laser therapy within the DHT curriculum is useful. It must focus primarily on depth of knowledge, which is grounded on evidence-based science and practice, amalgamated with practical training to build up DHT students with skills and judgment in the management of various clinical cases. Hopefully, this suggestion will encourage the regulatory bodies to address the need for additional DHT training.

Where Can You Learn More About Laser Therapy?

Academic Training Courses

Currently, University College London Eastman Dental Institute (UCL EDI) offers academic fellowship courses in laser dentistry for dentists and DHTs for one week and two days, respectively. These are continuing professional development courses. The attendees receive a certificate of attendance, including a certificate of core knowledge and health and safety. Also, UCL EDI currently offers online introductory courses in laser dentistry and PBM therapy.

Learning the science and its application to clinical practice is the key for successful health care professional training in utilising PBM therapy. Hence, it is of great importance to emphasise training and education, for example, in an online introductory laser in dentistry course (receptive to your theoretical and clinical needs).

Journals and Textbooks

Many journals focus on the field of PBM therapy in various disciplines, such as *Photobiomodulation, Photomedicine, and Laser Surgery* and *Lasers in Medical Science*. Both are evidence-based, peer-reviewed journals that are a tremendous resource for any practitioners utilising or thinking of including PBM in their daily practice. Two of the best PBM textbooks are *Handbook of Low-Level Laser Therapy* (Hamblin et al. 2017) and *The New Laser Therapy Handbook* (Turner and Hade 2010).

Scientific Associations

Associations include the MASCC/ISOO, mentioned earlier, and the Mucositis Study Group of the MASSC/ISOO.

Summary and Future Directions

The number of HNC survivors has increased due to the advances in therapeutic/preventive treatment modalities and supportive care. This growing population requires specialised oral care by trained DHTs in the management of various oral complications induced by HNC therapies. DHTs play a crucial role within a multidisciplinary team to optimise patients' oral care.

Recent advances in PBM technology as a safe, effective, and noninvasive treatment modality, with a better understanding of the mechanisms involved and dosimetry parameters, have lead to the management of a broader range of oral complications induced by HNC therapies. This will improve functionality and patients' QoL. The current laser parameter protocols are evolving to ensure continuous optimal clinical outcomes. Double-blind, multicentre, randomised controlled clinical trial studies are warranted.

An academic structured education and training in PBM for DHTs is imperative, allowing them to obtain competency in utilising PBM therapy in the management of patients with HNC to improve oral care and enhance QoL.

Education, nursing research, and evidence-based practice are the institutions for success in facilitating a positive outcome of oral care in patients with HNC. DHTs are and will continue to be the key players in achieving successful outcomes in management of this cohort of patients.

References

Abramoff, M.M., Lopes, N.N., Lopes, L.A. et al. (2008). Low-level laser therapy in the prevention and treatment of chemotherapy-induced oral mucositis in young patients. *Photomed. Laser Surg.* 26 (4): 393–400. http://dx.doi.org/10.1089/pho.2007.2144.

Amaroli, A., Ferrando, S., Hanna, R. et al. (2017). The photobiomodulation effect of higher-fluence 808-nm laser therapy with a flat-top handpiece on the wound healing of the earthworm Dendrobaena Veneta: a brief report. *Lasers Med. Sci.* 33 (1): 221–225. http://dx.doi.org/10.1007/s10103-016-2132-3.

Amaroli, A., Agas, D., Laus, F. et al. (2018). The effect of photobiomodulation of 808nm diode laser therapy at higher fluence on the in-vitro osteogenic differentiation of bone marrow stromal cells. *Front. Physiol.* 9 (123): 1–10. http://dx.doi.org/10.3389/fphys.2018.00123.

Anders, J.J., Lanzafame, R.J., and Arany, P.R. (2015). Low-level light/laser therapy versus photobiomodulation therapy. *Photomed. Laser Surg.* 33 (4): 183–184. http://dx.doi.org/10.1089/pho.2015.9848.

Andrade, F.D., Clark, R.M., and Ferreira, M.L. (2014). Effects of low-level laser therapy on wound healing. *Rev. Col. Bras. Cir.* 41 (2): 129–133. http://dx.doi.org/10.1590/s0100-69912014000200010.

Angiero, F., Ugolini, A., Cattoni, F. et al. (2020). Evaluation of bradykinin, VEGF, and EGF biomarkers in gingival crevicular fluid and comparison of photobiomodulation with conventional techniques in periodontitis: a split-mouth randomized clinical trial. *Lasers Med. Sci.* 35 (4): 965–970. http://dx.doi.org/10.1007/s10103-019-02919-w.

Ansari, M.A., Massudi, R., and Hejazi, M. (2009). Experimental and numerical study on simultaneous effects of scattering and absorption on fluorescence spectroscopy of a breast phantom. *Opt. Laser Technol.* 41 (6): 746–750.

Antunes, H.S., Herchenhorn, D., Small, I.A. et al. (2017). Long-term survival of a randomized phase III trial of head and neck cancer patients receiving concurrent chemoradiation therapy with or without low-level laser therapy (LLLT) to prevent oral mucositis. *Oral Oncol.* 71: 11–15. http://dx.doi.org/10.1016/j.oraloncology.2017.05.018.

Basu, T., Laskar, S.G., Gupta, T. et al. (2012). Toxicity with radiotherapy for oral cancers and its management: a practical approach. *J. Cancer Res. Ther.* 8 (Suppl 1): S72–S84. http://dx.doi.org/10.4103/0973-1482.92219.

Benedicenti, A. and Benedicenti, S. (ed.) (2016). *Atlas of Laser Therapy: State of the Art.* Villa Carcina, Italy: Teamwork Media SRL.

Bensadoun, R.J., Patton, L.L., Lalla, R.V. et al. (2011). Oropharyngeal candidiasis in head and neck cancer patients treated with radiation: update 2011. *Support. Care Cancer* 19: 737–744. http://dx.doi.org/10.1007/s00520-011-1154-4.

Bezinelli, L.M., Eduardo, F.P., Neves, V.D. et al. (2016). Quality of life related to oral mucositis of patients undergoing haematopoietic stem cell transplantation and receiving specialised oral care with low-level laser therapy: a prospective observational study. *Eur J Cancer Care (Engl)* 25 (4): 668–674. http://dx.doi.org/10.1111/ecc.12344.

Bjordal, J.M., Johnson, M.I., Iversen, V. et al. (2006). Low-level laser therapy in acute pain: a systematic review of possible mechanisms of action and clinical effects in randomized placebo-controlled trials. *Photomed. Laser Surg.* 24 (2): 158–168. http://dx.doi.org/10.1089/pho.2006.24.158.

Campos, T.M., do Prado Tavares Silva, C.A., Sobral, A.P.T. et al. (2020). Photobiomodulation in oral mucositis in patients with head and neck cancer: a systematic review and meta-analysis followed by a cost-effectiveness analysis. *Support. Care Cancer* 28: 5649–5659. http://dx.doi.org/10.1007/s00520-020-05613-8.

Cawley, M.M. and Benson, L.M. (2005). Trends in managing oral mucositis. *Clin. J. Oncol. Nurs.* 9 (5): 584–592. http://dx.doi.org/10.1188/05.CJON.584-592.

Chang, D.T., Sandow, P.R., Morris, C.G. et al. (2007). Do pre-irradiation dental extractions reduce the risk of osteoradionecrosis of the mandible? *Head Neck* 29: 528–536. http://dx.doi.org/10.1002/hed.20538.

Chang, C.C., Lee, W.T., Hsiao, J.R. et al. (2019). Oral hygiene and the overall survival of head and neck cancer patients. *Cancer Med.* 8 (4): 1854–1864. http://dx.doi.org/10.1002/cam4.2059.

Chung, H., Dai, T., Sharma, S.K. et al. (2012). The nuts and bolts of low-level laser (light) therapy. *Ann. Biomed. Eng.* 40 (2): 516–533. http://dx.doi.org/10.1007/s10439-011-0454-7.

Cooperstein, E., Gilbert, J., Epstein, J.B. et al. (2012). Vanderbilt head and neck symptom survey version 2.0: report of the development and initial testing of a subscale for assessment of oral health. *Head Neck* 34 (6): 797–804. http://dx.doi.org/10.1002/hed.21816.

Elad, S. and Zadik, Y. (2016). Chronic oral mucositis after radiotherapy to the head and neck: a new insight. *Support. Care Cancer* 24: 4825–4830. http://dx.doi.org/10.1007/s00520-016-3337-5.

Elting, L.S., Keefe, D.M., Sonis, S.T. et al. (2008). Patient-reported measurements of oral mucositis in head and neck cancer patients treated with radiotherapy with or without chemotherapy: demonstration of increased frequency, severity, resistance to palliation, and impact on quality of life. *Cancer* 113 (10): 2704–2713. http://dx.doi.org/10.1002/cncr.23898.

Epstein, J.B., Rea, G., Wong, F.L. et al. (1987). Osteonecrosis: study of the relationship of dental extractions in patients receiving radiotherapy. *Head Neck Surg.* 10 (1): 48–54. http://dx.doi.org/10.1002/hed.2890100108.

Epstein, J.B., Thariat, J., Bensadoun, R.J. et al. (2012). Oral complications of cancer and cancer therapy: from cancer treatment to survivorship. *CA Cancer J. Clin.* 62 (6): 400–422. http://dx.doi.org/10.3322/caac.21157.

de Freitas, L.F. and Hamblin, M.R. (2016). Proposed mechanisms of photobiomodulation or low-level light therapy. *IEEE J. Sel. Top Quantum Electron.* 22 (3): 7000417. http://dx.doi.org/10.1109/JSTQE.2016.2561201.

Gautam, A.P., Fernandes, D.J., Vidyasagar, M.S. et al. (2013). Effect of low-level laser therapy on patient reported measures of oral mucositis and quality of life in head and neck cancer patients receiving chemoradiotherapy – a randomized controlled trial. *Support. Care Cancer* 21 (5): 1421–1428. http://dx.doi.org/10.1007/s00520-012-1684-4.

Golpayegani, M.V., Ansari, G., and Tadayon, N. (2010). Clinical and radiographic success of low level laser therapy (LLLT) on primary molars pulpotomy. *Res. J. Biol. Sci.* 5: 51–55. http://dx.doi.org/10.3923/rjbsci.2010.51.55.

da Guarda, M.G., Paraguassu, G.M., Cerqueira, N. et al. (2012). Laser GaAlAs (lambda 860 nm) photobiomodulation for the treatment of bisphosphonate-induced osteonecrosis of the jaw. *Photomed. Laser Surg.* 30 (5): 293–297. http://dx.doi.org/10.1089/pho.2011.3219.

Hamblin, M.R., de Sousa, M.V.P., and Agrawal, T. (2017). *Handbook of Low-Level Laser Therapy*. Singapore: Pan Stanford.

Hanna, R., Agas, D., Benedicenti, S. et al. (2019). A comparative study between the effectiveness of 980nm photobiomodulation, delivered by Gaussian versus flattop profiles on osteoblasts maturation. *Front. Endocrinol. (Lausanne)* 20 (10): 92. http://dx.doi.org/10.3389/fendo.2019.0009.

Hanna, R., Dalvi, S., Benedicenti, S. et al. (2020). Photobiomodulation therapy in oral mucositis and potentially malignant oral lesions: a therapy towards the future. *Cancer* 12 (7): 1949. http://dx.doi.org/10.3390/cancers12071949.

Hanna, R., Dalvi, S., Amaroli, A. et al. (2021). Effects of photobiomodulation on bone defects grafted with bone substitutes: a systematic review of in vivo animal studies. *J. Biophotonics* 4 (1): e202000267. http://dx.doi.org/10.1002/jbio.2020 00267.

Hansen, H.J. and Thorøe, U. (1990). Low power laser biostimulation of chronic oro-facial pain: a double-blind placebo controlled cross-over study in 40 patients. *Pain* 43 (2): 169–179. http://dx.doi.org/10.1016/0304-3959(90)91070-Y.

He, M., Zhang, B., Shen, N. et al. (2018). A systematic review and meta-analysis of the effect of low-level laser therapy (LLLT) on chemotherapy-induced oral mucositis in pediatric and young patients. *Eur. J. Pediatr.* 177 (1): 7–17. http://dx.doi.org/10.1007/s00431-017-3043-4.

Hodgson, B.D., Margolis, D.M., Salzman, D.E. et al. (2012). Amelioration of oral mucositis pain by NASA near-infrared light-emitting diodes in bone marrow transplant patients. *Support. Care Cancer* 20 (7): 1405–1415. http://dx.doi.org/10.1007/s00520-011-1223-8.

Huang, Y.Y., Chen, A.C., Carroll, J.D. et al. (2009). Biphasic dose response in low level light therapy. *Dose-Response* 7 (4): 358–383. http://dx.doi.org/10.2203/dose-response.09-027.Hamblin.

Hunter, K.U., Schipper, M., Feng, F.Y. et al. (2013). Toxicities affecting quality of life after chemo-IMRT of oropharyngeal cancer: prospective study of patient-reported, observer-rated, and objective outcomes. *Int. J. Radiat. Oncol. Biol. Phys.* 85 (4): 935–940. http://dx.doi.org/10.1016/j.ijrobp.2012.08.030.

Jacques, S. (2013). Optical properties of biological tissues: a review. *Phys. Med. Biol.* 58: R37–R61. http://dx.doi.org/10.1088/0031-9155/58/11/R37.

Jensen, S.B., Mouridsen, H.T., Reibel, J. et al. (2008). Adjuvant chemotherapy in breast cancer patients induces temporary salivary gland hypofunction. *Oral Oncol.* 44: 162–173. http://dx.doi.org/10.1016/j.oraloncology.2007.01.015.

Joshi, P. (2017). A comparative evaluation between formocresol and diode laser assisted pulpotomy in primary molars – an in vivo study. *Eur. J. Pharm. Med. Res.* 4: 569–575.

Kagan, S.H. (2009). The influence of nursing in head and neck cancer management. *Curr. Opin. Oncol.* 21 (3): 248–253. http://dx.doi.org/10.1097/CCO.0b013e328329b819.

Karu, T.I. (2003). Low-power laser therapy. In: *Biomedical Photonics Handbook* (ed. T. Vo-Dinh), 48–41. CRC Press ISBN: 978-0-8493-1116-1117.

Kumaresan, D., Balasundaram, A., Naik, V.K. et al. (2016). Gingival crevicular fluid periostin levels in chronic periodontitis patients following nonsurgical periodontal treatment with low-level laser therapy. *Eur J Dent* 10 (4): 546–550. http://dx.doi.org/10.4103/1305-7456.195179.

Kwong, D.L., Sham, J.S., Chua, D.T. et al. (1997). The effect of interruptions and prolonged treatment time in radiotherapy for nasopharyngeal carcinoma. *Int. J. Radiat. Oncol. Biol. Phys.* 39: 703–710. http://dx.doi.org/10.1016/s0360-3016(97)00339-8.

Lalla, R.V., Sonis, S.T., and Peterson, D.E. (2008). Management of oral mucositis in patients who have cancer. *Dent. Clin. N. Am.* 52: 61–77. http://dx.doi.org/10.1016/j.cden.2007.10.002.

Lalla, R.V., Bowen, J., Barasch, A. et al. (2014). MASCC/ISOO clinical practice guidelines for the management of mucositis secondary to cancer therapy. *Cancer* 120 (10): 1453–1461. http://dx.doi.org/10.1002/cncr.28592.

Legouté, F., Bensadoun, R.J., Seegers, V. et al. (2019). Low-level laser therapy in treatment of chemoradiotherapy-induced mucositis in head and neck cancer: results of a randomised, triple blind, multicentre phase III trial. *Radiat. Oncol.* 14 (1): 83. http://dx.doi.org/10.1186/s13014-019-1292-2.

Lončar, B., Mravak, S.M., Baričević, M. et al. (2011). The effect of low-level laser therapy on salivary glands in patients with xerostomia. *Photomed. Laser Surg.* 29 (3): 171–175. http://dx.doi.org/10.1089/pho.2010.2792.

Louzeiro, G.C., Teixeira, D.D.S., Cherubini, K. et al. (2020). Does laser photobiomodulation prevent hyposalivation in patients undergoing head and neck radiotherapy? A systematic review and meta-analysis of controlled trials. *Crit. Rev. Oncol. Hematol.* 156: 103115. http://dx.doi.org/10.1016/j.critrevonc.2020.103115.

Maegawa, Y., Itoh, T., Hosokawa, T. et al. (2000). Effects of near-infrared low-level laser irradiation on microcirculation. *Lasers Surg. Med.* 27 (5): 427–437. http://dx.doi.org/10.1002/1096-9101(2000)27:5<427::AID-LSM1004>3.0.CO;2-A.

Mainali, A., Sumanth, K.N., Ongole, R. et al. (2011). Dental consultation in patients planned for/undergoing/post radiation therapy for head and neck cancers: a questionnaire-based survey. *Indian J. Dent. Res.* 22: 669–672. http://dx.doi.org/10.4103/0970-9290.93454.

Mastrangelo, F., Dedola, A., Cattoni, F. et al. (2018). Etiological periodontal treatment with and without low-level laser therapy on IL-1b level in gingival crevicular fluid: an in vivo multicentric pilot study. *J. Biol. Regul. Homeost. Agents* 32 (2): 425–431. PMID: 29577710.

Nair, R. and Bensadoun, R.J. (2016). *Mitigation of Cancer Therapy Side-Effects with Light*, 1–34. Morgan & Claypool Publishers.

National Institute for Health and Care Excellence (NICE) (2018). Low-level laser therapy for preventing or treating oral mucositis caused by radiotherapy or chemotherapy [NICE interventional procedures guidance IPG615]. www.nice.org.uk/guidance/ipg615/chapter/1-Recommendations (accessed 3 September 2021).

Nemeth, L., Groselj, M., Golez, A. et al. (2020). The impact of photobiomodulation of major salivary glands on caries risk. *Lasers Med. Sci.* 35 (1): 193–203. http://dx.doi.org/10.1007/s10103-019-02845-x.

Palma, L.F., Gonnelli, F.A.S., Marcucci, M. et al. (2017). Impact of low-level laser therapy on hyposalivation, salivary pH, and quality of life in head and neck cancer patients post-radiotherapy. *Lasers Med. Sci.* 32 (4): 827–832. http://dx.doi.org/10.1007/s10103-017-2180-3.

Palmier, N.R., Madrid, C.C., Paglioni, M.P. et al. (2018). Cracked tooth syndrome in irradiated patients with head and neck cancer. *Oral Surg. Oral Med. Oral Pathol. Oral Radiol.* 126: 335–341. http://dx.doi.org/10.1016/j.oooo.2018.06.005.

de Pauli Paglioni, M., Palmier, N.R., Prado-Ribeiro, A.C. et al. (2020). The impact of radiation caries in the quality of life of head and neck cancer patients. *Support. Care Cancer* 28: 2977–2984. http://dx.doi.org/10.1007/s00520-019-05171-8.

Porter, S.R., Fedele, S., and Habbab, K.M. (2010). Xerostomia in head and neck malignancy. *Oral Oncol.* 46: 460–463. http://dx.doi.org/10.1016/j.oraloncology.2010.03.008.

Prindeze, N.J., Moffatt, L.T., and Shupp, J.W. (2012). Mechanisms of action for light therapy: a review of molecular interactions. *Exp. Biol. Med. (Maywood)* 237 (11): 1241–1248. http://dx.doi.org/10.1258/ebm.2012.012180.

Romeo, U., Del, V.A., Capocci, M. et al. (2010). The low level laser therapy in the management of neurological burning mouth syndrome: a pilot study. *Ann. Stomatol* 1: 14–18.

Romeo, U., Galanakis, A., Marias, C. et al. (2011). Observation of pain control in patients with bisphosphonate-induced osteonecrosis using low level laser therapy: preliminary results. *Photomed. Laser Surg.* 29 (7): 447–452. http://dx.doi.org/10.1089/pho.2010.2835.

Scoletta, M., Arduino, P.G., Reggio, L. et al. (2010). Effect of low-level laser irradiation on bisphosphonate-induced osteonecrosis of the jaws: preliminary results of a prospective study. *Photomed. Laser Surg.* 28 (2): 179–184. http://dx.doi.org/10.1089/pho.2009.2501.

Seefeldt, V.B., Alvarenga, M.P., and Soares, L.E.S. (2020). Low-level gallium-aluminum-arsenide (GaAlAs) diode laser irradiation (λ 830 nm) associated with and without fluoridated gel in the prevention of enamel erosion. *Lasers Dent. Sci.* 4: 145–155. http://dx.doi.org/10.1007/s41547-020-00100-z.

Silva, L.C., Sacono, N.T., Freire, M.d.C.M. et al. (2015). The impact of low-level laser therapy on oral mucositis and quality of life in patients undergoing hematopoietic stem cell transplantation using the Oral Health Impact Profile and the Functional Assessment of Cancer Therapy-Bone Marrow Transplantation questionnaires. *Photomed. Laser Surg.* 33 (7): 357–363. http://dx.doi.org/10.1089/pho.2015.3911.

da Silva, T.M.V., Melo, T.S., de Alencar, R.C. et al. (2021). Photobiomodulation for mucosal repair in patients submitted to dental extraction after head and neck radiation therapy: a double-blind randomized pilot study. *Support. Care Cancer* 29 (3): 1347–1354. http://dx.doi.org/10.1007/s00520-020-05608-5.

Simoes, A., Nicolau, J., de Souza, D.N. et al. (2008). Effect of defocused infrared diode laser on salivary flow rate and some salivary parameters of rats. *Clin. Oral Investig.* 12 (1): 25–30.

Simoes, A., de Campos, L., de Souza, D.N. et al. (2010). Laser phototherapy as topical prophylaxis against radiation-induced xerostomia. *Photomed. Laser Surg.* 28 (3): 357–363.

Simunović-Soskić, M., Pezelj-Ribarić, S., Brumini, G. et al. (2010). Salivary levels of TNF-alpha and IL-6 in patients with denture stomatitis before and after laser phototherapy. *Photomed. Laser Surg.* 28 (2): 189–193.

Sonis, S.T. (2004a). A biological approach to mucositis. *J. Support. Oncol.* 2: 21–32.

Sonis, S.T. (2004b). Oral mucositis in cancer therapy. *J. Support. Oncol.* 2 (6 Suppl 3): 3–8.

Sonis, S.T., Oster, G., Fuchs, H. et al. (2001). Oral mucositis and the clinical and economic outcomes of hematopoietic stem-cell transplantation. *J. Clin. Oncol.* 19: 2201–2205. http://dx.doi.org/10.1200/JCO.2001.19.8.2201.

Soto, M., Lalla, R.V., Gouveia, R.V. et al. (2015). Pilot study on the efficacy of combined intraoral and extraoral low-level laser therapy for prevention of oral mucositis in pediatric patients undergoing hematopoietic stem cell transplantation. *Photomed. Laser Surg.* 33 (11): 540–546. http://dx.doi.org/10.1089/pho.2015.395.

Sroussi, H.Y., Epstein, J.B., Bensadoun, R.J. et al. (2017). Common oral complications of head and neck cancer radiation therapy: mucositis, infections, saliva change, fibrosis, sensory dysfunctions, dental caries, periodontal disease, and osteoradionecrosis. *Cancer Med.* 6 (12): 2918–2931. http://dx.doi.org/10.1002/cam4.1221.

Tenis, C.A., Martins, M.D., Gonçalves, M.L.L. et al. (2018). Efficacy of light-emitting diode (LED) photobiomodulation in pain management, facial edema, trismus, and quality of life after extraction of retained lower third molars: a randomized, double-blind, placebo-controlled clinical trial. *Medicine (Baltimore)* 97 (37): e12264. http://dx.doi.org/10.1097/MD.0000000000012264.

Turner, J. and Hode, L. (2010). *The New Laser Therapy Handbook: A Guide for Research Scientists, Doctors, Dentists*. Veterinarians and Other Interested Parties Within the Medical Field: PRIMA Books.

Verdonck-de Leeuw, I.M., Buffart, L.M., Heymans, M.W. et al. (2014). The course of health-related quality of life in head and neck cancer patients treated with chemoradiation: a prospective cohort study. *Radiother. Oncol. J. Eur. Soc. Ther. Radiol. Oncol.* 110 (3): 422–428. http://dx.doi.org/10.1016/j.radonc.2014.01.002.

Vescovi, P., Giovannacci, I., Merigo, E. et al. (2015). Tooth extractions in high-risk patients under bisphosphonate therapy and previously affected with osteonecrosis of the jaws: surgical protocol supported by low-level laser therapy. *J. Craniofac. Surg.* 26 (3): 696–699. http://dx.doi.org/10.1097/SCS.0000000000001665.

Vlacic, J., Meyers, I.A., and Walsh, L.J. (2007). Laser-activated fluoride treatment of enamel as prevention against erosion. *Aust. Dent. J.* 52 (3): 175–180. http://dx.doi.org/10.1111/j.1834-7819.2007.tb00485.x.

Walker, J. (1983). Relief from chronic pain by low power laser irradiation. *Neurosci. Lett.* 43 (2–3): 339–344. http://dx.doi.org/10.1016/0304-3940(83)90211-2.

Wang, Y., Huang, Y.Y., Wang, Y. et al. (2017). Photobiomodulation of human adipose-derived stem cells using 810nm and 980nm lasers operates via different mechanisms of action. *Biochim. Biophys. Acta Gen. Subj.* 1861 (2): 441–449. http://dx.doi.org/10.1016/j.bbagen.2016.10.008.

Whelan, H.T., Connelly, J.F., Hodgson, B.D. et al. (2002). NASA light-emitting diodes for the prevention of oral mucositis in pediatric bone marrow transplant patients. *J. Clin. Laser Med. Surg.* 20 (6): 319–324. http://dx.doi.org/10.1089/104454702320901107.

Wieneke, S. and Gerhard, C. (2018). *Tissue Optics and Laser–Tissue Interactions*, 3-1–3-42. IOP Publishing Ltd.

World Health Organization (WHO) (1979). *Handbook for Reporting Results of Cancer Treatment*. Geneva, Switzerland: WHO.

Yifru, T.A., Kisa, S., Dinegde, N.G. et al. (2021). Dysphagia and its impact on the quality of life of head and neck cancer patients: institution-based cross-sectional study. *BMC. Res. Notes* 14: 11. http://dx.doi.org/10.1186/s13104-020-05440-4.

Zadik, Y., Arany, P.R., Fregnani, E.R. et al. (2019). Systematic review of photobiomodulation for the management of oral mucositis in cancer patients and clinical practice guidelines. *Support. Care Cancer* 27: 3969–3983. http://dx.doi.org/10.1007/s00520-019-04890-2.

Zanin, T., Zanin, F., Carvalhosa, A.A. et al. (2010). Use of 660-nm diode laser in the prevention and treatment of human oral mucositis induced by radiotherapy and chemotherapy. *Photomed. Laser Surg.* 28 (2): 233–237. https://doi.org/10.1089/pho.2008.2242.

Zecha, J.A., Raber-Durlacher, J.E., Nair, R.G. et al. (2016). Low-level laser therapy/photobiomodulation in the management of side effects of chemoradiation therapy in head and neck cancer: part 2: proposed applications and treatment protocols. *Support. Care Cancer* 24 (6): 2793–2805. http://dx.doi.org/10.1007/s00520-016-3153-y.

23

The Hologram, a New Imaging Modality in Head and Neck Cancer

Mark McGurk

Head & Neck Academic Centre, University College London, London, UK

The practice of medicine has been transformed by the advent of computers and their slow but powerful ingress into it. Nowhere is there a more obvious example than in imaging the body structures. It is now forgotten that in the 1980s CT scanners were just starting to be introduced to the NHS. They were so scarce they were restricted to specialist groups like neurosurgeons.

Now the landscape has been transformed, with every accident and emergency department let alone hospital having access to a CT scanner. The new generation of machines has improved, and they are much quicker, more refined, and more accurate. Paralleling the development of the CT scanner has been huge advances in MRI technology. With the advent of 3 tesla magnets, the size of the voxel (unit of image captured) has reduced from 5 mm thickness to 0.8 mm, so new MRI scans demonstrate much more soft tissue detail. These scans are also dynamic in nature, which bring new information on perfusion and other tissue parameters. The explosion in application of computer technology has also extended to nuclear medicine images. Here radiation hotspots generated by injecting radioactive tracers into the body can be visualised and then colocalised into CT or MRI scans, producing anatomical detail to what was before a mere shadow.

What is the next leap forward? Development is exponential, and now we are being introduced to virtual reality (VR – a 3D environment distinct from your surroundings, like a game show) and augmented reality (AR – where 3D images are projected onto objects in the room). These will have a huge influence on medicine as the technology matures. VR is likely to transform teaching. Students will be able to participate in educational games that are interactive and very real to the participant. AR is already finding a place in treatment.

It is now possible to take the data captured by electronic (digital) imaging and reformat it to produce 3D objects This applies to CT, MRI, PET, and single photon emission computed tomography (SPECT)/CT imaging modalities. Independent from the great medical companies that are developing the CT/MRI machines, companies such as Google and Microsoft are pushing the boundaries on how the world will communicate and interact in the future. These two worlds are now starting to interact. One of the developments is the Microsoft HoloLens (Figure 23.1). This headset can take the segmented imaging data and transform it into a hologram in front of the operator. This image can be constructed to contain all of the anatomical detail that is relevant to the patient and the operation. This transforms the ability to appreciate the body in 3D. Previously, surgeons worked in the dark, feeling their way forward and carefully looking for their objective. Now it is projected in front of them.

A very important development has occurred in head and neck surgery with the management of salivary tumours. This has been helped by a collaboration of a charity Head & Neck Cancer Foundation with the Head & Neck Academic Centre at University College London. Most of the salivary tumours occur in the parotid gland. Unfortunately, a very important nerve that animates the face (facial nerve) runs through the gland. Up until now we only had a general idea where the nerve lay, and it could easily be displaced by tumours. Now with the new high-definition MRI scans the facial nerve can be traced and visualised as it passes through the parotid gland (Figure 23.2). The nerve's relationship with the tumour can be identified before surgery.

Technology introduces personalised surgery for the first time to parotid disease. An operation can be planned specially for the individual patient rather than a general operation performed. There are many applications of this technology to the salivary glands, finding parathyroid lumps, tracing sentinel nodes (Figure 23.3) in the neck, and planning surgery in the

Care of Head and Neck Cancer Patients for Dental Hygienists and Dental Therapists, First Edition. Edited by Jocelyn J. Harding.

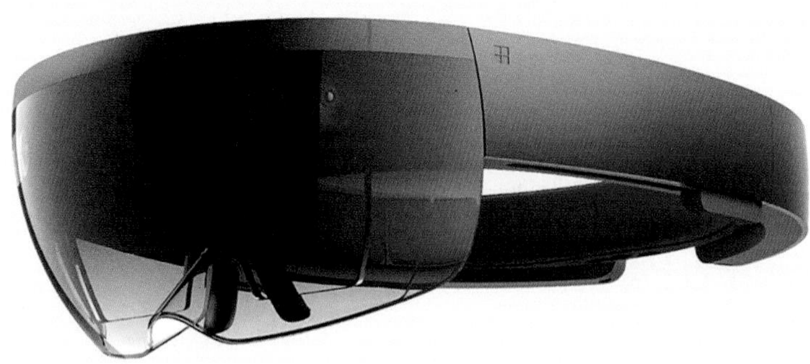

Figure 23.1 Image of the Microsoft HoloLens that is worn like glasses. *Source:* Microsoft Corporation.

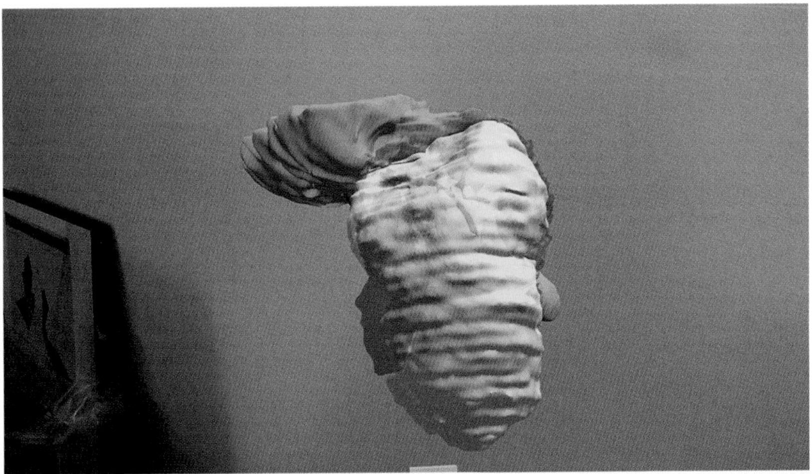

Figure 23.2 A large lipoma with the facial nerve showing through the structure.

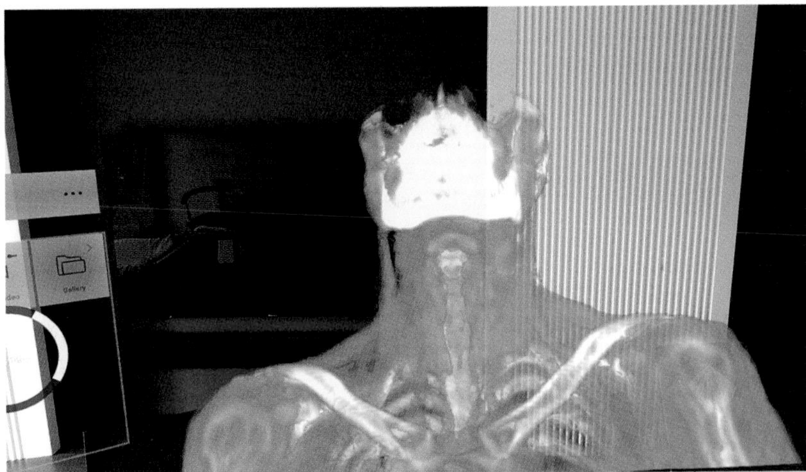

Figure 23.3 SPECT CT scan of the upper body demonstrating two hot sentinel nodes in the neck.

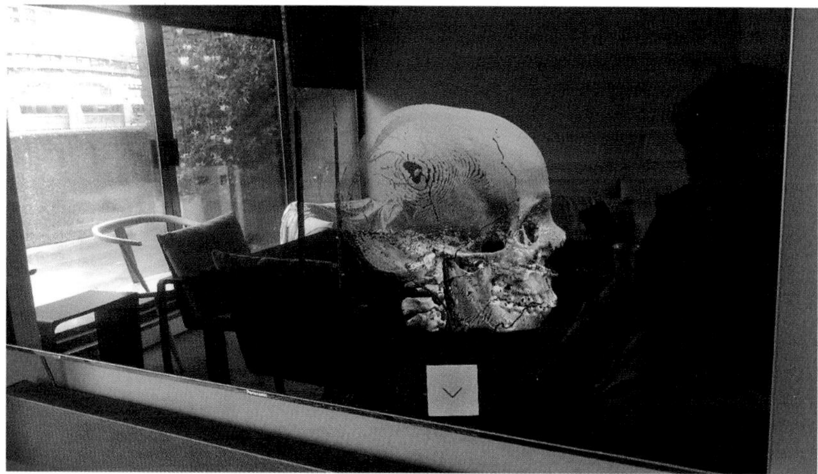

Figure 23.4 Data taken from a CT scan showing the skull and its vessels in preparation for surgery.

ear and skull base (Figure 23.4). The application of this technology is on the cusp of another breakthrough. In the very near future, the AR anatomical images will be accurately projected onto patients. Then doctors can wear these headsets and effectively look through the skin into the body. The technology has still to be developed, but this will usher in more and more minimally invasive procedures as operators will be able to target structures deep in the body percutaneously. This is a tribute to the impact of modern computers on our medical lives.

24

Laryngectomy Care: What Is Required?

Lauren Smallwood

Highly Specialist Speech and Language Therapist, Newcastle-upon-Tyne, UK

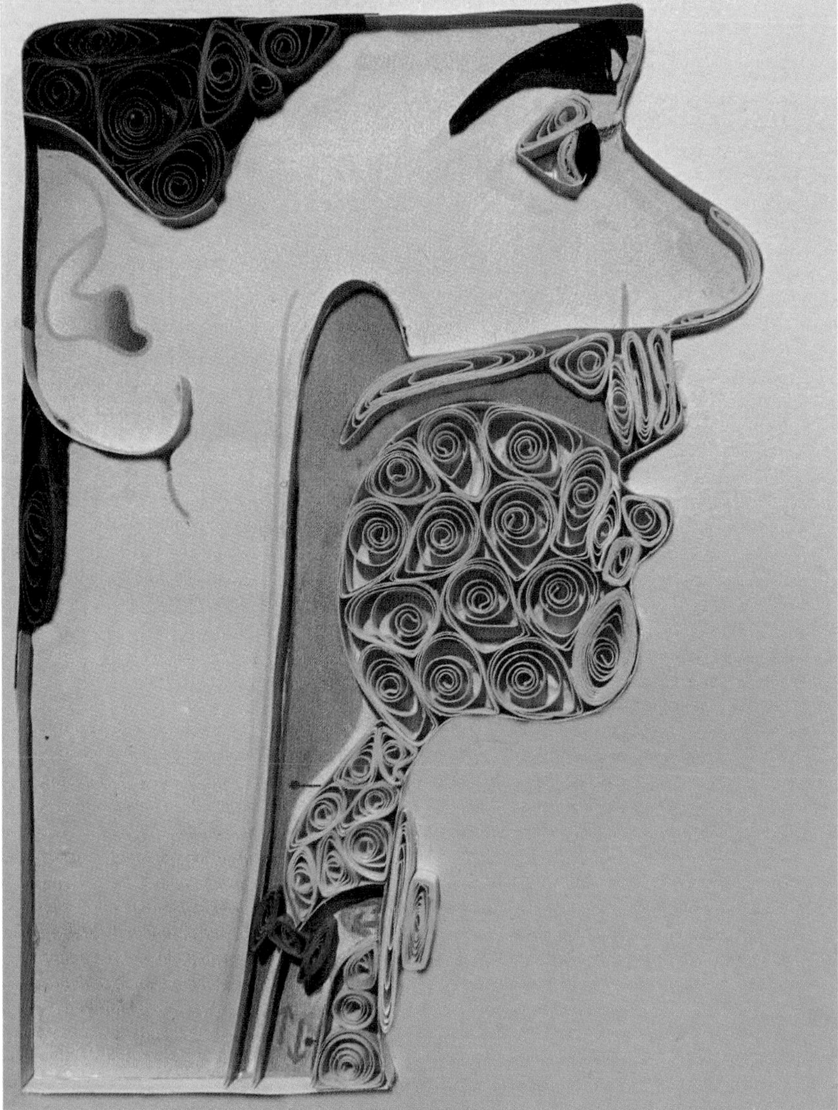

Image by Lisa Kyle.

Care of Head and Neck Cancer Patients for Dental Hygienists and Dental Therapists, First Edition. Edited by Jocelyn J. Harding.

A laryngectomy is a surgical procedure performed on people who may have laryngeal cancer that cannot be treated through less invasive procedures alone, e.g. radiotherapy and chemotherapy. A laryngectomy may also be required after a traumatic event involving the neck and its internal structures (Consalici and Dall'Olio 2010).

Following the surgery, an opening is created in the front of the neck; this is known as a stoma. The trachea (airway) is separated from the upper respiratory/digestive tract and redirected to the front of the neck via the stoma. The word 'stoma' was used in ancient Greek times to mean 'mouth', and in modern times it is used in medicine to indicate a small opening in the body.

People with a laryngectomy may also have undergone surgical voice restoration at some stage in their treatment, as they will no longer have their own vocal cords to produce voice. This involves a small puncture being placed between the tracheal and oesophageal walls to allow for a medical-grade silicone rubber voice prosthesis to be inserted. Once in place, the voice prosthesis (sometimes referred to as a 'speaking valve') can help direct air from the lungs up into the upper oesophageal tract, which can then enable speech production. The one-way valve should also then prevent diet or liquids from the oesophageal side entering the person's airway if the device is working correctly.

Not all people with a laryngectomy will have surgical voice restoration; they may use a hand-held vibratory device called an electrolarynx that they place on the side of their neck or cheek whilst speaking. They may even use oesophageal speech, where they learn to inhale air into their oesophagus and expel the air whilst speaking. Finding out how people are communicating can be very important, and the method they are using may not always be immediately obvious.

A Voice Prosthesis and Stoma Care

Looking after the stoma site is important for a person who has a laryngectomy, as it will help one to remain healthy. To keep the stoma patent, you may find people wear a laryngectomy tube at certain periods during the day or overnight. This helps to ensure the stoma does not become too narrow, which will also make changing a voice prosthesis much easier.

The skin around the stoma site can often be delicate, especially if the person has undergone radiotherapy treatment for cancer. This can cause inflammation of the skin and make it tender to touch in the early days, which can persist for some time afterwards. Stomas will come in all different shapes and sizes: regular, round, oval, deep set, large, or small. Caring for the stoma is vitally important, as it connects directly to the lungs, allowing the person to breathe (see Figures 24.1–24.3).

Good levels of care can help to reduce trauma to the skin around the stoma (especially if a baseplate is worn) and allow the person to closely monitor any change in the shape, size, or colour of the stoma.

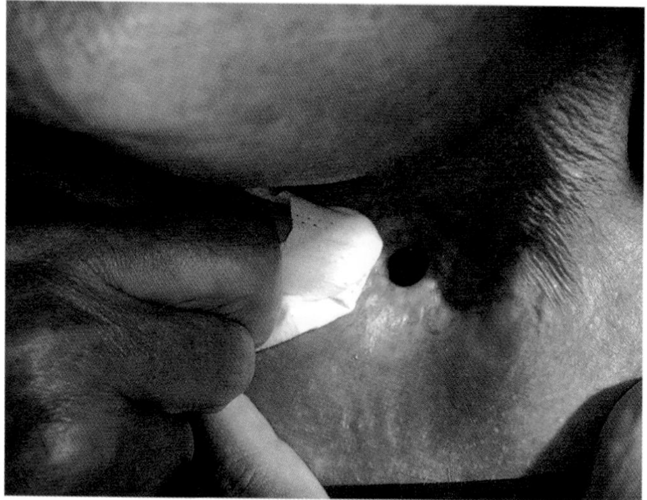

Figure 24.1 Cleaning the stoma site with a cleaning wipe.

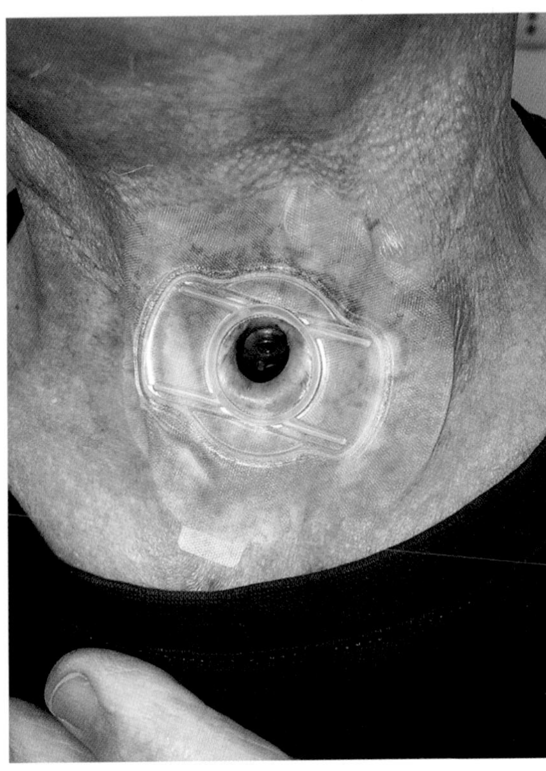

Figure 24.2 Wearing a convex baseplate.

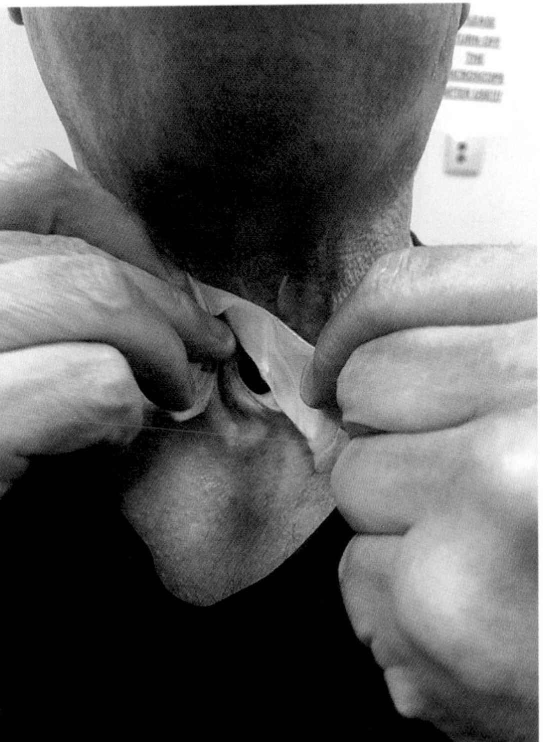

Figure 24.3 Removing the baseplate using an adhesive remover wipe.

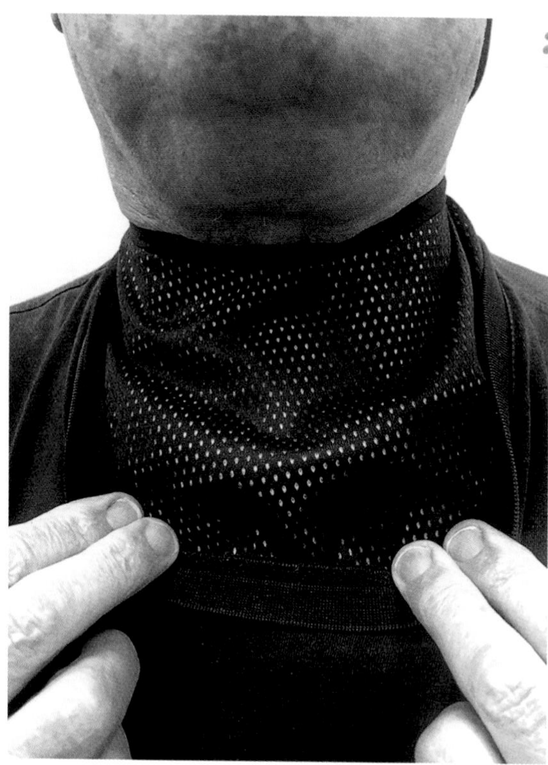

Figure 24.4 Example of a laryngectomy bib.

Routine advice provided to people with a laryngectomy may include (see Figure 24.4):

- Help maintain skin integrity: check the stoma is clean and clear of any mucous or secretions that may have built up throughout the day. Specially designed stoma wipes or dampened lint-free gauze are available for this purpose. People need to be careful not to fully occlude their airway whilst cleaning around the site.
- Avoid material entering the airway: keeping the stoma protected 24 hours a day is advised to reduce the risk of chest infections and foreign bodies entering the airway, for example, water, sand, dust, and insects (Ackerstaff et al. 2003). If material does enter the airway, it may elicit a cough – this is the body's protective reflex to try to expel any inhaled material.
- Protection from viruses: ensuring adequate protection of the stoma will not only protect people with a laryngectomy but also people they meet, to help reduce the transmission of airborne viruses. A surgical mask placed lightly over their heat moisture exchange (HME) device will provide an additional barrier (Kligerman et al. 2020).

If a voice prosthesis is in situ (see Figure 24.5), it will require daily care and monitoring to ensure optimum functionality and reduce the risk of bacteria building up inside the device. Due to the levels of care and safety precautions involved after someone has had a laryngectomy, you may find that a person with a laryngectomy will always keep spare equipment close to hand (there are also specially designed bags provided by health care companies for this purpose). This is so any laryngectomy needs can be attended to quickly and whilst on the go; for example, if the HME filter needs replacing throughout the day or the person notices a build-up of secretions around the stoma site that need clearing away.

Baseplates and HMEs

Wearing a baseplate with an HME filter helps the lungs to work effectively and generates a good seal for directing the required airflow for voicing. The baseplate is a device that is designed to be worn directly on the skin and then allows an HME filter to be attached.

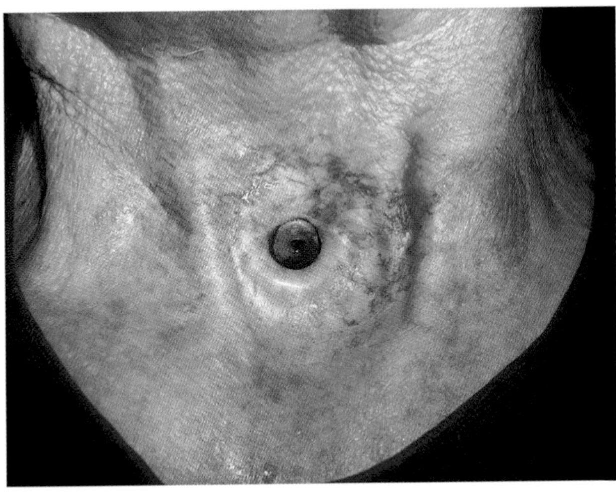
Figure 24.5 A surgical voice prosthesis in situ.

Most baseplates come in different shapes, and some have a convex baseplate to ensure the best seal. Baseplates can be designed for use on sensitive skin and therefore will be less sticky, which is easier for the person to remove. However, once the skin is less sensitive, more adhesive baseplates are available that can last longer throughout the day. People who use hands-free valve systems may find they require more durable baseplates to help deal with the increased air pressure leaving their stoma site. This is because they are not using their finger to occlude the stoma, which would usually provide additional pressure to keep the baseplate in situ.

The weather can also affect the amount of secretions a person produces; for example, warm, dry air can dry/irritate the stoma and create more mucous, just as much as cold, damp weather. Environmental factors like being in a warm kitchen and then opening the door of the fridge/freezer can also have an effect. The production of this mucus is natural and the body's way to protect the lungs (similar to a productive cough or cold), but with the right stoma protection the amount of secretions can be greatly reduced.

Equipment

Here are some key pieces of equipment that a person with a laryngectomy may need throughout the day (based on St George's University Hospitals NHS Foundation Trust 2022) (see Figures 24.6 and 24.7):

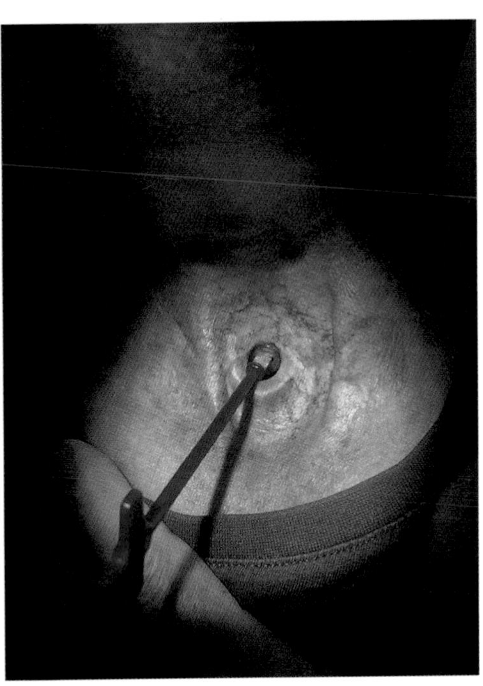
Figure 24.6 Cleaning the voice prosthesis.

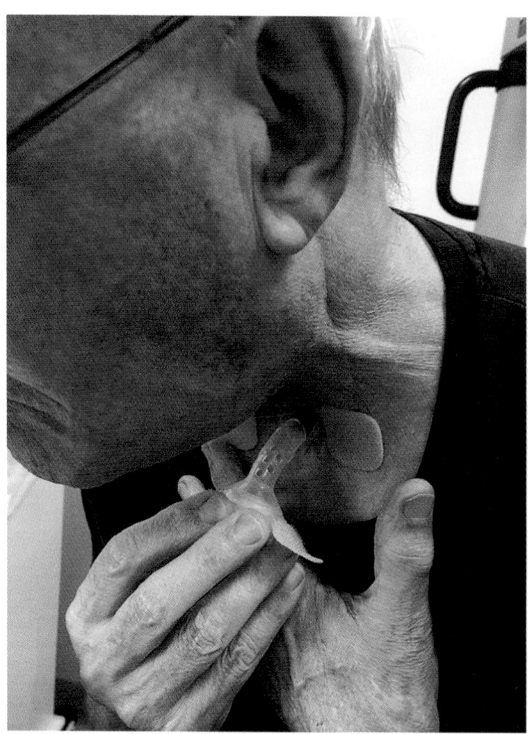

Figure 24.7 Inserting a fenestrated laryngectomy tube.

Equipment	Purpose
Small hand-held torch/good light source	This will allow the area to be cleaned more thoroughly, especially when cleaning a voice prosthesis.
Mirror	To make sure the person who is cleaning can see the entrance of the voice prosthesis clearly and avoid causing accidental trauma.
Dilator/catheter	People may change their own voice prosthesis at home and require a dilator to keep their tract patent whilst they complete the change. If the voice prosthesis is ever dislodged, it is important that people can keep their tract open until they are able to seek medical advice.
Voice prosthesis cleaning brush	A specially designed brush will be provided by the voice prosthesis manufacturer to ensure the centre of the valve can be kept free of debris and secretions. It is important the correct brush is selected for the valve in situ.
Warm water and lint-free gauze or cleaning wipes	These will help keep the area around the stoma clean and make removing any dried secretions less traumatic to the skin underneath.
Clean hands and waste disposal bags	People should avoid touching the stoma or the HME filter with unwashed hands. Thorough hand hygiene should be commenced prior to cleaning the stoma and after the process is finished. Any soiled items should be placed in a suitable disposable waste bag.
Barrier creams	Specially designed creams can be used to help ensure the skin around the stoma does not become too dry or irritated, especially if regularly wearing baseplates or laryclips.
Laryngectomy tube	A laryngectomy tube may be worn for long periods immediately after the surgery to help keep the stoma site patent. After a while, the time this device is worn may reduce if the stoma size remains stable. Many people will choose to intermittently insert a laryngectomy tube every now and again to ensure the stoma size has remained the same. They may be fenestrated, which will allow a person with a surgical voice prosthesis to still produce voice whilst wearing the tube.

Protection

People may choose to protect their stoma in various ways. Keeping the stoma covered can help to restore some humidification, which is important to keep the lungs healthy, but it also helps to prevent foreign materials from entering the airway.

Here are some examples of how a person may protect the stoma:

- HME cassettes (see Figures 24.8–24.10)
- Shower aid (see Figure 24.11)
- Bib/neck covering (see Figure 24.12).

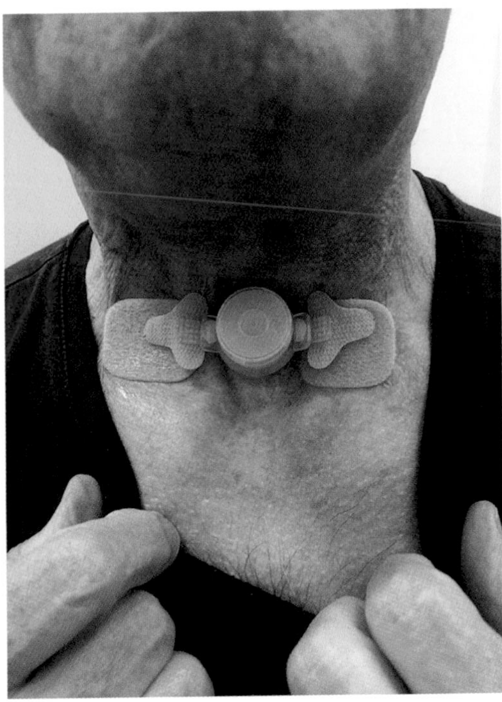

Figure 24.8 HME cassette used with a laryngectomy tube and laryclips to keep in situ.

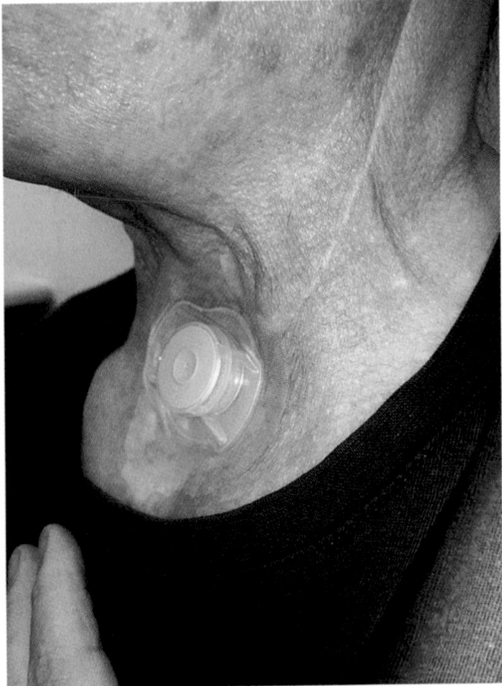

Figure 24.9 HME cassette and baseplate.

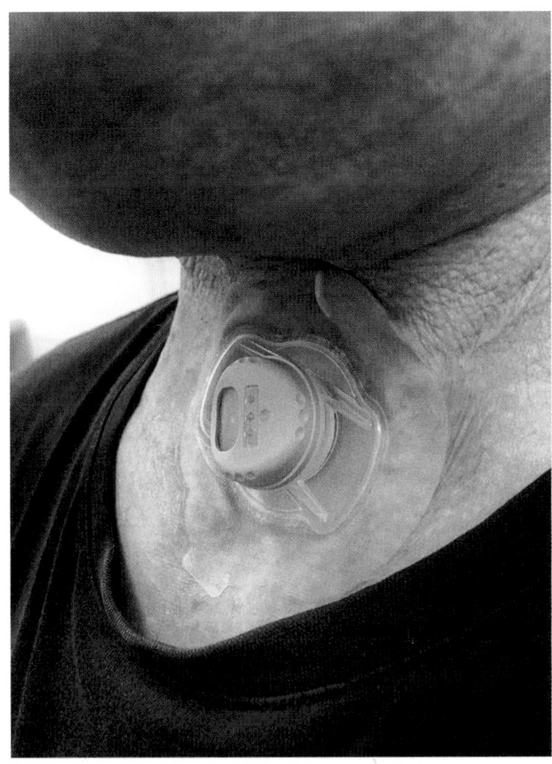

Figure 24.10 Using a hands-free HME cassette and baseplate.

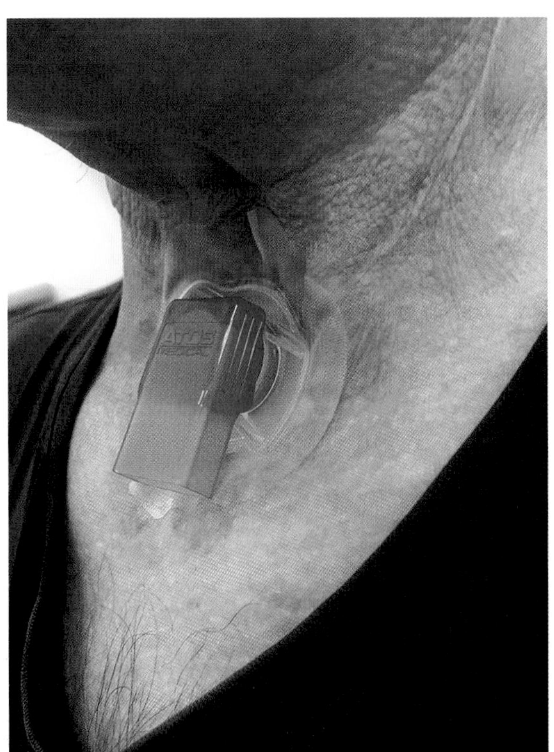

Figure 24.11 Example of a shower aid.

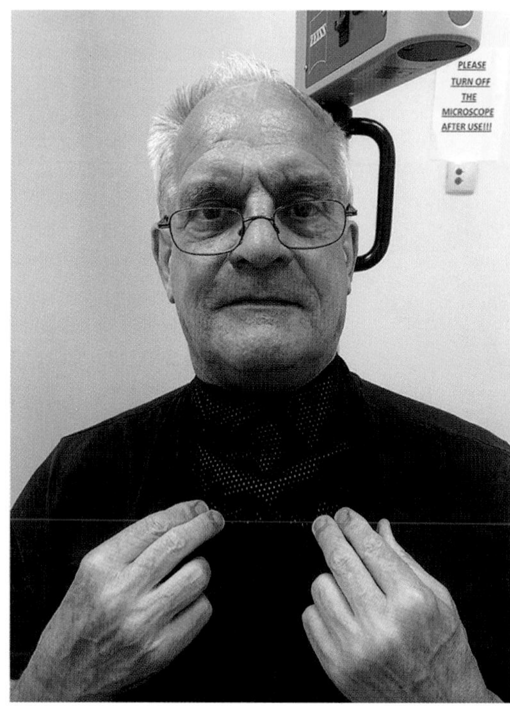

Figure 24.12 Wearing a laryngectomy bib.

Summary

Advice on how people should look after their laryngectomy should be given as soon as possible to allow for independent and optimal care of the site. If they need additional help to complete this daily care regime, a family member, friend, or community nurse can be trained to support with the care. Remember, this is the person's sole airway now, so any changes to the skin or tissues around the site need to be carefully monitored and cared for.

References

Ackerstaff, A.H., Fuller, D., Irvin, M. et al. (2003). Multicenter study assessing effects of heat and moisture exchanger use on respiratory symptoms and voice quality in laryngectomized individuals. *Otolaryngol. Head Neck Surg.* 129 (6): 705–712. https://doi.org/10.1016/S0194-59980301595-X.

Consalici, R. and Dall'Olio, D. (2010). Severe laryngeal fracture treated by supracricoid laryngectomy. *J. Laryngol. Otol.* 124 (11): 1239–1241. https://doi.org/10.1017/S0022215110001374.

Kligerman, M.P., Vukkadala, N., Tsang, R. et al. (2020). Managing head and neck cancer patients with tracheostomy or laryngectomy during the COVID-19 pandemic. *Head Neck* 42 (6): 1209–1213. https://doi.org/10.1002/hed.26171.

St George's University Hospitals NHS Foundation Trust. (2022). Caring for a stoma and voice prosthesis after a total laryngectomy - Speech and Language Therapy information for patients and carers. https://www.stgeorges.nhs.uk/wp-content/uploads/2022/01/SLT_SVP_01.pdf (accessed 27 July 2021)

25

Mental Health and Well-Being during Treatment

Lauren Barry

York and Scarborough Teaching Hospitals NHS Foundation Trust, York, UK

Treatment regimens differ depending on the stage and location of the cancer. Each treatment brings its own challenges and issues for the person living through it, and while for some patients this can be a very difficult stage, for others it can be the most positive. Surgery, chemotherapy, and radiotherapy are commonly used and will be explored in more detail elsewhere in this book. Often they are used in combination, which means that patients are dealing with the collective effects of many medical interventions.

Many patients seem to find it easier to cope emotionally during this time. It is often very busy, with many appointments. The treatment schedule can be very demanding in terms of time and will be set in stone. The patient will encounter a whole host of medical professionals at each visit, all of them regularly checking how the person is feeling. In addition, patients will need someone to accompany them to and from appointments.

This increased level of social support, routine, and professional input can have a positive impact on some at a time when the medical interventions are likely to be making them feel very unwell. Indeed, for some this will be the first time they will have actually felt unwell, and for some this will be the first time that they have really believed that they are ill, that they do have cancer.

For others, this loss of control, being told what to do, and having to run to someone else's timetable can be very frustrating. This can amplify the loss of control that a cancer diagnosis can bring. Practically, planning anything becomes a huge task and life is determined by the next appointment or waiting for the next treatment.

The treatments themselves can have immediate and very restrictive side effects. These side effects also have wide-reaching consequences for the patient. Nausea, for example, can be a side effect of chemotherapy. When it affects a patient's ability to eat, the patient may have to rely on medical intervention, such as a nasogastric tube, to meet nutritional requirements. If patients are not getting adequate nutrition, they are likely to suffer from fatigue, which can exaggerate the loss of well-being. Tube feeding also takes away the pleasure that many people gain from eating and drinking. Coupled with the possible loss of the ability to smell, the whole sensory experience of eating is taken away.

Chemotherapy can also cause mucositis. This debilitating condition not only affects nutritional intake but also comes with intense pain. Pain significantly affects a person's well-being and the ability to deal with everyday challenges, much less the challenges of going through life-changing treatment. It can make speaking very difficult, leading to isolation, and can disturb sleep, further reducing resourcefulness and well-being. In addition, simple everyday tasks such as oral hygiene become impossible for the person.

Radiotherapy brings with it xerostomia, making the mouth uncomfortable, altering taste, affecting sleep (patients often wake up due to oral dryness), and limiting speech. For some patients the need for a radiotherapy mask brings psychological challenges. They are very restrictive apparatuses and can bring feelings of claustrophobia or bring back traumatic memories and experiences. A psychology referral may be required to try to support patients with this area of treatment.

If patients are not able to eat or sleep well, this has huge implications for their mental health and well-being. Sleep and nutrition are the cornerstones of recuperation.

Depression and anxiety can understandably be experienced by patients undergoing treatment. Those with a pre-existing diagnosis of depression can find it is exacerbated (Kar et al. 2020). Radiotherapy may even result in hypothyroidism, which

Care of Head and Neck Cancer Patients for Dental Hygienists and Dental Therapists, First Edition. Edited by Jocelyn J. Harding.

leads to depressive symptoms. This is in addition to the general impacts of treatment leading to low mood, fear, and worry seen in depression and anxiety.

Any surgery is a daunting prospect. It comes with a complete surrendering of control to the surgical team and then to the ward staff. Being in hospital itself is a stressful time for many. Following surgery, patients are likely to need a period of recovery where normal routine is suspended. They may be completely reliant on others, especially with more invasive surgery affecting not just the head or neck but arms, legs or back due to reconstruction.

For some patients the treatment part of their journey brings with it new relationships with others going through a similar experience. Some patients meet others who go on to be lifelong friends, and they can bond over their shared experience. It may also strengthen already existing relationships with friends and family, bringing new closeness in the face of a life-changing event. Sadly, some people feel like a burden during their treatment and may find it difficult to ask for help or feel they are asking too much. Some of us are not naturally comfortable being cared for or supported by others, and this can be exacerbated.

It is unlikely that the dental hygienist or dental therapist would see patients during this time, as the nature of treatment means that patients are unable to undergo dental treatment. However, being available as a source of advice is important. Some may be part of a wider multidisciplinary team and able to give advice to patients themselves or other professionals. Those working in general practice may have patients whose family members are undergoing treatment or may have been instrumental in the detection of the cancer in the first place.

As with pretreatment, a general message of kindness to the self is important. Given how the patient is feeling both physically and psychologically during this time, what is realistic in terms of oral health is going to change. Patients will need reassurance as there is the potential for additional long-term problems, regular appointments with the dental team can help in supporting with problems that may surface.

Reference

Kar, A., Asheem, M.R., Bhaumik, U., and Rao, V.U.S. (2020). Psychological issues in head and neck cancer survivors: need for addressal in rehabilitation. *Oral Oncol.* 110: 104859.

Section 4

Head and Neck Cancer Treatment Complications

26

Chemotherapy and Risk Assessment in Dental Treatment Planning

StJohn Crean

University of Central Lancashire, Preston, UK

Dental practice provides a necessary and consequential service to the general public. Professionals are trained to a high standard overseen by a regulatory body. Those standards demand that professionals of the twenty-first century embrace the concept of not 'treating teeth in patients' but treating 'patients with teeth'. The dental profession thus occupies a key position as one of the pillars of the health industry. With this role comes challenges. One of those is the requirement to provide treatments based on risk assessments for the outcome journeys.

One emergent area of clinical challenge is the complexity in medications available to patients. Amongst those are chemotherapeutic agents. These are provided for cancer patients to support either in-patient care or increasingly within the community environment. These drugs come with a number of challenges and side effects of which the patients are given significant warnings. However, their impact on dental care should not be underestimated and should form part of any risk assessment discussion prior to treatment planning (Kumar and Clark 2017, 596–599).

The range of medication is large, but this short chapter will address the headline examples that may provide guidance for the required approach to adopt to minimise unpredictable outcomes (Specialist Pharmacy Service 2020).

An important principle to adhere to is that prior to any treatment being agreed and commencing, the dental professional must, if in any doubt, consult with colleagues in the oncology clinics. This is to ensure that any dental treatments proposed can be delivered safely within the dental clinical environment, striving to deliver predictable outcomes.

A range of chemotherapeutic medications are prescribed in the battle to contain and remove cancerous cells. Their aim is to damage DNA (or RNA) so conclusively that it results in the death of the malignant cells. The challenge for the dental professional is the effect on the nonmalignant cell population.

Toxicity side effects are combated by coadministration of such agents as granulocyte colony stimulating factor and stem cell preparations, and also by combining relatively low pro-apoptotic agents with more general cytotoxic agents. Drug resistance is also addressed by adopting the principle of intermittent combination chemotherapy, relying on normal cell recovery outstripping that of malignant programmed tissue.

However, an additional challenge for the dental professional lies in those patients who have been discharged from hospital care but continue in part of their treatment. Their attendance for dental care demands that dental clinicians understand the relevance and impact of such outpatient chemotherapy medication.

The range of drugs patients may be taking is classically grouped as

- DNA damaging agents, for example, cyclophosphamide, chlorambucil, cisplatin
- Antimetabolites, for example, 5-fluorouracil, mercaptopurine, methotrexate
- DNA repair inhibitors, for example, etoposide, bleomycin
- Antitubulin agents, for example, paclitaxel.

Modern pharmaceutical developments have, however, increased the list as reviewed recently (Cancer Research UK 2019). Newer groups include

- Monoclonal antibodies, for example, denusomab and adalimumab
- Tyrosine kinase inhibitors, for example, sunitinib, imatinib
- mTOR inhibitors (inhibit the mechanistic target of rapamycin), for example, everolimus and sirolimus

Care of Head and Neck Cancer Patients for Dental Hygienists and Dental Therapists, First Edition. Edited by Jocelyn J. Harding.

- Histone deacetylase inhibitors, for example, vorinostat
- PI3K inhibitors, for example, delalisib
- Sonic hedgehog pathway inhibitors, for example, vismodegib and sonidegib.

Time spent capturing an accurate medical history may reveal one of these pharmacological groups within the patient medication list. In this situation, the dental clinician should consider a number of possible side effects and reflect their impact on the outcome of the treatment.

General Side Effects

There are a number of common side effects that should be understood in order for the dental clinician to assess the impact of the treatment undergone/undergoing by the patient. These include hair loss, nausea, and fatigue. In addition, during the acute stages of the treatment mucositis can manifest itself.

However, it is the issue of *myelosuppression* (bone marrow suppression) that poses the most daunting of clinical issues. Every dental professional should understand the impact of such a side effect, no more so than prior to embarking on treatment, especially if invasive in nature (Lopez et al. 2011). Myelosuppression arises as a result of the toxic effects of the drugs on the normal cell production in the bone marrow. This means that the synthesis of white cells, red cells, and platelets is put at risk. Some or all of these cell syntheses may be affected, leading to pancytopenia. These effects usually arise within two weeks of treatment and could take at least another month to recover on treatment completion. (Lopez et al. 2011; Cancer Research UK 2019).

The level of myelosuppression achieved may reflect the extent to which disease cure is being pursued. Patients who are in the community imply a level of suppression aimed to facilitate as much as possible the activities of daily living. But the outpatient administration of medication whilst not achieving the same degree of suppression can still realise a significant impact in the development of (i) anaemia, (ii) leukopenia (reduced white cells), and (iii) thrombocytopenia (reduced platelets).

The key message for the dental professional is that each clinician should have evidence that the patient's bone marrow has recovered sufficiently for treatment to be planned accordingly and safely. These patients will be used to undergoing regular blood checks. Failure to have an up-to-date blood result assessment could lead to effects such as fungal and dental infections, excessive or prolonged bleeding after invasive procedures, mucositis, and a reduction in salivary flow leading to sore mouth and disturbed taste (King et al. 2020; Royal College of Surgeons 2018; Radfar et al. 2015).

An issue that may trouble the dental professional is who to ask for some up-to-date blood results. The author would recommend that the patient, having spoken with their general medical practitioner, shares the latest blood results. An agreement to communicate them securely to the dental practice should be agreed, taking into account the General Data Protection Regulation laws around transfer of personal medical data. These regulations are outlined in articles 6 and 9 of the Data Protection Act (2018) (National Health Service 2018). It is not unusual for there to be times when the patient's hospital team may need contacting. It is clear that no invasive treatment should be embarked upon outside of the hospital environment if the blood results are not available or are outside the normal parameters.

Another issue is, what are normal blood results? It is not unusual for the blood results to be accompanied by a normal range in parentheses. Dental professionals having sight of the figures can make the quantitative judgement alongside the clinical status of the patient. However, for guidance, the following are good indicators (Kumar and Clark 2017, 519).

For the full blood count:

1) Hgb should be above 13–15 g/dl, the mean corpuscular volume (size of red cells) above 80 fl (up to 96 fl), and the number of red cells above 3.9×10^{12}/l for females and 4.5×10^{12}/l for males.
2) Neutrophils (myeloid white cells, not lymphocytes) should be above 2×10^{9}/l. The total white cell count (WCC) should be above 4.0×10^{9}/l. Disturbance in the neutrophil level may necessitate discussion with the patient's hospital consultant as to whether antibiotic coverage would be of benefit.
3) Platelets should be above 150×10^{9}/l or in a range up to 450×10^{9}/l. Even in the hospital environment, a platelet count less than 50×10^{9}/l would require a platelet transfusion and treatment within a very short period.

Additional blood results to be aware of:

1) Coagulation tests. The international normalised ratio (INR) should normally be 1.0. Any increase would raise the suspicion of disturbed clotting function and perhaps liver disturbance. But if this is all that is disturbed, then it would be satisfactory to adhere to advice on patients with raised INR and employ the advised haemostatic procedures. Good advice is provided by the Scottish Dental Clinical Effectiveness Programme document 'Management of Dental Patients Taking Anticoagulants or Antiplatelet Drugs' (Scottish Dental Clinical Effectiveness Programme 2015). Clinicians must, however, be sure there are no other disturbed haematological indices.
2) Liver function. The practitioner should always ask the patient on chemotherapy whether there has been any issue with liver function during or after chemotherapy. This is important as the liver is the course of the body's clotting factors. Measures that would raise concern include
   a) Alanine transaminase (ALT) above 56 u/l and
   b) Aspartate transaminase (AST) above 40 u/l.

Dental professionals must always have these issues to the front of their thinking when treating such patients. Doubt should always be allayed by consultation with colleagues or specialists. Never take risks based on ignorance.

References

Cancer Research UK (2019). Infection during or after treatment. https://www.cancerresearchuk.org/about-cancer/coping/physically/fever/causes/infection/during-or-after-treatment.

King, R., Zebic, L., and Patel, V. (2020). Deciphering novel chemotherapy and its impact on dentistry. *Br. Dent. J.* 228: 415–421. https://doi.org/10.1038/s41415-020-1365-5.

Kumar, P. and Clark, M. (2017). *Kumar and Clark's Clinical Medicine*, 9e. Edinburgh: Elsevier.

Lopez, B., Esteve, C., and Perez, M. (2011). Dental treatment considerations in the chemotherapy patient. *J. Clin. Exp. Dent.* 3 (1): 31–42.

National Health Service (2018). Protecting patient data. https://digital.nhs.uk/services/national-data-opt-out/understanding-the-national-data-opt-out/protecting-patient-data#data-protection-act-2018.

Radfar, L., Admadabadi, R., Masood, F., and Scofield, R. (2015). Biological therapy and dentistry: a review paper. *Oral. Surg. Oral. Med. Oral. Pathol. Oral. Radiol.* 120: 594–601.

Scottish Dental Clinical Effectiveness Programme (2015). Management of dental patients taking anticoagulants or antiplatelet drugs. Available at https://www.scottishdental.org/library/management-of-dental-patients-taking-anticoagulants-or-antiplatelet-drugs/.

Specialist Pharmacy Service (2020). How should adults with cancer be managed by general dental practitioners if they need dentaltreatment? https://www.sps.nhs.uk/articles/how-should-adults-with-cancer-be-managed-by-general-dental-practitioners-if-they-need-dental-treatment.

Royal College of Surgeons of England (2018). The oral management of oncology patients requiring radiotherapy, chemotherapy and/or bone marrow transplantation: clinical guidelines. www.rcseng.ac.uk/-/media/files/rcs/fds/publications/rcs-oncology-guideline-update-v36.pdf.

27

Xerostomia, from the Greek (Xero = Dry, Stoma = Mouth) = Dry Mouth

Leigh Hunter

Growing Smiles, UK

Reduced salivary flow can impair basic oral functions and increase the risk of dental caries, periodontal disease, tooth wear, and opportunistic infections, directly influencing patients' QoL (Gonnelli et al. 2016). Xerostomia is one of the most disturbing side effects of HNC therapy. It can result in discomfort, dysgeusia (bad taste), dysphagia (difficulty swallowing), and dysphonia (hoarseness) (Djaali et al. 2020).

The consequences of xerostomia can compromise oral health, nutrition, general health, and QoL. It not only affects the patient but also family and carers. Xerostomia is one of the most common, most unpleasant, and debilitating side effects of HNC treatment. There is a wealth of information in the scientific literature on xerostomia and its assessment, causes, and treatment modalities. With ever-evolving management and treatment strategies, further reading is recommended.

It is important to continually update and develop knowledge and skills for successful management of the xerostomia patient. Lack of saliva flow is pathological rather than physiological, that is, it is not an automatic consequence of ageing (Xu et al. 2019). Prevention is key to maintain oral health for a patient's xerostomia – no matter the cause.

Xerostomia is a lot more common than many realise and should be considered part of oral health assessment for *all* patients. Many are unaware that their saliva flow or composition is compromised and that it may affect their oral health. Fluid intake should be a component of dietary and nutritional assessment and reviewed regularly. Diet and/or fluid advice should be considered using the COM-B model for behaviour change (Michie et al. 2014), which suggests that three conditions must exist for a new behaviour to occur: capabilities (C), opportunities (O), and motivation (M).

'You can't understand someone until you've walked a mile in their shoes' is very apt with xerostomic patients. Take the dry cracker challenge (Harding 2018), then imagine your mouth like that for long periods – potentially for life.

Background

Xerostomia is not a disease but a symptom. It is the subjective feeling of dry mouth, measured by directly questioning patients. It is different from salivary gland hypofunction (SGH), where people have lower-than-normal salivary output (flow rate). Xerostomia is the most common salivary problem and is described as the sensation of oral dryness (Wolff et al. 2017), with symptoms ranging from mild discomfort to significant disease. It is due to reduced salivary flow (hyposalivation) and/or changed salivary composition (Felix et al. 2012). For the general population it may be short or long term, but chemotherapy and radiotherapy for HNCs can result in both acute and chronic complications. Xerostomia in HNC patients is often compounded by an associated physiological cause of dry mouth, for example anxiety, age, mouth breathing, a medical condition such as diabetes, or medication. Dry mouth is reported more in women than men.

A systematic review in 2018 by Agostini et al. concluded an overall global estimated incidence of xerostomia of 22%, and despite diverse approaches to measuring the condition, just over one in four people suffer from xerostomia. It may affect any age, but xerostomia is most common in the older population. Very rarely, salivary glands may be absent at birth (salivary gland aplasia or agenesis), but the majority of salivary gland dysfunction is acquired. The prevalence and consequences of xerostomia are increasing, largely due to the ageing population who are at least partially dentate and polypharmacy relating to age-related medical conditions. Hundreds of over-the-counter (OTC) and prescribed medications

Care of Head and Neck Cancer Patients for Dental Hygienists and Dental Therapists, First Edition. Edited by Jocelyn J. Harding.

contribute or exacerbate oral dryness. These include antihistamines (for allergy or asthma), antihypertensive medications, analgesics, decongestants, pain medications, diuretics, muscle relaxants, and antidepressants.

A thorough medical and dental history is crucial to assess and manage xerostomia before, during, and after HNC diagnosis and treatment. Maxfacts notes that along with the aforementioned drugs, cytotoxic drugs used in chemotherapy, along with recreational drugs such as caffeine, cocaine, or nicotine and OTC herbal remedies (e.g. gingko and capsicum extracts or St. John's wort preparations), are all known to cause or exacerbate xerostomia (Maxfacts 2018). Malignancies of the salivary glands are rare, but they may present with xerostomia as one of the early symptoms.

Chemotherapy drugs can change the nature and amount of saliva produced. Cancer chemotherapy causes acute problems that generally resolve after therapy and damaged tissue heals; radiotherapy can cause both acute and chronic damage that may leave patients with lifelong problems. Sialadenitis (infection of the salivary gland) may also be a consequence of chemo-/radiotherapy. Both quality and quantity of saliva flow can be affected by chemotherapy affecting saliva components, for example amylase and immunoglobulin A (IgA). This can lead to complications with dryness and the consequences related to severe xerostomia.

Radiotherapy is one of the most common treatment modalities for HNC. It may be used alone or in combination with chemotherapy and/or surgery. Radiation therapy may lead to a rapid decline in salivary flow during the first week of radiation, with eventual reduction of 95% in the region. Five weeks after treatment both stimulated and unstimulated (resting) flow are inhibited, virtually ceasing, and complete recovery is rare. Significant progress has been made to spare salivary gland function chiefly due to advances in radiation techniques, for example IMRT. Other strategies have also been developed, such as radioprotectors, identification and preservation/expansion of salivary stem cells by stimulation with cholinergic muscarinic agonists, and application of new lubricating or stimulatory agents, surgical transfer of submandibular glands, and acupuncture (see Table 27.1).

It is thought that the oral mucosa is more vulnerable to the effects of radiation on DNA, and that this may be why the salivary glands are so vulnerable to the effects of high-energy radiation and why there is little recovery long term once the glands are damaged. Xerostomia can be severe and last months, years, and, in some cases, a lifetime. The peak of salivary-gland damage occurs typically around six months after radiotherapy, with chemotherapy in addition to irradiation known to exacerbate xerostomia. A review in the *Annals of Palliative Medicine* in 2020 (Snider and Paine 2020) estimated 81–100% of patients experience clinically significant xerostomia during radiotherapy. The majority of patients reported or were objectively found to have xerostomia from one month up to two years and beyond following treatment. Children report less xerostomia with cancer therapy than adults. Xerostomia is a major QoL issue for this group of patients.

Saliva and Its Role in Oral Health

Saliva is a complex oral fluid comprising a mixture of secretions from major and minor salivary glands, with additional contributions by crevicular fluid. Saliva promotes health in the mouth via lubrication and protection. Saliva flow varies depending on stimulation. At rest, for example when sleeping, there is a small continuous flow that coats the soft and hard tissues of the oral cavity. Around 80–90% of daily saliva produced is in response to some mechanical, gustatory, olfactory, or pharmacological stimulation.

Normal daily saliva production varies between 0.5 and 1.5 l. Saliva is produced by three pairs of major salivary glands – parotid, submandibular, and sublingual – and hundreds of minor salivary glands that are found throughout the mouth – especially the lips and soft palate. Saliva is 99% water (hence the importance of hydration). The remaining 1% is composed of organic and inorganic compounds, that is electrolytes, enzymes, and proteins. The loss of salivary proteins and electrolytes accelerates the caries process, affects the development and tenacity of plaque biofilm, and increases the risk of periodontal inflammation and potential oral infections. Saliva flow can be affected by one gland hypofunction or a number/all salivary glands.

Comparison of Stimulated and Unstimulated Saliva Flow in Healthy and Xerostomic Individuals

Unstimulated and stimulated saliva flow for persons with normal health and with xerostomia is as follows:

	Normal health	Xerostomia
Unstimulated saliva flow	0.3–0.5 ml/minute	0.7–0.1 ml/minute
Stimulated saliva flow	1–2 ml/minute	<0.1 ml/minute

Table 27.1 HNC treatment modalities.

Treatment modifications to prevent occurrence of xerostomia as a long-term side effect of HNC treatment.	IMRT irradiation schemes have the potential to spare crucial structures (e.g. salivary glands) from exposure to high radiation doses while being able to better shape the high-level irradiation to the target volume. IMRT schemes have been shown to reduce long-term problems with xerostomia. Relocate the submandibular salivary gland. Customised mouth-opening devices (intraoral stents). Protectants, that is chemical or biochemical agents that help to prevent or reduce radiation damage to healthy cells and tissues. Preclinical research: autologous stem cell transplantation has been proposed as a prevention of long-term xerostomia caused by radiation damage to salivary glands.	All aim to reduce damage and side effects including dry mouth. Amifostine is the most clinically used chemical radioprotector, but its effect in patients treated with radiation is not consistent. Systematic review showed that amifostine significantly reduced serious mucositis, acute/late xerostomia, and dysphagia without protection of the tumour in HNSCC patients treated with radiotherapy. There is evidence to suggest that amifostine prevents the feeling of dry mouth in people receiving radiotherapy to the head and neck (with or without chemotherapy) in the short term (end of radiotherapy) to medium term (three months postradiotherapy). However, it is less clear whether or not this effect is sustained to 12 months postradiotherapy.	
Use of prescribed medication to *increase saliva production* (for those with residual saliva flow) – often accompanied by side effects.	Pilocarpine hydrochloride: Tablets are licensed for the treatment of xerostomia following radiation therapy for HNC in the UK. Pilocarpine acts by opening the inefficient drainage channels in the trabecular meshwork. It is only effective in those with some residual salivary gland function. A review by Mercadante at UCL (Mercadante et al. 2017) concluded that pilocarpine and cevimeline should represent the first line of therapy in HNC survivors with radiotherapy-induced xerostomia and hyposalivation.	Available studies suggest that approximately half of patients will respond, but side effects can be problematic. Side effects usually are the result of generalised parasympathomimetic stimulation (e.g. sweating, headaches, urinary frequency, vasodilatation). Side effect rates were dose dependent. See full British National Formulary (BNF) guidance on use (https://bnf.nice.org.uk/drug/pilocarpine.html).	Contraindications include many lung conditions, such as asthma, cardiac problems, epilepsy, and Parkinson's disease; side effects include flushing, increased urination, increased perspiration, and GI disturbances.
	Malic and ascorbic acid.		Not suitable for anyone with natural teeth as they cause demineralisation.
	SalivaMAX (available by prescription in the US) is a supersaturated calcium phosphate powder that when dissolved in water becomes a solution with high electrolyte concentration.		
	Cevimeline *is not currently licensed for use in the* UK.		
	Some studies report that low-level laser therapy may be effective in mitigating salivary hypofunction and increasing salivary pH in HNC radiotherapy patients with benefits to QoL.		

A reduction in saliva flow reduces buffering action and increases the number of pathogenic microorganisms in the oral cavity. Saliva maintains neutral pH between 6 and 7.4, buffering, remineralising (calcium and phosphate), and neutralising acids and sugars in the mouth – both ingested and regurgitated. Saliva's buffering capacity and flow are directly related to the rate and extent of demineralisation. It promotes remineralisation by providing calcium, phosphate, and fluoride to enamel and dentine. Critical pH for enamel demineralisation is 5.5, for dentine 6.4.

Saliva contributes to pellicle formation, aids the self-cleansing mechanism, and plays a protective role via its many antimicrobial, antiviral, and antifungal properties (mucin, histatins, lysozyme, and lactoferrin) to maintain a healthy microflora. Reduced saliva affects microbial colonisation and proliferation in the oral cavity, increasing dysbiosis of bacterial plaque biofilm.

Saliva aids speech (formation of sounds), digestion (amylase), mastication, and deglutition. It is essential for taste perception and plays a role in and aids sensory perception, for example for pain and texture. A 2020 study identified a significant decrease in both unstimulated and stimulated salivary flow rate with the severity of progression of chronic periodontitis (Vallabhan et al. 2020). It is important to recognise an individual's oral health status at HNC diagnosis to identify potential risks to oral health and plan preventative strategies.

Diagnosis of xerostomia is based on history and clinical examination. HNC therapy will exacerbate xerostomia if present at diagnosis or because of HNC treatment. Xerostomia should be addressed both by home care/management and appropriate professional support and treatment. The aim is to obtain and maintain oral health, prevent disease, and avoid QoL issues.

Assessment

Assessment is by a combination of patient-reported questionnaire and clinical inspection: ALF – ask, look, feel. Clinically, there needs to be a visual examination of the soft and hard tissues and quantitative saliva flow (sialometry). Sialometry is the objective measurement of saliva flow, stimulated and unstimulated.

There are several assessment and diagnostic tools available. The Challacombe Scale of clinical oral dryness (clinical oral dryness score, or CODS) is reliable and easy to use for assessment of severity of dry mouth (Das and Challacombe 2016). A light source and mouth mirror are all that is required. The scale works as an additive score from 1 to 10, 1 being the least, 10 most severe. Clear images and descriptors aid assessment with guidance offered on recommended treatment.

CODS is closely related to both the unstimulated salivary flow and the thickness of the mucin layer over the epithelium (mucosal wetness), suggesting a physiological basis to the feeling of xerostomia. A low CODS (1–3) indicates mild dryness manageable normally in general practice, whereas a high CODS (7–10) is an indication for referral for further investigation and/or specialist care.

A simple index for symptoms of xerostomia (Bother Index CCMed Ltd 2018; see Figure 27.1) has also been developed and correlates well with CODS and more objective measures of hyposalivation. The Xerostomia Bother Index was developed in conjunction with health care professionals to help indicate the severity to which a patient's QoL is being affected by xerostomia. It is a simple, easy-to-use tool that can be completed by the patient, a clinician, a carer, or a family/friend. A five-point scale is used to illustrate the extent to which the patient is affected by the symptom.

Examples of other assessment tools for assessing xerostomia include Regional Oral Dryness Inventory (RODI) and Xerostomia Inventory (with modifications).

Treatment

Treatment for HNC aims to reduce impact on salivary glands when possible. Treatment for xerostomia and salivary hypo function mainly consists of palliative care.

HNC treatment modalities are constantly under review to remove or reduce complications and side effects of treatment. Some of these can be seen in Table 27.1.

Oral Health Care for HNC Patients with Xerostomia

Aim to start HNC treatment from a state of optimal oral health. This will reduce side effects of treatment. Following HNC diagnosis patients should be encouraged to visit their dentist and tell them when HNC treatment is due to start. Extraction of teeth with questionable prognosis should be completed before radiotherapy as extractions afterwards may result in osteoradionecrosis. An appointment with a dental hygienist/therapist should be made as soon as possible. These visits are important to

Xerostomia Bother Index

The **Xerostomia Bother Index** was developed in conjunction with Healthcare Professionals. It helps to indicate how severely a persons their quality of life is effected by their Dry Mouth symptoms.

The form can be completed by a clinician, carer, family/friend, or by the patient themselves.

Circle the number on the scale that best illustrates the severity of the symptom. Score all symptoms. If you do not suffer from the symptom still score it, as 0.

Name: Date: / /

		None				Severe
1	Dry / Cracked Lips	0	1	2	3	4
2	Cracked corners of the mouth	0	1	2	3	4
3	Burning rough tongue	0	1	2	3	4
4	Halitosis (bad breath)	0	1	2	3	4
5	Thick sticky saliva in the corners of the mouth	0	1	2	3	4
6	Frequent thirst	0	1	2	3	4
7	Difficulty eating, swallowing, talking	0	1	2	3	4
8	Increase in plaque and/or decay	0	1	2	3	4
9	Sore bleeding gums	0	1	2	3	4
10	Difficulty wearing dentures	0	1	2	3	4
11	Disturbed sleep (due to dry mouth)	0	1	2	3	4
12	Other	0	1	2	3	4

The Xerostomia Bother Index is a subjective tool. Inevitably there will be a degree of inter-observer variability. However, it can help identify areas for further investigation and possible clinical intervention.

A.S SALIVA ORTHANA Dry Mouth Relief

CCMed Ltd, BN21 3TE - Tel: 01264 332172
Emaill: info@CCMed.co.uk - www.CCMed.co.uk
Twitter: @DryMouth_Relief - Facebook: Saliva Orthana

A.S SALIVA ORTHANA Dry Mouth Relief

Figure 27.1 The Xerostomia Bother Index (CCMed.co.uk 2018). *Source:* Xerostomia Bother Index/CCMed Ltd.

assess the current oral health status of the patient, educate and motivate the patient, gather baseline data as a benchmark to monitor oral health throughout treatment, and develop a preventive plan for disease and to support the patient's oral health throughout and beyond cancer diagnosis. Professional dental care should be accessible, timely, and flexible. Does the patient have the knowledge, skills, and motivation to implement the necessary oral health care? A multidisciplinary approach will enable the best care for the patient to manage and reduce short- and long-term consequences of xerostomia.

Big picture thought: Address funding issues for patients to access appropriate dental services. Consider the use of a 'voucher' scheme for patients to use locally, for example at dental practices if tertiary care does not offer access (distance travelled/time etc.) to suitable care – for example hygiene therapy.

HNC patients are managed by a multidisciplinary team. Get to know them and build good working relationships. Sharing knowledge and skills is important so patients get clear, unambiguous advice – 'everyone singing from the same hymn sheet'. Keep in mind that these multidisciplinary team members may well change through a patient's cancer journey. Be flexible and prioritise care plans. Retain contemporaneous records. Patient education should reflect the COM-B model of behaviour change. These patients are often overloaded with information and advice – some will need more frequent attendance than others and require more support. Involve the patient and carer/family as appropriate. Some patients may not have visited a dental practice for many years and may not grasp the significance of good oral health in the context of their diagnosis of HNC. Follow up verbal advice with written material/useful links for the patients'/carers' future reference and review.

Develop an oral care plan and communicate with the patient, carers, and other team members. Be prepared to modify to suit symptoms as they develop or diminish. The aim of treatment is to reduce and limit complications in terms of preventing disease, controlling symptoms, maintaining function, and comfort. It is important to explain what to expect in terms of oral health with an HNC diagnosis and advise how to manage symptoms. One size does not fit all.

Treatment for xerostomia may be divided into categories:

Category	Example	Options
Identification and treatment of pre-existing disease/condition that contributes to xerostomia	Uncontrolled diabetes Sjogren's syndrome HIV/AIDS Parkinson's disease Gastroesophageal reflux disease	Improve management/control Liaise with GP, specialist, other health care providers, for example diabetes nurse
Identification and management of any medications that contribute to xerostomia. prescribed and OTC	High blood pressure medication Antidepressants Decongestants	Is there an alternative? Liaise with prescriber Discuss with patient re use of OTC medications
Identification and management of lifestyle factors that contribute to xerostomia	Smoking Alcohol Caffeine, for example tea, coffee, soft drinks Mouth breathing Recreational drugs, for example medicinal cannabis	The dental team has a key role supporting patients to mitigate lifestyle factors

Patient Education

The Mouth Cancer Foundation has published a booklet for patients that can be downloaded at https://www.mouthcancerfoundation.org/wp-content/uploads/2021/02/mouth-cancer-foundation-handbook.pdf (Mouth Cancer Foundation 2021).

A combination of treatment strategies is necessary for short and long-term management of xerostomia.

Home Self-Care

A 2019 study concluded that poor oral hygiene is both a risk and a prognostic factor of HNC (Chang et al. 2019). Excellent oral hygiene and effective personal mouth care reduce complications both short and long term from xerostomia.

The HNC cancer patient may require frequent supportive hygiene therapy. Invasive treatment must be in conjunction with the medical team and specialists to ensure it is safe to provide treatment at that time. Professional mechanical plaque removal (PMPR) with a toothbrush will not create any more bacteraemia than would be created by the patient at home. This may be appropriate if for whatever reason the patient is unable to carry out daily plaque removal. These visits enable clinicians to monitor oral health, modify treatment plans, and offer support.

Visit https://maxfacts.uk/help/oral-hygiene/practical-guide (Maxfacts 2020).

The aim of personal oral hygiene is to remove plaque biofilm effectively and regularly to maintain health without damaging the hard or soft tissues.

Toothbrushing

Toothbrushing should be done at least two times/day, at night plus at least one other time. Focus on technique and effectiveness over tools. Some oral hygiene aids can be adapted for dexterity issues. An electric or manual toothbrush may be used – if electric select rechargeable. Heads should be changed regularly, and storage of all oral hygiene kits should be out of contact with anyone else's oral care brushes to reduce risk of cross infection. A 360 toothbrush can be an effective tool to remove dried debris and secretions from the soft tissues. (In conjunction with an antimicrobial rinse it can make a significant difference to comfort.) If mucositis or soreness is experienced, a supersoft toothbrush may be required initially, for example TePe Special Care, Curaprox ATI, or a supersoft head for an electric brush – Curaprox Hydrosonic Pro brush; the single tuft head and narrow neck of the small sensitive soft standard head may help with trismus or limited opening. A single tuft brush or a toothbrush with a child-sized head may make brushing easier for anyone with limited opening. A sonic suction brush is also now available for home use (G100) for anyone at risk of aspiration.

Toothpaste

A pea-sized amount of high fluoride toothpaste (at least 1450 ppm) should be used. Spread around the teeth first before brushing each surface of all teeth. Use SLS-free low abrasive fluoride toothpaste – sodium lauryl sulphate is a foaming agent in many toothpastes that can aggravate ulceration or mucositis. There are a number of SLS-free fluoride toothpastes available OTC, for example Sensodyne Pronamel. Some patients will not tolerate mint flavour, finding it too 'stingy'. OraNurse toothpaste is SLS and flavour free with 1450 ppm fluoride. Oralieve is ultra-mild mint and SLS free. Others are also available, for example Biotene and Xerostom. A very high fluoride toothpaste may be indicated for anyone suffering xerostomia at high risk of caries. These are prescription-only medicines that can be prescribed by either a doctor or dentist. Both are mild mint and contain SLS: Duraphat 2800 ppm and Duraphat 5000. These patients should continue use while they remain high risk – in particular root caries risk.

Interdental Cleaning

Interdental cleaning (IDC) is a key part of biofilm control and should be established before HNC treatment starts, using previously established IDC methods in conjunction with an oral care professional. Avoid trauma. A waterflosser may be an option for IDC, and/or general debridement with or without the use of an appropriate mouthwash.

Tongue Cleaning

Tongue cleaning as part of an oral hygiene routine will reduce plaque and debris buildup on the dorsum of the tongue and can help reduce the risk of candida infection and oral malodour. A tongue scraper is generally accepted as more effective than a toothbrush. The tongue should be cleaned daily from the posterior to anterior to reduce trauma to papilla. An inverted teaspoon may also be used to clean the dorsum of the tongue.

Use of Disclosing Agents

Use of disclosing agents can be beneficial in improving plaque biofilm removal. Tablets, liquids, and toothpaste are available. Use in conjunction with a mouth mirror.

Prosthesis Care

Leave a prosthesis, for example dentures, out at night and follow cleaning, disinfecting, and storage according to professional advice. Denture/prosthesis/appliance care guidelines can be found at https://www.dentalhealth.org/pages/faqs/category/downloads (Oral Health Foundation 2022).

Rinsing with water before replacing in mouth or use of lubricant improves comfort. Use a small amount of fixative if necessary. Leave denture out at night unless otherwise advised. Candida infections are common – monitor and treat if present. NB Some patients may have other types of oral appliances that will also require thorough hygiene.

After Use Care

After use all oral hygiene brushes should be cleaned under running water – this includes denture care tools.

Excellent oral hygiene as a starting point pre-HNC treatment significantly reduces the risk of mucositis and other unwanted and unpleasant complications during treatment.

Use of Adjuncts

Use of adjuncts for home care should be on an individual risk-based approach and modified as required. The patient may be unable to complete or tolerate personal mechanical plaque removal. Alternatives need to be acceptable and effective and limited in use until mechanical plaque biofilm control can be re-established.

The increased risk of dental caries in HNC patients is due to accumulation of tenacious plaque biofilm and frequent and prolonged exposure to sugars (often in the effort to relieve symptoms of xerostomia). The use of sugar-free chewing gum and/or sucking sugar-free sweets (preferably with xylitol) can reduce caries risk. Dentate patients should be aware of acidic potential of some sugar-free products.

Adjuncts may include mouthwash, although it is not an alternative to physical plaque biofilm disruption. As alcohol has a drying effect on the soft tissues, select alcohol-free varieties with beneficial active ingredients for the individual patient. Use at a different time of day to toothbrushing unless advised. Alcohol-free chlorhexidine may be used short term when any form of physical plaque removal is impossible. This should be used on recommendation of a dental professional. Use of alcohol-free fluoride mouth rinse at a different time of day to brushing is recommended for high caries risk patients.

Adjuncts may also include remineralising products for home use for high caries risk patients, or use of topical amorphous calcium phosphate/casein phosphopeptide (ACP/CCP) products or fluoride gels – either applied topically or in custom trays, for example GC MI Paste Plus or GC Tooth Mousse.

Food and Drink

See https://hncf.org.uk/patient-friendly-recipes for recipes (Head & Neck Cancer Foundation 2022). A healthy diet is import for recovery, maintaining the integrity of oral hard and soft tissues, and aiding resistance to infection and wound healing. Dietician/nutritional guidance in relation to oral and overall health should be in line with the Eatwell guide (Public Health England 2016) and in conjunction with a dietician as necessary.

For oral health, advice should be personal, practical, and positive and in line with Delivering Better Oral Health (DBOH) guidance. The following are some important points and suggestions:

- Keep mouth moist.
- Ensure adequate hydration – take sips of water frequently (or other sugar-free, neutral-pH fluids). Consider alternatives to sugar in tea/coffee if taken, for example granulated xylitol. (NB Not all products suitable for vegans/vegetarians/others on selective diets.)
- Suck ice chips.
- Rinse with water after eating and keep water at bedside when sleeping.
- Drink water or nonalcoholic/sugar-free liquid when eating. Avoid dry, hard, crunchy foods or soften in liquids.
- Take small bites and eat slowly. Choose soft, high-liquid foods and moisten foods. Avoid spicy and salty food.

- Diet advice specific to oral health (i.e. DBOH) – reduce amount and frequency of sugary and acidic food and drinks. Don't eat/drink sugar or acidic food/drink last thing at night or before sleeping.
- Suggest alternatives – collaborate with dietician as necessary.
- Sugar-free sweets/candies and chewing gums that contain xylitol are intended to stimulate salivary flow and can provide transient relief of xerostomia. Xylitol and in some cases erythritol added to such products helps prevent caries. Such products have been shown to have more positive effects than lubricants in post-RT and haemodialysis patients. NB Some sugar-free sweets may be acidic and increase risk of dental erosion and use should be on a risk/benefit basis.
- Saliva aids digestion, buffering, remineralisation, lubrication, tissue coating and is antimicrobial.
- Explain what and why.

Compromised quality and quantity of saliva flow can result in some or all the following:

Sign/symptom	Consequences – oral, dental, and QoL	Mitigation - aim to prevent, control, and maintain integrity of hard and soft tissues	
Oral cavity		**Patient/carer**	**Professional**
Viscous, sticky, frothy saliva	Poor or no buffering capacity increasing risk of caries, erosion, and gingival and periodontal inflammation	Sips of water Use of sugar-free gum, candies (look for those with xylitol). Check potential acidic challenge	Recommend products and advise on use, which can vary by brand Review regularly and modify as necessary
Atrophic mucosa			
Oral mucositis			
Candidiasis	Increased bulk and tenacity of plaque biofilm	Regular tongue cleaning	Perform regular PMPR as appropriate
Mouth ulcers			
Dry cracked lips and commissures		Regular lip moisturising/balm	
	Increased risk of infection and trauma		Product example - Oralieve Nourishing Lip Care
Loss of surface papilla; erythema of tongue; rough, fissured tongue, often coated	Difficulty eating, which may impact nutritional status	Alternative oral hygiene procedures, for example use of alcohol-free chlorhexidine mouth rinse for short term until personal plaque control can be performed	Guided biofilm therapy, where plaque biofilm is removed from soft and hard tissues using erythritol, may have benefits in maintaining a healthy oral microflora and reducing complications
Parotid gland enlargement	Difficulty speaking	Extra-soft toothbrush	
(Sialadenitis) Salivary gland infection	Ineffective self-cleansing mechanism	Products that reduce pain and promote healing, for example those with hyaluronic acid, such as Gengigel First Aid, Oracoat Renewing Melts, Oracoat XyliMelts	
Mouth 'sore' painful	Inability to maintain adequate oral hygiene	Dry mouth gels – various manufacturers	
Poor sleep patterns	Abrasion/trauma to soft tissues as they may become very friable	Use of humidifier – especially at nighttime Keep water at bedside to sip	Recommend short-term use of chlorhexidine mouthwash/gel until mechanical plaque removal can be performed Product example – Corsodyl, Curasept ADS Implant
	Tiredness, irritability, poor motivation to comply with self-care routines		
			Increase frequency of PMPR

Sign/symptom	Consequences – oral, dental, and QoL	Mitigation - aim to prevent, control, and maintain integrity of hard and soft tissues	
Oral cavity		**Patient/carer**	**Professional**
Feeling of dryness or burning sensation Increased thirst Dysphonia (hoarseness) Speaking – voice disturbances, tongue sticks to palate leading to 'clicky' speech Dysgeusia (bad taste) Diminished/altered sense of taste Oral malodour (halitosis)	Trauma to soft tissues Dentures and prosthesis 'rubbing'. Inability to maintain adequate plaque control. Lack of lubrication of soft tissues. Increased risk of infection	Identify and resolve any roughness on prostheses, restorations, or teeth that may increase trauma Use of fixatives to aid retention Rinse before placing in mouth Massage gels/lubricants with finger or 360 brush IDC – use waterflosser, extra-soft interdental brush as advised Tongue cleaning Products specific to oral malodour, for example Ultradex mouth rinse/spray	Examples of products that may ease symptoms: those with hyaluronic acid, such as Gengigel First Aid, Oracoat Renewing Melts, Oralieve gel, Biotene gel, XyliMelts, Bioxtra gel, Xerostom gel Product examples – CB12 Sugar-free gums and sweets, for example Chewsy, Peppersmith, Dr Heff's mints, Dr John's range, some Wrigley's
Sensitive to spicy, salty foods	Mint oral hygiene products may not be tolerated	Mint-free toothpastes, for example OraNurse Mild mint pastes, for example Oralieve, Biotene, Xerostom, and others	
Dysphagia - difficulty swallowing especially dry foods Difficulty chewing Residual food debris	Increased risk of caries, oral malodour	360 brush to aid cleaning sulcus, palate, and other soft tissues. Rinse after eating. Sip water when eating. Avoid hard, dry foods Avoid sugar-containing food and drink - keep to mealtimes/avoid before sleeping.	Dr. John's fresh breath pops (contain ascorbic and citric acid, increasing risk of erosion) Sugar-free gum and sweets
Teeth			
Caries - rapid increase in incidence. Atypical sites, for example cervical, incisal edges, cusps Dental erosion Dentine hypersensitivity	Exposed tooth and root surfaces are at high risk of rampant caries	Daily use of high-fluoride toothpaste 1450 ppm or prescribed 2800 ppm or 5000 ppm Alcohol-free fluoride mouth rinse, OTC or prescribed Sodium fluoride mouthwash 0.05% or sodium fluoride mouthwash 2%. Topical fluoride and/or ACP/CCP for home (direct application or in trays) Xylitol products Desensitising toothpaste use	Regular dental care to monitor and support home care, including dental hygiene visits. Product example – Duraphat toothpaste 2800/5000 Sugar-free chewing gum with xylitol, for example Chewsy, Peppersmith Topical fluoride varnish application, up to four/year Topical fluoride/xylitol gel/mousse application four/year in trays in surgery, for example Flairesse Professional application of desensitiser, for example chlorhexidine varnish, fluoride varnish
Difficulty wearing dentures - removing and/or replacing	Long-term removal and long-term inability to wear. Can impact diet nutritional status, loss of confidence, and other QoL factors	Use of fixative advice and care of remaining teeth, periodontium Treatment and control of denture stomatitis and other candida infection	Denture hygiene Possible refit/replace dentures long term

(Continued)

Sign/symptom	Consequences – oral, dental, and QoL	Mitigation - aim to prevent, control, and maintain integrity of hard and soft tissues	
Oral cavity		**Patient/carer**	**Professional**
Periodontium			
Gingival inflammation – gingivitis /periodontitis	Increased risk of gingival inflammation and periodontal destruction	Daily effective plaque biofilm control using suitable IDC, toothbrush, and toothpaste with suitable adjunct, for example mouthwash as appropriate	Oral hygiene instruction – COM-B Increase frequency of PMPR
Teeth don't feel 'clean'	Difficulty controlling plaque biofilm - effectiveness and motivation	Focus on what can be done, encourage and seek assistance from carer if necessary	Adjunctive use of antimicrobials Increased frequency of PMPR

Dry Mouth Relief

Dry mouth relief aims to stimulate saliva flow and/or maintain the integrity of the soft tissues, that is saliva replacements, lubricants, and stimulants. Saliva stimulants (sialagogues) are suitable for anyone with residual saliva gland function. Sugar-free chewing gum, candies, and mints can be used to stimulate salivary output.

A 2011 Cochrane review found that there is no strong evidence that any topical preparation is better than simple measures for treatment of xerostomia (Furness et al. 2011). Artificial saliva is frequently used and may help to relieve symptoms. For many, trial and error may be the only way to identify what works for a specific patient. Some manufacturers have trial size products that can be useful, for example Oralieve and Xerostom.

Saliva substitutes should simulate natural human saliva and provide long-lasting hydration of the oral mucosa. They should be inexpensive, edible and easy to swallow, and retainable in the mouth to reduce the number of reapplications. Saliva substitutes contain agents to increase viscosity (cellulose derivatives), such as carboxymethylcellulose or hydroxyethyl cellulose, mucins, xanthan gum, linseed oil, polyethylene oxide, buffering agents such as calcium, phosphate, and fluoride ions, preservatives such as methyl or propyl paraben, flavouring such as xylitol or sorbitol, and related agents. It is important that they also contain salivary enzymes such as lactoperoxidase, lysozyme, and lactoferrin, which help protect the mouth from bacterial and fungal infections.

Saliva substitutes are available on prescription and OTC in various forms. These may be liquids, sprays, gels, oils, lozenges, mouth rinses, chewing gums, toothpastes, and mucoadhesive disks. Many are not available on prescription with cost for some patients, proving prohibitive for long-term use. Products and instructions differ between manufacturers. Patients should follow instructions on each to maximise benefit.

The following are all listed in the BNF and available on prescription for the treatment of xerostomia. Check local prescribing guidance.

Name	Detail	Dose	Availability
AS Saliva Orthana® lozenges Do not contain fluoride	Mucin 65 mg, xylitol 59 mg, in a sorbitol basis, pH neutral	One lozenge as required, allow to dissolve slowly in the mouth	
AS Saliva Orthana oral spray may be prescribed	Gastric mucin (porcine) 3.5%, xylitol 2%, sodium fluoride 4.2 mg/l, with preservatives and flavouring agents, pH neutral	Apply two to three sprays as required, spray onto oral and pharyngeal mucosa	Dental practitioners' formulary
Biotene Oralbalance® Replacement Gel may be prescribed as artificial saliva gel	Lactoperoxidase, lactoferrin, lysozyme, glucose oxidase, xylitol in a gel basis pH 6.0–7.5	Apply as required, apply to gums and tongue	Dental practitioners' formulary

Name	Detail	Dose	Availability
BioXtra® gel may be prescribed	Lactoperoxidase, lactoferrin, lysozyme, whey colostrum, xylitol and other ingredients	Apply as required, apply to oral mucosa	Dental practitioners' formulary
Glandosane® Aerosol Spray may be prescribed	Carmellose sodium 500 mg, sorbitol 1.5 g, potassium chloride 60 mg, sodium chloride 42.2 mg, magnesium chloride 2.6 mg, calcium chloride 7.3 mg, and dipotassium hydrogen phosphate 17.1 mg/50 g, pH 5.75	Apply as required, spray onto oral and pharyngeal mucosa	Dental practitioners' formulary
Oralieve gel moisturising gel	Contains traces of milk protein and egg white protein	Apply as required, particularly at night, to oral mucosa	
Oralieve Moisturising Mouth Spray	Aqua, glycerin, xylitol, poloxamer 407, sodium benzoate, monosodium phosphate, xanthan gum, aroma, disodium phosphate, benzoic acid, whey protein, lactoferrin, lactoperoxidase, potassium thiocyanate, glucose oxidase, SLS free, alcohol free, pH 5.8	One spray as required, on the inside of each cheek, gums, and tongue	
Saliveze® oral spray may be prescribed	Carmellose sodium (sodium carboxymethylcellulose), calcium chloride, magnesium chloride, potassium chloride, sodium chloride, and dibasic sodium phosphate, pH neutral	Apply one spray as required, spray onto oral mucosa	Dental practitioners' formulary
Salivix® may be prescribed as artificial saliva pastilles	Sugar free, reddish-amber, acacia, malic acid, and other ingredients	One unit as required, suck pastille	Dental practitioners' formulary
SST® May be prescribed as saliva stimulating tablets	Sugar free, citric acid, malic acid, and other ingredients in a sorbitol base	One tablet as required, allow tablet to dissolve slowly in the mouth	Dental practitioners' formulary
Xerotin Oral Spray may be prescribed as artificial saliva oral spray	Sugar free, water, sorbitol, carmellose (carboxymethylcellulose), potassium chloride, sodium chloride, potassium phosphate, magnesium chloride, calcium chloride, and other ingredients, pH neutral.	One spray as required.	Dental practitioners' formulary

Source: https://bnf.nice.org.uk/treatment-summary/dry-mouth.html.

Some of the above are also available OTC. As new products are developed it is incumbent that anyone caring for HNC patients stay abreast of options available.

NB The pH of some saliva substitute and stimulant products may increase risk of acid erosion, and this should be considered in dentate patients. Do the benefits outweigh the risk? Can the risks be managed or countered, for example increasing fluoride exposure. Lemon and glycerine swabs should *NOT* be used as the acidity causes oral problems after short periods of use.

A wide range of subjective reports appear in the literature on which is the 'best' saliva substitute. Saliva substitutes, for example SalivaMAX, are used to replace saliva, with most offering relatively short-term relief. They need to be reapplied regularly. Artificial saliva can be used as required, but as it is swallowed swiftly, the moisturising and lubrication also have a limited time span.

Xerostomia is a subjective measurement of oral dryness and as such what will ease symptoms for one may not have the same impact for another. Treatment should focus on patient lifestyle modification and creating an environment conducive to health and well-being. A combination of products, for example gel and mucoadhesive disk or mouthwash and gel, often proves most beneficial.

Alternative Therapies

Alternative therapies and treatments for dry mouth that have been cited in the literature include:

- *Acupuncture* following radiotherapy has been used to relieve xerostomia symptoms for some time. Many patients achieve relief, even for symptoms refractory to pilocarpine therapy. A regimen of three to four weekly treatments followed by monthly sessions is now recommended, although some patients achieve lasting response without further therapy.

- *Botulinum toxin* is reported in the literature as a promising pharmacological approach for xerostomia induced by HNC treatments. To date no established protocols for its use could be found.
- Topical lycopene-enriched *virgin olive oil* showed an improvement in QoL scores and reduction in xerostomia symptoms.
- A novel edible saliva substitute in the form of an *oral moisturising jelly* (OMJ) has shown promising results over a saliva gel. Various disciplines including dentistry, nursing, medicine, and food sciences collaborated to develop OMJ. OMJ is a ready-to-eat gel with a semisolid appearance that dissolves in the mouth.
- As hydrogel technology and buccal mucoadhesive polymers that allow continuous substance release advance, new and more novel treatment options will become available. *Mucoadhesive disks* are available in the UK and can be stuck to the palate or buccal mucosa/tooth. They contain lubricating agents, flavouring, and antimicrobial agents.

Patients will find many alternative therapies and home care remedies when searching for treatment for xerostomia. These can be relatively cost effective and easy to use, for example small spray bottles purchased at larger chemists and filled with water to spray as required. Others include Chinese herbal medicine – herbs such as aloe, ginger, or spilanthes have all claimed to be of some benefit for xerostomia. Pineapple juice or its extracts are often recommended, claiming to improve subjective oral dryness. With a pH between 3.2 and 4 the negative consequences of long term use become obvious.

When faced with questions from patients, consider the potential benefit versus the cost in terms of increased risk of oral disease and expense.

Summary

Xerostomia is a common and unpleasant side effect of HNC therapy. The consequences of xerostomia can compromise oral health, nutrition, and general health and impact QoL. Management involves patient education to control symptoms and prevent complications, along with professional support to create and maintain an oral environment that is conducive to health and well-being.

Patient education:

Ask – is there something that can be done to improve oral health and/or QoL?

Advise – ensure advice is personal, practical, and positive.

Act – in the best interests of the patient, providing an oral care plan that will prevent disease and promote oral health, overall health, and well-being.

Support – acknowledge, empathise, and consider capability, opportunity, and motivation.

References

Agostini, B.A., Cericato, G.O., Silveira, E.R.D. et al. (2018). How common is dry mouth? Systematic review and meta-regression analysis of prevalence estimates. *Braz. Dent. J.* 29 (6): 606–618.

CCMed.co.uk (2018). Xerostomia Bother Index. www.ccmed.co.uk/wp-content/uploads/2018/02/Bother-index_CCMed.pdf.

Chang, C.C., Lee, W.T., Hsiao, J.R. et al. (2019). Oral hygiene and the overall survival of head and neck cancer patients. *Cancer Med* 8 (4): 1854.

Das, P. and Challacombe, S.J. (2016). Dry mouth and clinical oral dryness scoring systems. https://www.researchgate.net/publication/322009020_Dry_Mouth_and_Clinical_Oral_Dryness_Scoring_Systems.

Djaali, W., Simadibrata, C.L., and Nareswari, I. (2020). Acupuncture therapy in post-radiation head-and-neck cancer with dysgeusia. *Med Acupunct* 32 (3): 157–162.

Felix, D.H., Luker, J., and Scully, C. (2012). Oral medicine: 4. Dry mouth and disorders of salivation. *Dent. Update* 39 (10): 738–743.

Furness, S., Worthington, H.V., Bryan, G. et al. (2011). Interventions for the management of dry mouth: topical therapies. *Cochrane. Database. Syst. Rev.* 12: (Article No.: CD008934).

Gonnelli, F.A.S., Palma, L.F., Giordani, A.J. et al. (2016). Low-level laser therapy for the prevention of low salivary flow rate after radiotherapy and chemotherapy in patients with head and neck cancer. *Radiol. Bras.* 49 (2): 86–91.

Harding, J. (2018). The cracker challenge – how it feels to have a dry mouth. *Dent. Nurs.* 14 (8): 402–405.

Head & Neck Cancer Foundation (2022). Patient-friendly recipes. https://hncf.org.uk/patient-friendly-recipes.

Maxfacts (2018). Dry mouth. https://maxfacts.uk/diagnosis/a-z/xerostomia/detailed.
Maxfacts (2020). Practical guide to oral hygiene. https://maxfacts.uk/help/oral-hygiene/practical-guide.
Mercadante, V., Arwa, A. H., Giovanni, L., et al. (2017). Interventions for the management of radiotherapy-induced xerostomia and hyposalivation: a systematic review and meta-analysis. https://discovery.ucl.ac.uk/id/eprint/1539876/1/Mercadante_Manuscript%20with%20authors.pdf.
Michie, S., Atkins, L., and West, R. (2014). *The Behaviour Change Wheel: A Guide to Designing Interventions*. Bream, UK: Silverback Publishing.
Mouth Cancer Foundation (2021). Supporting head & neck cancers. https://www.mouthcancerfoundation.org/wp-content/uploads/2021/02/mouth-cancer-foundation-handbook.pdf.
Oral Health Foundation (2022). Downloads and resources. https://www.dentalhealth.org/pages/faqs/category/downloads.
Public Health England (2016). The Eatwell Guide. https://www.gov.uk/government/publications/the-eatwell-guide.
Snider, J.W. and Paine, D.C. (2020). Sticky stuff: xerostomia in patients undergoing head and neck radiotherapy – prevalance, prevention, and palliative care. *Ann Palliat Med* 9 (3): 1340–1350.
Vallabhan, C.G., Sivarajan, S., Shivkumar, A.D. et al. (2020). Assessment of salivary flow rate in patients with chronic periodontitis. *J. Pharm. Bioall. Sci.* 12 (S1): 308–312.
Wolff, A., Joshi, R.K., Ekstrom, J. et al. (2017). A guide to medications inducing salivary gland dysfunction, xerostomia, and subjective sialorrhea: a systematic review sponsored by the World Workshop on Oral Medicine VI. *Drugs R. D.* 17 (1): 1–28.
Xu, F., Laguna, L., and Sarkar, A. (2019). Aging-related changes in quantity and quality of saliva: where do we stand in our understanding? *J. Texture Stud.* 50 (1): 27–35.

Further Reading

Abdollahi, M., Radfar, M., and Rahimi, R. (2008). Current opinion on drug-induced oral reactions: a comprehensive review. *J. Contemp. Dent. Pract.* 9 (3): 1–15.
American Dental Association (2021). Xerostomia (dry mouth). https://www.ada.org/en/member-center/oral-health-topics/xerostomia.
Assy, Z., Bots, C.P., Arisoy, H.Z. et al. (2021). Differences in perceived intra-oral dryness in various dry-mouth patients as determined using the regional oral dryness inventory. *Clin. Oral. Invest.* 25 (6): 4031–4043.
Bültzingslöwen, I., Sollecito, T.P., Fox, P.C. et al. (2007). Salivary dys-function associated with systemic diseases: systematic review and clinical management recommendations. *Oral. Surg. Oral. Med. Oral. Pathol. Oral. Radiol. Endod.* 103 (S57): 1–15.
Cohen-Brown, G. and Ship, J.A. (2004). Diagnosis and treatment of salivary gland disorders. *Quintessence. Int.* 35 (2): 108–123.
Davies, A.N. and Thompson, J. (2015). Parasympathomimetic drugs for the treatment of salivary gland dysfunction due to radiotherapy. *Cochrane. Library* https://doi.org/10.1002/14651858.cd003782.pub3.
de Almeida, P.D.V., Gregio, A.M.T., Machado, M.A.N. et al. (2008). Saliva composition and functions: a comprehensive review. *J. Contemp. Dent. Pract.* 9 (3): 72–80.
Effinger, K.E., Migliorati, C.A., Hudson, M.M. et al. (2014). Oral and dental late effects in survivors of childhood cancer: a Children's Oncology Group report. *Support. Care Cancer* 22 (7): 2009–2019.
Furness, S., Bryan, G., McMillan, R. et al. (2013). Interventions for the management of dry mouth: non-pharmacological interventions. *Cochrane Database Syst. Rev.* (9): (Article No.: CD009603).
Ghazzaoui, S.F. et al. (2016). Acupuntura para xerostomia e hipofluxo salivar: revisão de literatura. *Revista. Brasileira. De. Odontologia.* 73 (4): 340.
Gu, J., Zhu, S., Li, X. et al. (2014). Effect of amifostine in head and neck cancer patients treated with radiotherapy: a systematic review and meta-analysis based on randomized controlled trials. *PLoS One* 9 (5): e95968.
Humphrey, S.P. and Williamson, R.T. (2001). A review of saliva: normal composition, flow, and function. *J. Pros. Dent.* 85 (2): 162–169.
Iorgulescu, G. (2009). Saliva between normal and pathological: important factors in determining systemic and oral health. *J. Med. Life.* 2 (3): 303–307.
Jager, D.H.J., Bots, C.P., Forouzanfar, T., and Brand, H.S. (2018). Clinical oral dryness score: evaluation of a new screening method for oral dryness. *Odontol.* https://doi.org/10.1007/s10266-018-0339-4.
Johnstone, P., Niemtzow, R., and Riffenburgh, R. (2002). Acupuncture for xerostomia: clinical update. *Cancer* 94 (4): 1151–1156.

Llena-Puy, C. (2006). The role of saliva in maintaining oral health and as an aid to diagnosis. *Medicina. Oral, Patologia. Oral y. Cirugia. Bucal.* 11 (5): E449–E455.

Mese, H. and Matsuo, R. (2007). Salivary secretion, taste and hyposalivation. *J. Oral Rehabil.* 34 (10): 711–723.

Palma, L.F., Gonnelli, F.A.S., Marcucci, M. et al. (2017). Impact of low-level laser therapy on hyposalivation, salivary pH, and quality of life in head and neck cancer patients post-radiotherapy. *Lasers. Med. Sci.* 32 (4): 827–832.

Riley, P., Glenny, A.M., Hua, F. et al. (2017). Pharmacological interventions for preventing dry mouth and salivary gland dysfunction following radiotherapy. *Cochrane Library.* https://doi.org/10.1002/14651858.cd012744.

Thomson, M.W. (2007). Measuring change in dry-mouth symptoms over time using the xerostomia. *Invent. Gerodontol.* 24: 30–35.

28

The Role of Acupuncture in Radiotherapy-Induced Xerostomia

Andrea N. Beech

Gloucestershire Royal Hospital, Gloucester, UK

Background

Acupuncture involves the insertion of needles at specific points of the skin and is widely used for a range of illnesses and ailments as a complementary or alternative medicine. It is estimated that one million treatments are given in England each year. Acupuncture is commonly used to induce an analgesic effect and also to release muscular spasm through pressure point needle insertion. Neuroimaging research studies have shown acupuncture modulates activities in areas of the brain involved with pain signal processing.

As well as for analgesic effect, acupuncture can be used as a stimulant, and it is this application that could have use in improving saliva production. Despite this, the physiological effects have not been well studied with neuroimaging. The exact mechanism of action of acupuncture in the stimulation of saliva production is unknown. The following scientific possibilities exist as to how acupuncture may improve xerostomia:

1) Acupuncture at points in the head and neck area directly stimulates the nerves that stimulate the major salivary glands (parotid, submandibular, and sublingual glands).
2) The action of acupuncture interacts with certain components of the neuronal network involved in salivation.
3) There is a placebo effect through the expectation that acupuncture *will* increase salivary flow, as in Pavlovian conditioning.

In addition to scientific theories, other theories exist, including the use of a more holistic management of the body after radiotherapy and other cancer treatment, with acupuncture having been used in Chinese medicine for more than 3000 years. The stimulation of inserting the needles in to specific points on the skin to free the flow of energy, called ‘Qi’, is believed to encourage a healthy body state. It also is thought to improve blood flow of the skin overlying important structures such as the salivary glands.

The holistic theory in the use of acupuncture to stimulate saliva production can be emphasised by the calming environment and feeling of well-being whilst receiving acupuncture treatment following the insult of gruelling cancer treatment. The patient can also perceive that acupuncture is an attractive and minimally invasive treatment, showing as an improvement in saliva production that is not necessarily a ‘true’ improvement. Over the 12–18 month period after completion of radiotherapy, the body naturally recovers itself both physically and emotionally and regains its balance as a whole, therefore there is a strong indication that the use of acupuncture has a psychological impact to the feeling of improved saliva flow.

Care of Head and Neck Cancer Patients for Dental Hygienists and Dental Therapists, First Edition. Edited by Jocelyn J. Harding.

Evidence and true understanding of how acupuncture works is limited in the available literature. What is clear is that it can help some patients and is a useful and cost-effective treatment modality whether used exclusively or in conjunction with Western medical treatments.

Patient Assessment

It is a patient's perception of how dry the mouth is, rather than diagnostically proven saliva amount or radiotherapy dose or treatment duration – that is important. Patients who may benefit from acupuncture treatment are those who report a severely dry mouth with difficulty speaking, eating, and swallowing because of the lack of mouth wetting. Those who also have a very reduced taste, related to their low saliva amount, could also benefit.

Patients will often have tried drugs to stimulate salivary flow, such as a cholinergic agonist – for example, pilocarpine. Either these have been ineffective for them, the side effects such as stomach cramps and excess sweating are too troublesome for them to persevere, or they are reluctant to take medication at all.

It is useful to record how dry a patient's mouth is from 0 to 10 on a scale such as a visual analogue scale (VAS). It is also good practice to record separate scales for general mouth comfort, taste, difficulty eating, and difficulty swallowing on a questionnaire form. Following acupuncture treatment this can be helpful to see the amount of response each patient has had by getting the person to complete the same questionnaire at various points in treatment.

General assessment of the patient including medical and social history and medication history is important when planning any treatment. Contraindications to acupuncture treatment are needle phobia and any breaks in the skin or sores where the needles need to be placed. Anticoagulant or antiplatelet therapy is not contraindicated due to the size of the needles to be used. There is a time commitment to the treatment, and the patient must be prepared for weekly visits to the clinic, therefore a patient who is unable to commit to the treatment timetable is not suitable to embark on acupuncture.

It is important that patients have tried an exhaustive list of the topical options available to improve mouth wetting as described elsewhere in this publication. Not all patients will need acupuncture, and in most units access may be limited with long waits or unavailable. In addition it is important that patients appreciate that they will probably still need topical assistance for their dry mouth long term even if they find acupuncture useful.

Treatment

The recognised regime for treatment is every week for four weeks, then once monthly. If at three months (six treatment sessions) after commencing treatment there is no improvement, it is unlikely to begin to work at that point, and treatment may be abandoned. The total length of treatment is different for each person and depends on individual response.

The patient is positioned either in a dental chair or a bed. The needles are positioned after cleaning of the skin with an alcohol wipe. Needles are left in situ for 15 minutes while the patient is left in a quiet room with lights dimmed. At 15 minutes the needles can be rotated to provide further stimulation and left for a further 15 minutes before being removed.

Needle Position

The number of needles placed is eight – three in each ear and one in each forefinger in 'L1 – L2' position on both index fingers in the radial aspect. The exact position of each is demonstrated in Figures 28.1 and 28.2 (Johnstone et al. 2002). A sugar-free lozenge or sugar-free chewing gum can also be used whilst treatment takes place. *It is important to note that practitioners can vary with their positioning of acupuncture needles depending on their own training.*

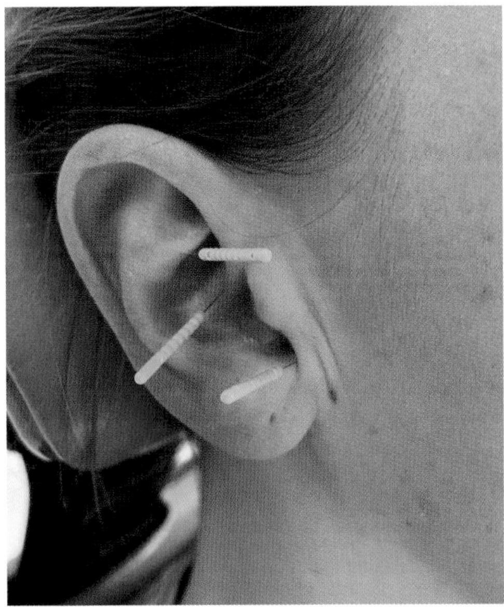
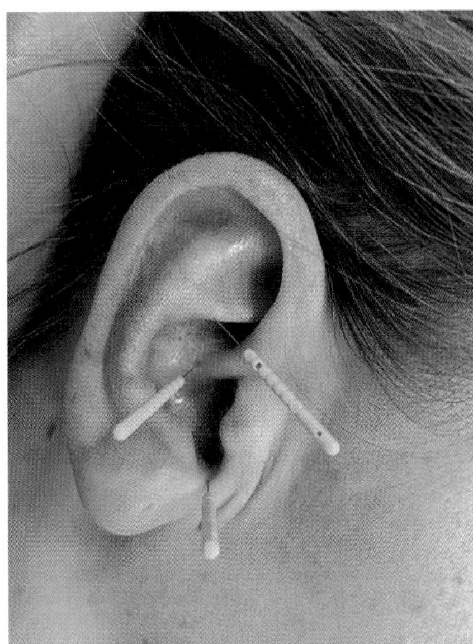

Figure 28.1 Needles in position in the ear.

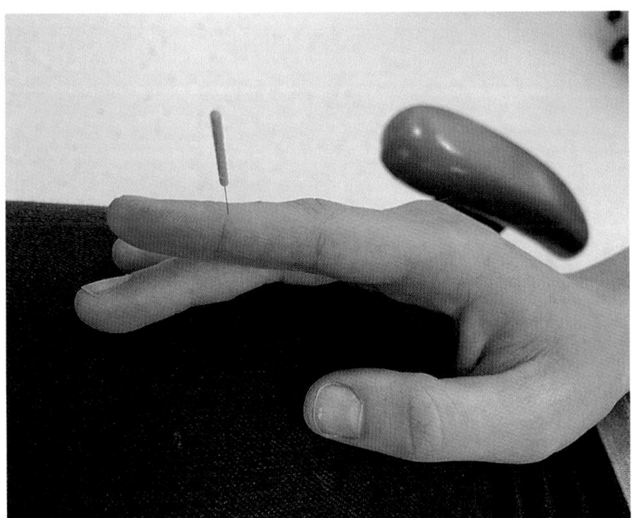

Figure 28.2 Position of needle in the forefinger.

Reference

Johnstone, P.A., Niemtzow, R.C., and Riffenburgh, R.H. (2002). Acupuncture for xerostomia: clinical update. *Cancer* 94: 1151–1156.

29

Oral Ulceration, Viral Infection, and Candidosis

Mike Lewis

Cardiff University, Cardiff, UK

Oral Ulceration

Recurrent aphthous stomatitis (RAS), which presents as characteristic painful round ulcers (Figure 29.1), is the most frequent cause of oral ulceration. Although RAS has been categorised into three subtypes, namely minor, major, and herpetiform, based on the different clinical features, the management of all types is the same. To date, no single causative aetiology for RAS has been identified, although a variety of factors have been proposed, in particular haematinic deficiency (iron, vitamin B_{12}, or folate), stress, and a hypersensitivity reaction to benzoate-based preservatives in foods or sodium lauryl sulphate in toothpaste. Management should aim to eliminate any predisposing factor and the provision of topical preparations, such as chlorhexidine spray, doxycycline mouthwash, beclomethasone inhaler, betamethasone mouthwash, or hydrocortisone oromucosal tablets.

Recurrent Herpes Simplex Infection

Almost all adults have antibody evidence of having had primary infection with herpes simplex type 1 (HSV-1) in early life and can therefore suffer from orofacial symptoms due to reactivation of latent virus. The most frequent manifestation of recurrent HSV-1 infection is herpes labialis (cold sore), which predominantly affects the mucocutaneous junction of the lip. Alternatively, recurrent clusters of ulcers may develop in the hard palate (Figure 29.2). Factors that may trigger the reactivation include emotional stress, local trauma, menstruation, systemic illness, and immuno-suppression. Aciclovir or penciclovir cream can be applied topically for treatment of herpes labialis. Systemic aciclovir can be used for frequent or severe outbreaks of HSV-1 infection.

Pseudomembranous Candidosis (Thrush)

Pseudomembranous candidosis consists, as its name suggests, of an extensive pseudomembrane of fungi, desquamated epithelial cells, and fibrin (Figure 29.3). Diagnosis is straightforward from the clinical signs, although the presence of candida can be confirmed microbiologically by culture of a swab. Oral candidosis is an opportunistic infection due to a range of underlying local and systemic predisposing factors, in particular inhaled steroids, systemic steroids, immune suppression, and systemic illness. Treatment involves the elimination of any predisposing factor and provision of systemic fluconazole. (Do not use fluconazole in a patient on warfarin or statin).

Care of Head and Neck Cancer Patients for Dental Hygienists and Dental Therapists, First Edition. Edited by Jocelyn J. Harding.

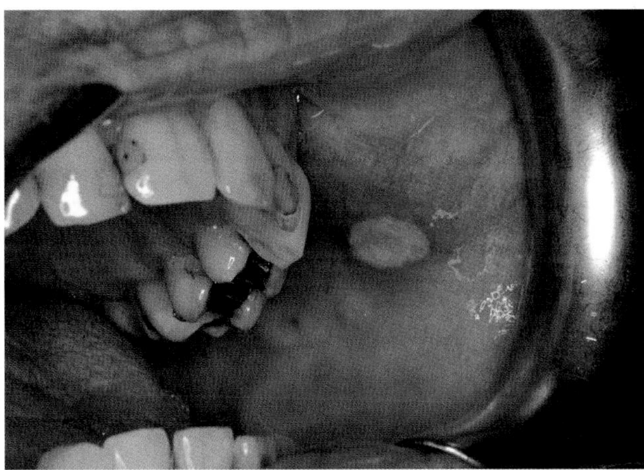

Figure 29.1 Ulceration characteristic of recurrent aphthous stomatitis.

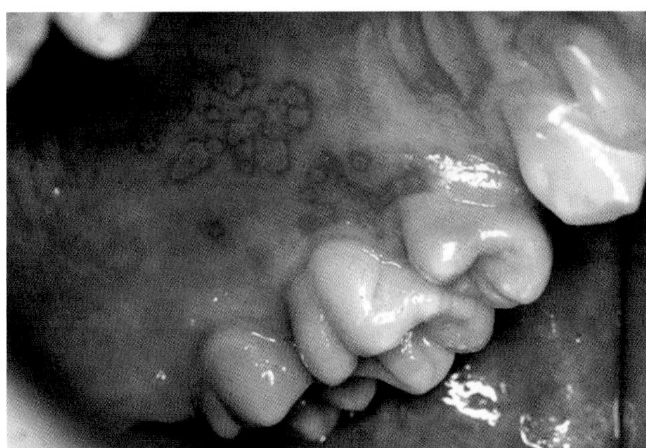

Figure 29.2 Multiple ulcers due to reactivation of latent HSV-1.

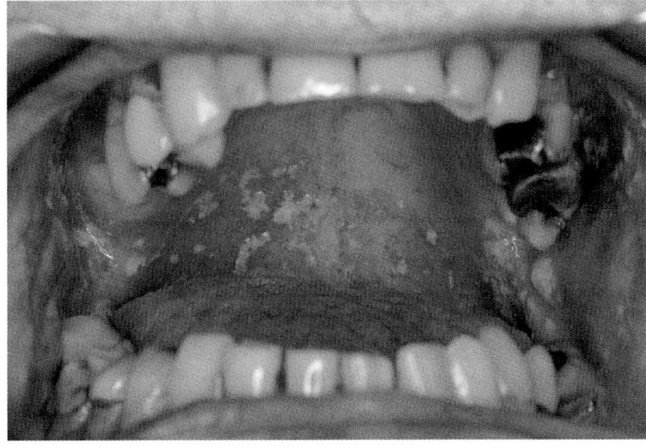

Figure 29.3 Pseudomembranous candidosis in the soft palate.

Chronic Erythematous Candidosis

Chronic erythematous candidosis (CEC) is associated with the wearing of a partial or full denture. The presentation of CEC is characteristic and involves a distinct pattern of painless erythema of the palatal mucosa confined to the area covered by the denture (Figure 29.4). The candidal infection is primarily on the denture rather than the oral mucosa, and therefore treatment is focused on establishing adequate denture hygiene. A major factor is wearing of the denture whilst sleeping.

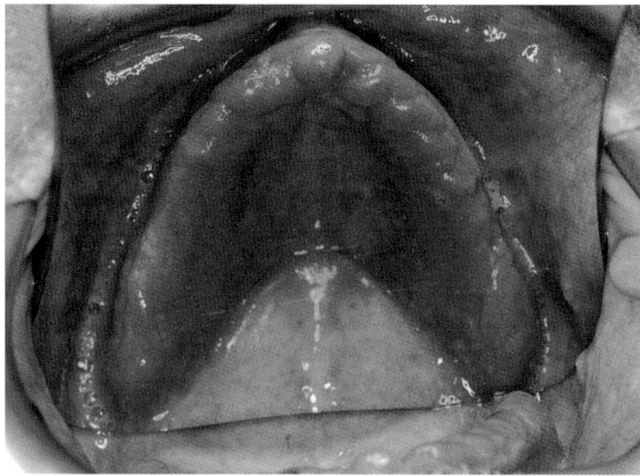

Figure 29.4 Erythema of the palatal mucosa due to denture-associated candidal infection.

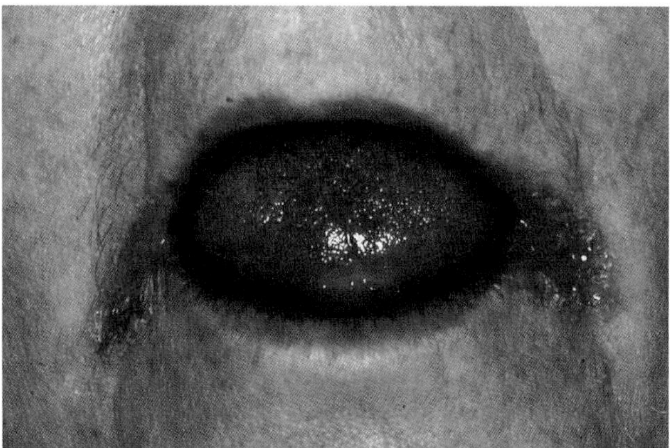

Figure 29.5 Erythema due to angular cheilitis.

The denture should be removed at this time and placed, if acrylic, in a dilute hypochlorite solution for up to three weeks. A denture with any metal component needs to be placed in chlorhexidine. In addition, sugar-free miconazole gel should be applied to the fitting surface of the denture whilst being worn. (Do not use miconazole in a patient on warfarin or statin.)

Angular Cheilitis

The inflammation of angular cheilitis presents as erythema and discomfort at the angles of the mouth (Figure 29.5) due to the presence of *Candida* species and/or *Staphylococcal* species. The patient's dental status often provides a guide to the nature of the infection. An individual who wears a denture is likely to have oral candida that spread to the angles, whilst a nondenture wearer is likely to have infection involving staphylococci. Haematological investigations should include full blood count, corrected whole blood, folate, vitamin B_{12}, ferritin, and haemaglobin A1c (HbA1c). Treatment is based on correcting the underlying predisposing factor and provision of a topical antimicrobial. Miconazole cream or miconazole combined with hydrocortisone, in either cream or ointment, is effective. (Do not use miconazole in a patient on warfarin or statin.)

Further Reading

Lewis, M.A.O. and Lamey, P.-J. (2019). *Oral Medicine in Primary Dental Care*, 4e. Springer.

Scottish Dental Clinical Effectiveness Programme (2016). Drug prescribing for dentistry, 3e. Available as free app for mobile devices. www.sdcep.org.uk.

30

Halitosis

Charlotte M. Carling

Dental Hygienist/Therapist, London, UK

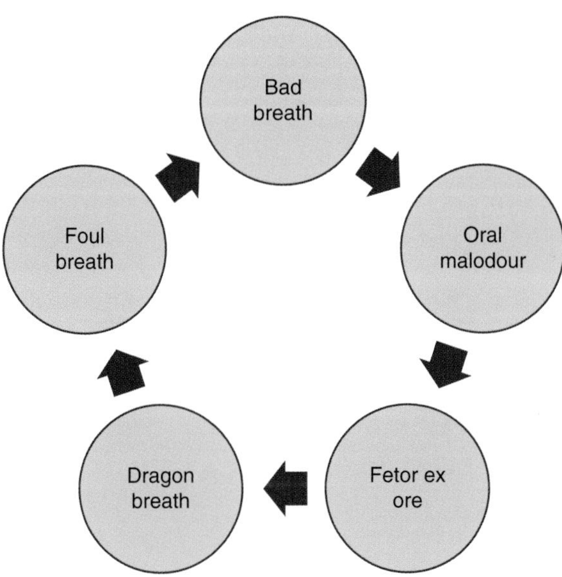

Introduction

This chapter provides a concise review of the complex nature of halitosis. The literature search has focused on the aetiology, prevalence, diagnosis, and current treatment strategies to furnish dental professionals with the knowledge base and practical clinical assessment skills to implement an effective individualised therapeutic approach. Halitosis is a common problem with psychological implications, affecting individuals of all ages (Scully and Greenman 2012). It is a prevalent complaint analogous to body odour (Lee et al. 2007) and is the most common reason for referral to dentists after dental caries and periodontal diseases (Bicak 2018; Scully and Greenman 2012). Therefore, this highlights the need for accurate diagnosis and appropriate management.

Halitosis

Halitosis (Latin halitus: breath, vapour) describes an offensive, unpleasant smell of the breath, independent of the cause (Zürcher et al. 2014). Bad breath can significantly impact a patient's quality of life, having negative connotations with associated stigma, leading to social, professional embarrassment, with individuals experiencing psychological

Care of Head and Neck Cancer Patients for Dental Hygienists and Dental Therapists, First Edition. Edited by Jocelyn J. Harding.

consequences and affective limitations (Zaitsu et al. 2011). Some patients remain entirely unaware of their oral emission, whereas others without oral malodour are convinced they are sufferers (Rosenberg et al. 1995).

Epidemiology

Available epidemiology data are based on subjective self-examination of malodour, limiting accuracy and sensitivity (Scully and Greenman 2012). There are limited studies documenting the prevalence of halitosis in population-wide community-based samples (Kapoor et al. 2016). However, there is an estimate that between 30% and 50% of the population has oral malodour from the available data (Outhouse et al. 2006a; Liu et al. 2006; Bornstein et al. 2009). In addition, oral malodour perception is different in culturally diverse populations (Rayman and Almas 2008).

Aetiopathogenesis and Classification

Oral malodour is classified as either genuine halitosis (Table 30.1), which includes both intraoral and extraoral and physiologic halitosis, known as transient, or nongenuine halitosis, which includes pseudo-halitosis and halitophobia (Scully and Greenman 2012; Bicak 2018). It is significant to highlight the necessity of an interdisciplinary method for the treatment of halitosis to prevent misdiagnosis or unnecessary treatment (Kapoor et al. 2016). A clinical evaluation of malodour on 2000 patients in Belgium showed that 76% of these patients had oral causes: tongue coating (43%), gingivitis/periodontitis (11%), or a combination of the two (18%). The authors concluded that although halitosis has a predominantly oral origin, a multidisciplinary approach remains necessary to identify ear, nose, and throat or extraoral pathologies and/or pseudo-halitosis/halitophobia (Quirynen et al. 2009). Other factors associated with intraoral halitosis include xerostomia, neoplasms, hyposalivation, odontogenic, stress, and age-related factors such as decreased oral mobility and poly-medication or the use of removable prostheses (Porter and Scully 2006). Halitosis can be considered to have an adverse effect on patients receiving radiotherapy, connected to hyposalivation and poor oral health (Albuquerque et al. 2010).

For ease of reference the leading causes of oral malodour are depicted in Table 30.2.

Table 30.1 Classification of halitosis.

Pathologic halitosis – intraoral	Genuine
Pathologic halitosis – extraoral	Genuine
Physiologic halitosis	Genuine – transient
Pseudo-halitosis	Nongenuine
Halitophobia	Nongenuine

Table 30.2 Leading causes of oral malodour.

Tongue-coating microorganisms	Poor oral hygiene, soft diet, smoking, alcohol
Plaque biofilm related disease – gingivitis, periodontitis, and other periodontal conditions	Gingivitis, periodontitis, pericoronitis, periodontal abscesses, acute necrotizing ulcerative gingivitis
Ulceration	Systemic disease Inflammatory/infectious disorders, gastrointestinal and haematological disease. Diabetes, malignancy, aphthae, and medication
Hyposalivation – dry mouth	Medication, Sjögren syndrome, and cancer treatment
Dentures, dental appliances –orthodontics	Poor hygiene and candidiasis
Odontogenic	Food packing
Bone diseases	Dry socket, osteomyelitis, osteonecrosis, and malignancy – neoplasm

Source: Adapted from Scully and Greenman (2012).

Origin

The mouth is home to hundreds of bacterial microbial species that produce several field substances as a result of protein degradation such as volatile sulphur compounds (VSCs) (Krespi et al. 2006). The main contributors that produce malodorous VSCs are hydrogen sulphide (H_2S), methyl mercaptan (CH_3SH), and dimethyl sulphide [$(CH_3)_2S$], which are mainly produced by proteolytic gram-negative anaerobic oral bacteria (Bollen and Beikler 2012). Other odoriferous components include diamines and short chain fatty acids, which also give rise to oral malodour. These bacterial interactions are most likely to occur in the gingival crevice and periodontal pockets, but oral malodour can also arise from the dorsum of the tongue, therefore this explains the reason why oral malodour can arise with patients that have good oral hygiene (Porter and Scully 2006). VSCs in the oral cavity and their emergence depend on many local factors. Contributory factors include reduced salivary production, decreased oxygen (O_2) concentration in the oral cavity, bacterial reproduction, and metabolism (Bicak 2018). When the salivary flow rate decreases, bacterial count and halitosis in the oral cavity increase (Kleinberg et al. 2002).

Diagnosis

A multidisciplinary stepwise approach is required for an accurate diagnosis (Figure 30.1), to discriminate between (i) anamnesis – medical/dental history, (ii) full-mouth oral screening, inclusive of periodontal assessment, (iii) evaluation of tongue coating – Winkel tongue coating index (WTCI), (iv) organoleptic scores (OLSs) – intensity of breath (defined below), (v) halimeter (sulphide monitoring) and gas chromatography, and (vi) oral malodour questionnaire of patient-reported outcomes measures (Renvert et al. 2020). Medications implicated can be referenced from Kapoor et al. (2016). Breath intensity – OLS (Rosenberg 1996) – is considered the 'gold standard' (Erovic Ademovski et al. 2012):

- 0 – Odour cannot be detected.
- 1 – Questionable malodour, barely detectable.
- 2 – Slight malodour, exceeds the threshold of malodour recognition.
- 3 – Malodour is definitely detected.
- 4 – Strong malodour.
- 5 – Very strong malodour.

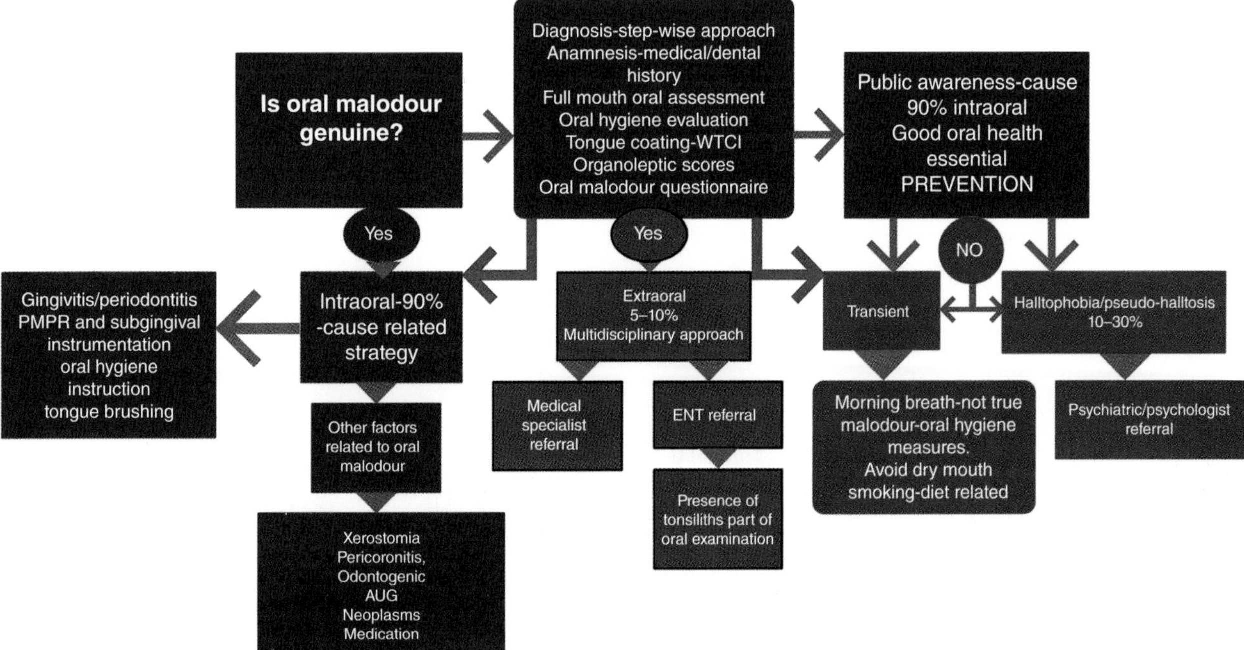

Figure 30.1 Diagnosis stepwise approach.

Extraoral Causes

Up to 10% of halitosis cases can originate from the ENT region, with a small percentage due to pathology of the tonsils (West and Tawhid 2019). Tonsillitis/tonsil stones (small collections of microbial and cellular debris that form in the crevices/crypts of the tonsils) are associated with a 10-fold increased risk of abnormal VSC levels (Fletcher and Blair 1988). Mouth breathing can be a cause of halitosis and typically takes place when nasal obstruction impedes normal nasal breathing at rest. Postnasal drip (mucus of the paranasal sinuses) onto the dorsum of the tongue can cause halitosis (Porter and Scully 2006). Carcinoma of the larynx, nasopharyngeal abscesses, asthma and lower tract infections, cystic fibrosis, bronchiectasis, intestinal lung diseases, and pneumonia have been known to cause halitosis (Kapoor et al. 2016; Aylıkcı and Colak 2013). Due to extraoral causes medical intervention is required to determine underlying cause.

Management of Oral Causes and the Dental Professional's Role

Treatment modalities are summarised and, for ease of reference, depicted in Figure 30.2. An accurate diagnosis is vital for the effectiveness of treatment. It should be individualised to manage it effectively, as it is essential to remember that the patient suffering from halitosis may be embarrassed and anxious (Kapoor et al. 2016). Empathy and sympathy are essential components in management of patients with halitosis, and support should be provided to both sufferer, family and friends (Porter and Scully 2006). Management strategies currently can be divided into professional mechanical plaque removal, oral hygiene advice, mechanical/chemical reduction of microorganisms, adjunctive masking products, and chemical neutralisation of VSCs (Armstrong et al. 2010).

Lifestyle

Lifestyle habits such as smoking, alcohol, and odoriferous foods can all contribute to oral malodour (Scully and Greenman 2012). The ingestion of foods such as onions, garlic, cauliflower, radishes, cabbage, and durian or species (Suarez et al. 1999) may be a consequence. However, incorporating a fibrous diet and drinking plenty of water has been advocated (Lenton et al. 2001).Tobacco smoke contains VSCs (Stedman 1968), and smoking also predisposes the patient to hyposalivation and has a critical link with periodontitis (Labriola et al. 2005: Chang et al. 2021). Alcohol intake may predict oral malodour (Rosenberg et al. 2007).

Physiological Halitosis

Morning breath is transient, is related to normal nocturnal hyposalivation, and is probably increased due to microbial metabolic activity during sleep, It is rarely of any significance (Outhouse et al. 2006b; Porter and Scully 2006; Fukui

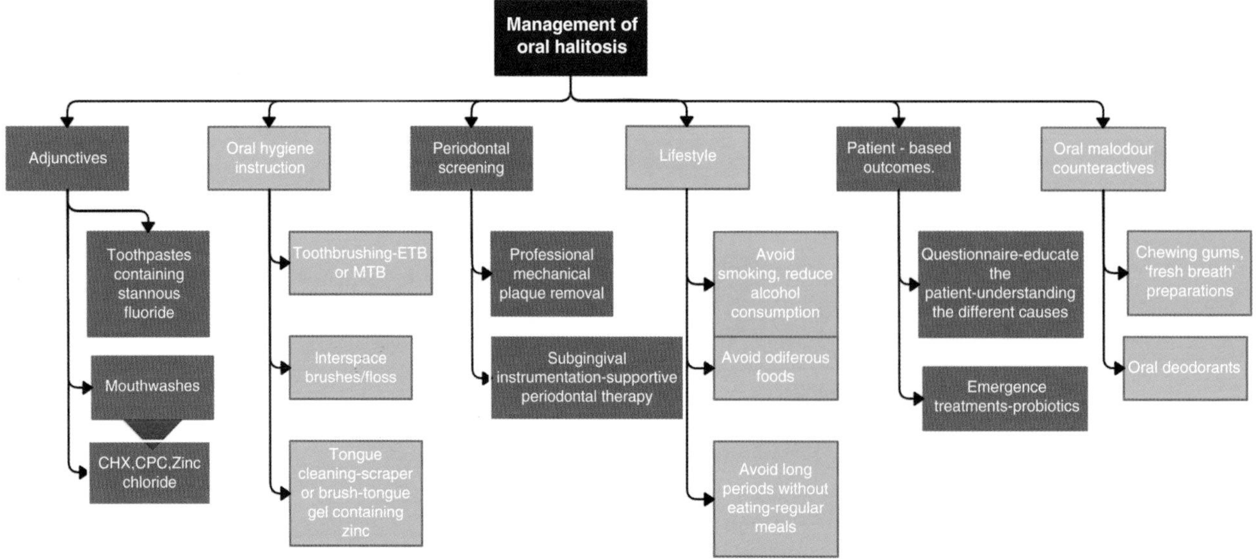

Figure 30.2 The management of oral halitosis.

et al. 2008; Scully and Greenman 2012). Starvation can lead to similar odour (Scully and Greenman 2012). Menstruation can also aggravate oral malodour (Kawamoto et al. 2010).

Patient-Based Outcomes

Patient-based outcomes are subjective measures that capture patients' perspectives of disease or therapy, complement conventional clinical measures, and are an integral part of treatment (Shanbhag et al. 2012). The systematic review looked at the impact of periodontal therapy on oral health-related quality of life in adults and the available evidence. The results of the studies concluded that oral hygiene instructions (OHI) + scaling and root planing (SRP) improved outcomes. Saito et al.'s two-centre clinical study in Japan highlighted that conventional nonsurgical periodontal therapy in patients with periodontitis has the potential to ameliorate patient perceptions of oral health (Saito et al. 2010).

Gingivitis and Periodontitis Disease

The treatment of periodontitis should follow the BSP UK Clinical Practice Guidelines for the Treatment of Periodontal Diseases to obtain the best clinical results. (British Society of Periodontology and Implant Dentistry 2021). Yaegaki and Sanada studies assessed the biochemical and clinical factors influencing oral malodour in peridontal patients. They concluded that the amount of VSCs in the mouth and the methyl mercaptan/sulphide ratio in mouth air from patient with periodontal involvement were eight times greater than those of control subjects (Yaegaki and Sanada 1992a).

Oral Hygiene Aids

Lack of interdental cleaning plays a significant high incidence in oral malodour, therefore interdental aids are an essential adjunct to toothbrushing and tongue cleaning (Froum and Rodriguez Salaverry 2013).

Tongue Biofilm

The dorsum of the tongue with its papillary structure, crypts, and furrows harbours a significant number of microorganisms, forming a unique ecological site with a large surface area (Danser et al. 2003). The resident microbes on the dorsum of the tongue, particularly the posterior third, should be either brushed or gently scraped. The morning is advocated to be on an empty stomach so that vomiting ensues, or gagging may be preferable to reduce retching (Danser et al. 2003). The purpose of tongue cleaning is to dislodge trapped food, cells, and bacteria between the filiform papillae, thus decreasing VSC concentrations (Danser et al. 2003). A systematic review by Van der Sleen et al. demonstrated that cleaning the tongue either by brushing or scraping can reduce oral malodour (Van der Sleen et al. 2010). A Cochrane review comparing brushes and tongue scrapers in adults for the effectiveness of reduction in VSCs concluded a small but significant difference favouring tongue scrapers (Outhouse et al. 2006b).

Toothpaste

Stannous-containing sodium fluoride dentifrice can reduce malodour (Feng et al. 2010). There is significant immediate antimalodour activity for 0.454% stabilised stannous fluoride sodium hexametaphosphate dentifrice (Chen et al. 2010).

Mouthwash

Mouthwashes are consumer accepted and widely available with a variety of ingredients. Mouthwashes containing chlorhexidine gluconate (CHX), cetylpyridinium chloride (CPC), or two-phase oil (Yaegaki and Sanada 1992b) may have some short-term benefit. Metal ions, hydrogen peroxide, and other oxidising agents are active in neutralising VSCs. Zinc chloride benefits are that it makes VSCs nonvolatile and at concentrations of at least 1% is effective (Yaegaki and Suetaka 1989).

Oral Malodour Counteractives

Over-the-counter nonpharmacological methods, such as chewing gum, stimulate salivary flow, therefore reducing malodour, but they merely have a temporary effect in just masking oral malodour (Tanaka et al. 2010). Foods that provide short-term relief are parsley, cloves, mint, or any breath-freshening preparations (Outhouse et al. 2006a).

Emerging Treatments

These include probiotics (Teughels et al. 2008) and other inhibitors of VSC production, including *Fusobacterium nucleatum* vaccines (Liu et al. 2009).

COVID-19 and Halitosis

The multifactorial impact of COVID-19 has had major implications affecting all aspects of life, initiating research in many fields. Riad et al. (2021b) investigated halitosis in a few confirmed cases while the patients were actively infected. The patients reported an offensive malodour that significantly affected their lives due to complaints from their spouses (Riad et al. 2021b). The findings suggest that possible epithelial alterations of the tongue dorsum may be caused by SARS-CoV-2 due to angiotensin-converting enzyme 2 receptors, which are profoundly located in abundance around the oral mucosa with the highest expression on the tongue dorsum (Xu et al. 2020). A 35-year-old female patient presented with severe halitosis adjacent to necrotising gingivitis, which suggested the impact of bacterial co-infection on COVID-19 severity (Patel and Woolley 2021).In addition, another plausible psychological impact of COVID-19 could be health-related behavioural change in individuals resulting in inadequate oral hygiene regime (Riad et al. 2021a; Riad et al. 2021b). Another indirect effect of COVID-19 on oral health is triggered by universal masking policies that may cause mouth breathing, yielding xerostomia and halitosis (Martel et al. 2020). It might also work vice versa, as mouth breathers are at a higher risk of getting infected by COVID-19 due to the decreased nitric oxide saturation, in addition to their vulnerability for developing xerostomia and halitosis (Martel et al. 2020). Conclusively, a further explanatory hypothesis for the diagnosis of halitosis in COVID-19 patients is that mask wearing has increased the public awareness of their own mouth odour (Riad et al. 2021b). Research is limited, and further investigative studies are needed to estimate the prevalence of halitosis among COVID-19 patients and its possible aetiologies that may be linked either directly, or indirectly, to SARS-CoV-2 infection (Riad et al. 2021a).

Summary

Dentists and dental care professionals should be the primary health professionals to screen and manage halitosis in complaining patients. They are in a niche position to educate the public that intraoral malodour is the leading cause of halitosis. The necessity of an interdisciplinary pathway for the treatment of halitosis is crucial to prevent misdiagnosis. The literature is scarce on this common phenomenon, especially randomised control trials; additional research is needed to support current concepts or advocate new ideas in the aetiology, diagnosis, assessment, and treatment strategies.

References

Albuquerque, D., Tolentino, E., Amado, F. et al. (2010). Evaluation of halitosis and sialometry in patients submitted to head and neck radiotherapy. *Medicina. Oral. Patologia. Oral. Cir. Bucal.* e850–e854.

Armstrong, B.L., Sensat, M.L., and Stoltenberg, J.L. (2010). Halitosis: a review of current literature. *Am. Dent. Hygien. Ass.* 84: 65–74.

Aylıkcı, B.U. and Colak, H. (2013). Halitosis: from diagnosis to management. *J. Nat. Sci., Biol. Med.* 4: 14–23.

Bicak, D.A. (2018). A current approach to halitosis and oral malodor – a mini review. *Open. Dent. J.* 12: 322–330.

Bollen, C.M. and Beikler, T. (2012). Halitosis: the multidisciplinary approach. *Int. J. Oral. Sci.* 4: 55–63.

Bornstein, M.M., Kislig, K., Hoti, B.B. et al. (2009). Prevalence of halitosis in the population of the city of Bern, Switzerland: a study comparing self-reported and clinical data. *Eur. J. Oral. Sci.* 117: 261–267.

British Society of Periodontology and Implant Dentistry (2021). Clinical guidelines in the treatment of peridontal diseases. https://emea01.safelinks.protection.outlook.com/?url=https%3A%2F%2Fwww.bsperio.org.uk%2Fassets%2Fdownloads%2FBSP_Treatment_Flow_Chart_16_For_Screen.pdf&data=04%7C01%7C%7Ce4cfbc3149af41357c6a08d9d46eef37%7C84df9e7fe9f640afb435aaaaaaaaaaaa%7C1%7C0%7C637774395181710631%7CUnknown%7CTWFpbGZsb3d8eyJWIjoiMC4wLjAwMDAiLCJQIjoiV2luMzIiLCJBTiI6Ik1haWwiLCJXVCI6Mn0%3D%7C3000&sdata=i6OjA1ElDtGSrtwgz8y9PPad1hqMmkJuQR5dwqwr%2FEc%3D&reserved=0.

Chang, J., Meng, H.W., Lalla, E., and Lee, C.T. (2021). The impact of smoking on non-surgical periodontal therapy: a systematic review and meta-analysis. *J. Clin. Periodontol.* 48: 60–75.

Chen, X., He, T., Sun, L. et al. (2010). A randomized cross-over clinical trial to evaluate the effect of a 0.454% stannous fluoride dentifrice on the reduction of oral malodor. *Am. J. Dent.* 23: 175–178.

Danser, M.M., Gómez, S.M., and Van der Weijden, G.A. (2003). Tongue coating and tongue brushing: a literature review. *Int. J. Dent. Hyg.* 1: 151–158.

Erovic Ademovski, S., Lingström, P., Winkel, E. et al. (2012). Comparison of different treatment modalities for oral halitosis. *Acta Odontol. Scand.* 70: 224–233.

Feng, X., Chen, X., Cheng, R. et al. (2010). Breath malodor reduction with use of a stannous-containing sodium fluoride dentifrice: a meta-analysis of four randomized and controlled clinical trials. *Am. J. Dent.* 23 Spec No B,: 27B–31B.

Fletcher, S.M. and Blair, P.A. (1988). Chronic halitosis from tonsilloliths: a common etiology. *J. La. State. Med. Soc.* 140: 7–9.

Froum, S.J. and Rodriguez Salaverry, K. (2013). The dentist's role in diagnosis and treatment of halitosis. *Compendium Contin. Educ. Dentistry (Jamesburg, N.J.: 1995)* 34: 670–677.

Fukui, Y., Yaegaki, K., Murata, T. et al. (2008). Diurnal changes in oral malodour among dental-office workers. *Int. Dent. J.* 58: 159–166.

Kapoor, U., Sharma, G., Juneja, M., and Nagpal, A. (2016). Halitosis: current concepts on etiology, diagnosis and management. *Europ. J. Dent.* 10: 292–300.

Kawamoto, A., Sugano, N., Motohashi, M. et al. (2010). Relationship between oral malodor and the menstrual cycle. *J. Periodontal. Res.* 45: 681–687.

Kleinberg, I., Wolff, M.S., and Codipilly, D.M. (2002). Role of saliva in oral dryness, oral feel and oral malodour. *Int. Dent. J.* 52 (Suppl 3): 236–240.

Krespi, Y.P., Shrime, M.G., and Kacker, A. (2006). The relationship between oral malodor and volatile sulfur compound-producing bacteria. *Otolaryngol. Head. Neck. Surg.* 135: 671–676.

Labriola, A., Needleman, I., and Moles, D.R. (2005). Systematic review of the effect of smoking on nonsurgical periodontal therapy. *Periodontol.* 2000 (37): 124–137.

Lee, S.S., Zhang, W., and Li, Y. (2007). Halitosis update: a review of causes, diagnoses, and treatments. *J. California Dent. Assoc.* 35: 258–264.

Lenton, P., Majerus, G., and Bakdash, B. (2001). Counseling and treating bad breath patients: a step-by-step approach. *J. Contemp. Dent. Pract.* 2: 46–61.

Liu, P.-F., Haake, S.K., Gallo, R.L., and Huang, C.-M. (2009). A novel vaccine targeting Fusobacterium nucleatum against abscesses and halitosis. *Vacc.* 27: 1589–1595.

Liu, X.N., Shinada, K., Chen, X.C. et al. (2006). Oral malodor-related parameters in the Chinese general population. *J. Clin. Periodontol.* 33: 31–36.

Martel, J., Ko, Y.-F., Young, J.D., and Ojcius, D.M. (2020). Could nasal nitric oxide help to mitigate the severity of COVID-19? *Microbes. Infect.* 22: 168–171.

Outhouse, T.L., Al-Alawi, R., Fedorowicz, Z., and Keenan, J.V. (2006a). Tongue scraping for treating halitosis. *Cochrane Database of Systematic. Reviews* (Art. No.: CD005519).

Outhouse, T.L., Fedorowicz, Z., Keenan, J.V., and Al-Alawi, R. (2006b). A Cochrane systematic review finds tongue scrapers have short-term efficacy in controlling halitosis. *Gen. Dent.* 54: 352–359.

Patel, J. and Woolley, J. (2021). Necrotizing periodontal disease: oral manifestation of COVID-19. *Oral Dis.* 27: 768–769.

Porter, S.R. and Scully, C. (2006). Oral malodour (halitosis). *BMJ.* 333: 632–635.

Quirynen, M., Dadamio, J., Van den Velde, S. et al. (2009). Characteristics of 2000 patients who visited a halitosis clinic. *J. Clin. Periodontol.* 36: 970–975.

Rayman, S. and Almas, K. (2008). Halitosis among racially diverse populations: an update. *Int. J. Dent. Hyg.* 6: 2–7.

Renvert, S., Noack, M.J., Lequart, C. et al. (2020). The underestimated problem of intra-oral halitosis in dental practice: an expert consensus review. *Clin. Cosmet. Investigat. Dent.* 12: 251–262.

Riad, A., Boccuzzi, M., Pold, A., and Krsek, M. (2021a). The alarming burden of non-communicable diseases in COVID-19 new normal: implications on oral health. *Oral Dis.* 27: 791–792.

Riad, A., Kassem, I., Hockova, B. et al. (2021b). Halitosis in COVID-19 patients. *Spec. Care Dent.* 41: 282–285.

Rosenberg, M. (1996). Clinical assessment of bad breath: current concepts. *J. Am. Dent. Assoc.* 127: 475–482.

Rosenberg, M., Knaan, T., and Cohen, D. (2007). Association among bad breath, body mass index, and alcohol intake. *J. Dent. Res.* 86: 997–1000.

Rosenberg, M., Kozlovsky, A., Gelernter, I. et al. (1995). Self-estimation of oral malodor. *J. Dent. Res.* 74: 1577–1582.

Saito, A., Hosaka, Y., Kikuchi, M. et al. (2010). Effect of initial periodontal therapy on oral health-related quality of life in patients with periodontitis in Japan. *J. Periodontol.* 81: 1001–1009.

Scully, C. and Greenman, J. (2012). Halitology (breath odour: aetiopathogenesis and management). *Oral Dis.* 18: 333–345.

Shanbhag, S., Dahiya, M., and Croucher, R. (2012). The impact of periodontal therapy on oral health-related quality of life in adults: a systematic review. *J. Clin. Periodontol.* 39: 725–735.

Stedman, R.L. (1968). The chemical composition of tobacco and tobacco smoke. *Chem. Rev.* 68: 153–207.

Suarez, F., Springfield, J., Furne, J., and Levitt, M. (1999). Differentiation of mouth versus gut as site of origin of odoriferous breath gases after garlic ingestion. *Am. J. Physiol.* 276: G425–G430.

Tanaka, M., Toe, M., Nagata, H. et al. (2010). Effect of eucalyptus-extract chewing gum on oral malodor: a double-masked, randomized trial. *J. Periodontol.* 81: 1564–1571.

Teughels, W., Van Essche, M., Sliepen, I., and Quirynen, M. (2008). Probiotics and oral healthcare. *Periodontol.* 2000 (48): 111–147.

Van der Sleen, M., Slot, D., Van Trijffel, E. et al. (2010). Effectiveness of mechanical tongue cleaning on breath odour and tongue coating: a systematic review. *Int. J. Dent. Hyg.* 8: 258–268.

West, M. and Tawhid, I. S. (2019). Halitosis: identifying the cause. https://www.gmjournal.co.uk/halitosis-identifying-the-cause.

Xu, H., Zhong, L., Deng, J. et al. (2020). High expression of ACE2 receptor of 2019-nCoV on the epithelial cells of oral mucosa. *Int. J. Oral. Sci.* 12: 8.

Yaegaki, K. and Sanada, K. (1992a). Biochemical and clinical factors influencing oral malodor in periodontal patients. *J. Periodontol.* 63: 783–789.

Yaegaki, K. and Sanada, K. (1992b). Effects of a two-phase oil-water mouthwash on halitosis. *Clin. Prev. Dent.* 14: 5–9.

Yaegaki, K. and Suetaka, T. (1989). The effect of zinc chloride mouthwash on the production of oral malodour, the degradations of salivary cellular elements, and proteins. *J. Dent. Health.* 39: 377–386.

Zaitsu, T., Ueno, M., Shinada, K. et al. (2011). Social anxiety disorder in genuine halitosis patients. *Health. Qual. Life Outcom.* 9: 94.

Zürcher, A., Laine, M.L., and Filippi, A. (2014). Diagnosis, prevalence, and treatment of halitosis. *Curr. Oral. Health. Rep.* 1: 279–285.

31

Oral Mucositis

Shemifhar Freytes[1] *and Alessandro Villa*[2]

[1] *Enlivity Corporation, Newton, Massachusetts, USA*
[2] *University of California San Francisco, San Francisco, California and Miami Cancer Institute, Baptist Health South Florida, USA*

Introduction

Oral mucositis (OM) is a common and debilitating side effect of cancer treatment caused by radiation therapy (RT) to the head and neck that involves the oral cavity or by certain types of chemotherapy agents (Harris 2006; Villa and Sonis 2015). OM is characterised by painful mouth sores (ulcerative lesions), redness, and damage along the mucosal lining. These ulcers usually develop on the lips, buccal mucosa, ventral tongue, and floor and roof of the mouth (see Figure 31.1), but they can also appear in other areas of the GI tract, anywhere from the mouth to the rectum (Camp-Sorrell 2000).

OM often affects oral function, including swallowing and speaking (Harris 2006). When severe enough this condition can limit nutritional intake requiring diet modifications and, in certain cases, total parenteral nutrition (TPN) (Sadasivan 2010). Mucosal damage can also increase the risk of infection and is frequently dose-limiting (Harris 2006). Patients with severe mucositis may require more hospitalizations or may need to modify or halt treatment altogether due to reduced quality of life and poor nutritional status (Lalla 2005; Duncan et al. 2005).

OM affects up to 40% of patients undergoing chemotherapy for solid tumours, about 80% of those receiving high-dose chemotherapy for stem cell transplant conditioning, and almost 100% of patients receiving RT for head and neck cancers (Lalla et al. 2019; Elad 2020; Logan et al. 2020). OM usually starts to develop 5–10 days after initial treatment in chemotherapy patients, peaking close to day 10 and improving slowly thereafter (Cheng 2007). In the case of RT patients, OM starts to appear within two weeks of initial treatment, and symptoms can last for more than six weeks after treatment has ended (Leenstra et al. 2014; Anderson and Lalla 2020; Villa and Sonis 2015). However, it is important to acknowledge that the duration of OM depends on the treatment schedule and the modality used. Some sources report OM may last 46–102 days after treatment (McCullough 2016).

OM Risk Factors

OM is frequently under-reported, particularly in patients undergoing chemotherapy (Boers-Doets et al. 2012). Early identification of patients at risk of developing this side effect can be critical to the successful management of this dose-limiting condition. Two categories of risk factors play a role in the severity and duration of OM: treatment-related risk factors and patient-related risk factors (Sonis 2004; Cawley and Benson 2005).

Treatment-related risk factors include:

- Combined modalities of chemotherapy and radiation
- Aggressive treatment schedules
- High-dose chemotherapy
- Specific chemotherapy agents such as antimetabolites, antitumor antibiotics, and alkylating agents (Anderson and Lalla 2020).

Care of Head and Neck Cancer Patients for Dental Hygienists and Dental Therapists, First Edition. Edited by Jocelyn J. Harding.

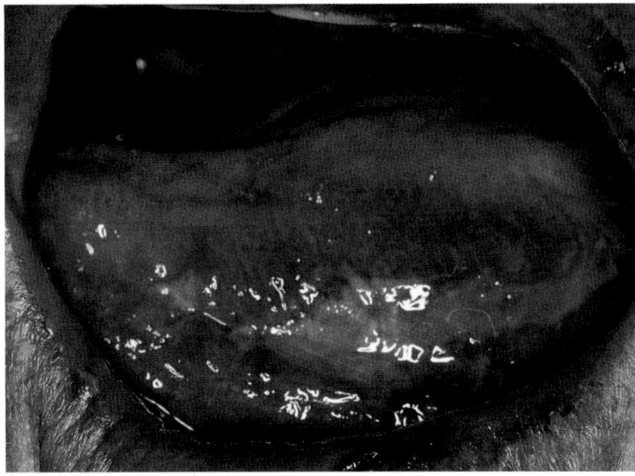

Figure 31.1 Large ulceration of the left ventral tongue (ulcerative mucositis).

Patient-related risk factors include:

- Genetic predisposition
- Sex (females may be more likely than males to develop OM, although conflicting evidence exists)
- Age (patients below the age of 20 and patients above 65 are more likely to develop OM)
- Low BMI
- Pre-existing dry mouth/xerostomia
- Poor dental health and oral hygiene
- Tobacco smoking
- Alcohol consumption
- Poor nutritional status
- Previous history of cancer treatment.

OM Assessment and Diagnosis

OM is diagnosed through a detailed inspection of the oral cavity along with an evaluation of patient-related factors such as pain, nutritional status, and quality of life (Naidu 2004). Several grading scales and assessment tools exist to evaluate the severity and progression of OM, which varies from mild, to medium, to severe.

Assessment tools and scales for the evaluation of OM include:

- Common terminology criteria for adverse events (CTCAE)
- Radiation therapy oncology oral mucositis grading system (RTOG)
- Oral mucositis assessment scale (OMAS)[1]
- Oral assessment guide (OAG)
- WHO grading of mucositis.

Among the available OM assessment tools, the WHO grading scale is the most widely used in both clinical trials and clinical practice (Wilkes 1998). Unlike the RTOG and OMAS tools, the WHO scale considers the patient's ability to eat and drink, which is an important aspect of OM morbidity.

Definition of Oral Mucositis by Grading Scale

In the WHO scale, OM is graded from 0 to 4: grade 0 (none) if there are no visual signs or symptoms; grade 1 (mild) if there is redness and the patient reports mild soreness; grade 2 (moderate) if the patient experiences soreness, redness, and ulceration but is still able to eat solid foods; grade 3 (severe) if ulcers with extensive redness are present, and the patient is

1 Sometimes referred to as the objective scoring system for site assessment.

Table 31.1 Definition of oral mucositis by grading scale.

	Grade				
Scale	**0 (none)**	**1 (mild)**	**2 (moderate)**	**3 (severe)**	**4 (life-threatening)**
WHO	No visual signs of mucositis	Soreness and erythema, no ulceration	Erythema, ulcers. Patient can swallow solids	Ulcers, extensive erythema. Liquid diet only, no solids	Severe ulceration, NPO
CTCAE 5.0	–	Asymptomatic or mild symptoms; intervention not indicated	Moderate pain or ulcer that does not interfere with oral intake; modified diet indicated	Severe pain, interfering with oral intake	Life-threatening consequences; urgent intervention indicated
RTOG	None	Erythema of mucosa	Patchy mucositis, <1.5 cm, noncontiguous	Fibrinous mucositis >1.5 cm, contiguous	Necrosis +/− hemorrhage
OMAS	Normal	Ulceration <1 sq. cm (not severe)	1–3 sq. cm (Severe)	> 3 sq. cm (N/A)	–

NPO, nothing by mouth.

unable to swallow solid foods; and grade 4 (life-threatening) if oral alimentation is impossible and TPN or enteral support is needed (Wilkes 1998). See Table 31.1.

Prevention and Management

OM is an associated toxicity of different treatment modalities, and it might be unavoidable for many patients. However, progressions and symptom management can be critical to treatment adherence and success.

OM mitigation and management is based on four key pillars:

1) Oral health and hygiene
2) Pain management
3) Nutrition
4) Healing.

Oral Health and Hygiene

The main preventative measures of OM are oral hygiene and oral health due to the risk of infection associated with this condition. When ulcers start to develop, they can quickly become populated by the patient's oral microflora, which can impair healing and lead to wound progression (Biswal 2008).

It is generally recommended that patients at high risk for OM see a dentist to address any dental caries, infections, or compromised teeth before the start of treatment. Prophylactic dental care can reduce the risk of OM by >25% in patients with non-head-and-neck malignancies (Sonis 1988).

Other recommended preventative measures include flossing and brushing at least twice per day with a soft toothbrush and mild-flavoured fluoridated toothpastes and rinsing with saline solutions, sodium bicarbonate, or water at least four times a day (Bensinger et al. 2008).

Pain Management

Pain is consistently reported as one of the most distressing symptoms of OM (Rose-Ped et al. 2002). Because healing takes time and the patient's ability to heal might be impaired due to treatment and infection, pain management should be addressed quickly in order to improve patient outcomes. Pain management can allow patients to continue eating and drinking without the need for TPN (Lalla et al. 2008).

Topical anesthetic rinses recommended include swish-and-spit viscous lidocaine, as well as benzydamine rinses in the case of RT-induced mucositis without concomitant chemotherapy (Galloway and Amdur 2018). However, in the case of hematopoietic stem cell transplantation patients, strong opioids, such as morphine, may be required (Barasch et al. 2006).

Other pain management strategies include the use of corticosteroids such as dexamethasone to treat inflammation, as well as the use of mucoadhesive rinses that soothe the mucosa and create a protective barrier (Rugo et al. 2017; Murdock and Reeves 2020). However, it is important to note that there is not enough evidence to support the use of corticosteroids.

Nutrition

Nutrition is an important aspect of cancer treatment and OM management. Patients who are unable to keep a good nutritional status may become too weak to withstand treatment. Patients at risk for mucositis should avoid foods that are hard/sharp, acidic, spicy, or irritating (Brown and Gupta 2020). They should also avoid tobacco and alcohol, including alcohol-containing mouthwashes (Gupta and West 2016). Patients can also opt to prophylactically have a PEG tube placed, to help with weight loss and dehydration (Bensinger et al. 2008). When possible, patients should be referred to a registered dietitian who can help monitor and manage their nutrition.

Healing

Healing occurs naturally, shortly after damage from treatment stops. However, studies suggest photobiomodulation therapy (PBMT)[2] and oral glutamine supplementation can promote healing during treatment, reducing the severity and duration of OM.

PBMT is the application of low-level, red, and near-red light (600–1000 nm) over injuries. Unlike surgical lasers, this approach has no heating effect. Studies suggest this approach can speed tissue repair by reducing oxidative stress and increasing ATP production around the affected areas (Legouté et al. 2019). Low-level laser therapy has been shown to prevent OM in patients receiving hematopoietic stem-cell transplantation (HSCT) conditioned with high-dose chemotherapy.

Oral glutamine supplementation has been evaluated in a number of clinical studies that suggest it can reduce the severity and duration of OM in patients with head and neck cancer who are receiving concomitant RT-CT by acting directly on epithelial cells, improving mucosal immune response, and increasing resistance to microbial invasion (Anderson and Lalla 2020; Peterson 2004). The recent MASCC guidelines for the prevention of oral mucositis suggests oral glutamine for the prevention of OM in head and neck cancer patients receiving RT-CT.

Additionally, it should be noted that palifermin, a class of keratinocyte growth factor, is currently being used outside of the European Union to prevent OM and speed the healing of severe sores in patients receiving high-dose chemotherapy and total body irradiation, followed by autologous stem-cell transplantation (SCT) (Galloway and Amdur 2018).

Additional Prevention and Management Options

Cryotherapy, an approach that consists of cooling of the mouth through the use of cold water, ice chips, or popsicles, has been effective in preventing chemotherapy-induced mucositis with 5-fluoruracil. This method stimulates vasoconstriction, which reduces the penetration of chemotherapy agents in the mucosal lining (Bensinger et al. 2008).

Honey has been studied in recent years as a potential adjuvant therapy agent. Honey appears to be safe and effective in patients with chemotherapy and RT-induced mucositis; however, further research is needed in this area (Xu et al. 2016).

The field of supportive care continues to evolve, particularly around OM where management has traditionally consisted of pain mitigation. The Multinational Association of Supportive Care in Cancer consistently performs systematic reviews and regularly puts forth updated clinical guidelines for the management of OM, as well as other conditions.[3]

2 PBMT was previously known as low-level laser therapy (LLLT).

3 Updated oral mucositis guidelines from the Multinational Association of Supportive Care in Cancer can be accessed through https://www.mascc.org/mucositis-guidelines.

References

Anderson, P.L. and Lalla, R.V. (2020). Glutamine for amelioration of radiation and chemotherapy associated mucositis during cancer therapy. *Nutrients* 12 (6): 1675. http://dx.doi.org/10.3390/nu12061675.

Barasch, A., Elad, S., Altman, A. et al. (2006). Antimicrobials, mucosal coating agents, anesthetics, analgesics, and nutritional supplements for alimentary tract mucositis. *Support Care Cancer* 14 (6): 528–532. http://dx.doi.org/10.1007/s00520-006-0066-1.Epub.

Bensinger, W., Schubert, M., Ang, K.-K. et al. (2008). NCCN Task Force report: prevention and management of mucositis in cancer care. *J. Natl. Compr. Cancer Netw.* 6 (1): S1–S24.

Biswal, B. (2008). Current trends in the management of oral mucositis related to cancer treatment. *Malaysian J. Med. Sci.* 15 (3): 4–13.

Boers-Doets, C.B., Epstein, J.B., Raber-Durlacher, J.E. et al. (2012). Oral adverse events associated with tyrosine kinase and mammalian target of rapamycin inhibitors in renal cell carcinoma: a structured literature review. *Oncologist* 17 (1): 135–144. http://dx.doi.org/10.1634/theoncologist.2011-0111.

Brown, T.J. and Gupta, A. (2020). Management of cancer therapy–associated oral mucositis. *JCO Oncol. Pract.* 16 (3): 103–109.

Camp-Sorrell, D. (2000). Chemotherapy: toxicity management. In: *Cancer Nursing Principles and Practice*, vol. 5 (ed. C.H. Yarbro, M.H. Frogge, M. Goodman, et al.), 444–486. Boston: Jones & Bartlett.

Cawley, M.M. and Benson, L.M. (2005). Current trends in managing oral mucositis. *Clin. J. Oncol. Nurs.* 9 (5): 584–592.

Cheng, K. (2007). Oral mucositis and quality of life of Hong Kong Chinese patients with cancer therapy. *Eur. J. Oncol. Nurs.* 11 (1): 36–42.

Duncan, G.G., Epstein, J.B., Tu, D. et al. (2005). Quality of life, mucositis, and xerostomia from radiotherapy for head and neck cancers: a report from the NCIC CTG HN2 randomized trial of an antimicrobial lozenge to prevent mucositis. *Head Neck* 27 (5): 421–442.

Elad, S. (2020). The MASCC/ISOO mucositis guidelines 2019: the second set of articles and future directions. *Support Care Cancer* 28 (5): 2445–2447.

Galloway, T. and Amdur, R.J. (2018). Management and prevention of complications during initial treatment of head and neck cancer. https://www.uptodate.com/contents/management-and-prevention-of-complications-during-initial-treatment-of-head-and-neck-cancer#!.

Gupta, A. and West, H.J. (2016). Mucositis (or stomatitis). *JAMA Oncol.* 2 (10): 1379. http://dx.doi.org/10.1001/jamaoncol.2016.2103.

Harris, D. (2006). Cancer treatment–induced mucositis pain: strategies for assessment and management. *Ther. Clin. Risk Manag.* 2 (3): 251–258. http://dx.doi.org/10.2147/tcrm.2006.2.3.251.

Lalla, R.P.D. (2005). Oral mucositis. *Dent. Clin. N. Am.* 49 (1): 67–84. ix.

Lalla, R.V., Sonis, S.T., and Peterson, D.E. (2008). Management of oral mucositis in patients who have cancer. *Dent. Clin. N. Am.* 52 (1): 61–77. http://dx.doi.org/10.1016/j.cden.2007.10.002.

Lalla, R.V., Brennan, M.T., Gordon, S.M. et al. (2019). Oral mucositis due to high-dose chemotherapy and/or head and neck radiation therapy. *J. Natl. Cancer Inst.* 53 (lgz011): http://dx.doi.org/10.1093/jncimonographs/lgz011.

Leenstra, J.L., Miller, R.C., Qin, R. et al. (2014). Doxepin rinse versus placebo in the treatment of acute oral mucositis pain in patients receiving head and neck radiotherapy with or without chemotherapy: a phase III, randomized, double-blind trial (NCCTG-N09C6 [alliance]). *J. Clin. Oncol.* 32 (15): 1571–1577.

Legouté, F., Bensadoun, R.J., Seegers, V. et al. (2019). Low-level laser therapy in treatment of chemoradiotherapy-induced mucositis in head and neck cancer: results of a randomised, triple blind, multicentre phase III trial. *Radiat. Oncol.* 14 (83): http://dx.doi.org/10.1186/s13014-019-1292-2.

Logan, R., Al-Azri, A.R., Bossi, P. et al. (2020). Systematic review of growth factors and cytokines for the management of oral mucositis in cancer patients and clinical practice guidelines. *Support Care Cancer* 28 (5): 2485–2498.

McCullough, R. (2016). Actual duration of patient-reported mucositis: far longer than 2 to 4 weeks and may be avoidable altogether. *Korean J. Clin. Oncol.* 13 (1): 1–6. http://dx.doi.org/10.14216/kjco.16001.

Murdock, J.L. and Reeves, D.J. (2020). Chemotherapy-induced oral mucositis management: a retrospective analysis of MuGard, Caphosol, and standard supportive care measures. *J. Oncol. Pharm. Pract.* 26 (3): 521–528. http://dx.doi.org/10.1177/107.

Naidu, M.U.R. (2004). Chemotherapy-induced and/or radiation therapy-induced oral mucositis – complicating the treatment of cancer. *Neoplasia* 6 (5): 423–431. http://dx.doi.org/10.1593/neo.04169.

Peterson, D.E. (2004). Novel therapies. *Semin. Oncol. Nurs.* 20 (1): 53–58. http://dx.doi.org/10.1053/j.soncn.2003.10.009.

Rose-Ped, A.M., Belim, L.A., Epstein, J.B. et al. (2002). Complications of radiation therapy for head and neck cancers. The patient's perspective. *Cancer Nurs.* 25 (6): 461–469. http://dx.doi.org/10.1097/00002820-20021200.

Rugo, H.S., Seneviratne, L., Thaddeus Beck, J. et al. (2017). Prevention of everolimus-related stomatitis in women with hormone receptor-positive, HER2-negative metastatic breast cancer using dexamethasone mouthwash (SWISH): a single-arm, phase 2 trial. *Lancet* 18 (5): 654–662. http://dx.doi.org/10.1016/S1470-2045(17)30109-2.

Sadasivan, R. (2010). Chemotherapy-induced oral mucositis. *US Oncol. Rev.* 6 (1): 13–16. http://dx.doi.org/10.17925/OHR.2010.06.0.13.

Sonis, S.K.A. (1988). Impact of improved dental services on the frequency of oral complications of cancer therapy for patients with non-head-and-neck malignancies. *Oral Surg. Oral Med. Oral Pathol.* 65 (1): 19–22.

Sonis, S. (2004). The pathobiology of mucositis. *Nat. Rev. Cancer* 4: 277–284. http://dx.doi.org/10.1038/nrc1318.

Villa, A. and Sonis, S. (2015). Mucositis: pathobiology and management. *Curr. Opin. Oncol.* 27 (3): 159–164. http://dx.doi.org/10.1097/CCO.0000000000000018.

Wilkes, J. (1998). Prevention and treatment of oral mucositis following cancer chemotherapy. *Semin. Oncol.* 25 (5): 538–551.

Xu, J.L., Xia, R., Sun, Z.-H. et al. (2016). Effects of honey use on the management of radio/chemotherapy-induced mucositis: a meta-analysis of randomized controlled trials. *Int. J. Oral Maxillofac. Surg.* 45 (12): 1618–1625. http://dx.doi.org/10.1016/j.ijom.2016.04.023.

32

Nausea and Tooth Erosion

Lucy Harrison

Royal London Dental Hospital, London, UK

Head and neck cancer patients can experience nausea pre-, during or posttreatment. This can be due to anxiety, medications, a side effect of the cancer treatment itself, or altered anatomy following treatment. Nausea can lead to voluntary or involuntary vomiting episodes, and if these frequently occur, this can cause tooth erosion.

Pathophysiology

There are three centres within the brain that coordinate the process of nausea and vomiting. The vomiting centre, which is located in the central medulla, can be triggered by fear, pain, or taste. This centre can also be stimulated by the chemoreceptor trigger zone (CTZ) and the nucleus tractus solitarius, which can be triggered by medications, surgery, and chemotherapy (Bhakta and Goel 2017). Nausea and vomiting are considered to be protective mechanisms and can be acute or chronic. Patients who have combined chemotherapy and radiotherapy are more like to experience nausea and vomiting.

Treatment for Nausea

Nausea and vomiting can be controlled with antisickness (antiemetic) medications. They are the most effective if they are taken regularly rather than once the symptoms occur. For the medical team to prescribe the appropriate medications it is important to determine the cause as different treatments work in different ways (Macmillan Cancer Support 2021).

Dental Erosion

If the patient's nausea cannot be controlled and persistent vomiting occurs, this is when the patient's dental health can be affected. Dental erosion is defined as the loss of enamel through acidic episodes that lead to pain and sensitivity due to the dentine becoming exposed. When someone vomits, it is the physical ejection of gastric contents that are very acidic. Saliva can slowly neutralise the acidity in the mouth; however, if someone vomits frequently the saliva does not have a chance to neutralise the mouth, and this is when the acid starts to breakdown the enamel of the teeth, which increases the risk of dental caries.

Dental Management

It is essential for dental professionals to work alongside these patients to try to minimise the dental damage from the vomiting episodes. Firstly, it is important to educate the patient about the relationship between vomiting and dental erosion and, in turn, tooth surface loss. Prevention of dental erosion should then be discussed; this can include liaising with the medical team about prescribing antisickness medications (Table 32.1). If the patient's vomiting episodes *still persist*, different dental

Care of Head and Neck Cancer Patients for Dental Hygienists and Dental Therapists, First Edition. Edited by Jocelyn J. Harding.

Table 32.1 Medications for nausea.

Drug	Brand name	Treatment use
5HT3 inhibitors	Kytril Zofran Navoban Aloxi	Chemotherapy/radiotherapy-related sickness and works best with steroids
Metoclopramide and domperidone	Mxolon Motilium	Help to empty the stomach, which can relieve the feeling of nausea
Lorazepam	Ativan	An antianxiety drug
Neurokin 1 (NK1) inhibitors	Emend Ivemend	Used alongside 5HT3 inhibitor and steroids

tips can be given. Patients should be advised to not brush their teeth following an episode, as this can mechanically brush in the gastric acids causing erosion. Instead encourage them to use fluoride mouthwash or sugar-free chewing gum, which can neutralise the mouth. Certain foods can be encouraged; cheese and milk can neutralise the pH in the patient's mouth following a vomiting episode. Head and neck cancer patients should be put on a high-fluoride toothpaste (Duraphat 2800/5000 ppm), which can be prescribed from the dentist or the patient's GP.

Patients with head and neck cancer need to have a multidisciplinary approach to their oral care. As dental professionals, it is important for us to be involved to ensure the patient's quality of life is not impacted by dental erosion caused by nausea and vomiting.

References

Bhakta, A. and Goel, R. (2017). Causes and treatment of nausea and vomiting. *Prescriber* 28 (7): 17–23.

Macmillan Cancer Support (2021). Nausea and vomiting. https://www.macmillan.org.uk/cancer-information-and-support/impacts-of-cancer/nausea-and-vomiting (accessed 3 May 2021).

33

Osteoradionecrosis

Imogen Fox

Dental Therapist, London, UK

Osteoradionecrosis (ORN) is one of the most serious complications of head and neck cancer treatment. It is very difficult to manage and can be very painful. The tumour size and location, radiation dose, local trauma, infection, immune defects, and malnutrition can predispose its development (Chrcanovic et al. 2010). Blood vessels that supply the bone in the area of radiotherapy are permanently damaged, meaning the healing ability of the area is decreased. When trauma happens in an area with reduced healing ability – for example, when teeth are extracted or when biopsies are taken – there is a risk that the socket may take longer or fail to heal. ORN occurs in around 7% of irradiated patients after tooth extraction (Nabil and Samman 2011).

Symptoms

The symptoms of ORN include the following:

- Swelling
- Infection
- Ulcers or sores inside the mouth or on the jaw
- Trismus
- Loosening of teeth or the development of a malocclusion
- Numbness or a feeling of heaviness in the jaw
- Development of exposed bone inside the mouth
- Bone sticking out through the skin, which is called sequestrum.

Grading

ORN is graded as follows:

Grade	Description
I	Soft tissue died, exposing the bone underneath it.
II	ORN that has not responded to treatment.
III	ORN affects the whole thickness of the bone, has caused a fracture, or both.

Source: Based on Chronopoulos et al. (2018).

Care of Head and Neck Cancer Patients for Dental Hygienists and Dental Therapists, First Edition. Edited by Jocelyn J. Harding.

Management of ORN

Treating a nonhealing area of soft tissue or bone can be extremely challenging. The first line of management should therefore be prevention.

Prior to Radiotherapy

Before the start of a course of radiotherapy, every patient should have a comprehensive dental assessment. It is at this point that many patients require extraction of symptomatic or very heavily restored teeth. Knowledge of the field of radiotherapy is vital in the decision for extraction. Higher-risk teeth that fall outside the field of radiotherapy may not require extraction at this time. It may therefore be more appropriate for the dental assessment to be completed within the hospital department, where this information will be readily available to the dentist conducting the assessment. This is also in line with the NICE guidelines, which suggest this should be completed by a specialist dentist/oral surgeon (National Institute for Health and Care Excellence 2004).

A multitude of factors need to be considered when deciding on a dental treatment plan prior to radiotherapy. It is ideal for the patient to be entirely dentally fit before beginning treatment (including periodontal health). This will not only reduce the risk of ORN but also ensure the patient is unlikely to suffer any other dental complications during treatment. Serious infections or pain could delay the patient's cancer treatment plan.

It is important that we allow a window of healing time after extractions before the start of the course of radiotherapy. Often the hospital team will plan to take teeth out during any surgery they may already have planned. If no other surgery is planned, then an appointment will need to made be to facilitate this. Extractions are usually done under a general anaesthetic to make sure the patient is as comfortable as possible, as it is common for patients to require multiple molar extractions at one time.

The patient should also start following an oral hygiene regime and use of daily fluoride treatments, as recommended by the dental team.

During and After Radiotherapy

The good practice of oral care allows for the best chance of successful healing. Following a healthy diet, including foods and beverages that are low in sugar, will also help reduce the risk of dental complications.

During the treatment phase many patients find their diet needs to be dramatically adapted. A dietician can work with the patient to help manage weight and nutrition, but this should also take into account sugar frequency where possible.

The risk of ORN does not reduce as time passes. Once an area of the mouth and jaw has been exposed to high-dose radiation, the risk of failed healing remains for the lifetime of the patient. For this reason, the patient must have ongoing, regular support for dental care.

Early caries and periodontal disease detection and management can help to minimise a patient's chances of future extraction. A minimally invasive restorative approach should be taken where possible. Complex or advanced treatment plans such as implants should be carefully weighed, with thought towards radiation fields. If an extraction is required, this should be completed in the least traumatic way possible, and a course of antibiotics should also be considered.

Treatment and Management of ORN

If ORN is diagnosed, there are a number of treatments that can be attempted. Pharmaceutical treatments have mixed success rates but can be attempted or used alongside surgery and/or hyperbaric oxygen therapy.

Surgery

Surgical debridement can sometimes be completed. This means removing dead or infected tissue from around a wound. The area of necrotic bone may also need to be removed. This procedure is known as a sequestrectomy. Bone and soft tissue grafting is often used to replace the removed structure. Microvascular reconstruction of the area may then need to be completed to help restore the blood flow to the area. This is done to maximise the chance of healing in the area.

Hyperbaric Oxygen Therapy

This treatment method is usually used in combination with surgery. It requires a course of treatments both before and after the surgery. Hyperbaric oxygen therapy involves breathing pure oxygen in a pressurized room. The higher pressure increases the amount of oxygen that enters the blood, which could to help heal damaged and infected tissues (Oral Cancer Foundation 2020).

References

Chrcanovic, B., Reher, P., Sousa, A., and Harris, M. (2010). Osteoradionecrosis of the jaws – a current overview – part 1. *Oral Maxillofac. Surg.* 14 (1): 3–16.

Chronopoulos, A., Zarra, T., Ehrenfeld, M., and Otto, S. (2018). Osteoradionecrosis of the jaws: definition, epidemiology, staging and clinical and radiological findings. A concise review. *Int. Dental J.* 68 (1): 22–30.

Nabil, S. and Samman, N. (2011). Incidence and prevention of osteoradionecrosis after dental extraction in irradiated patients: a systematic review. *Int. J. Oral Maxillofac. Surg.* 40 (3): 229–243.

National Institute for Health and Care Excellence. (2004). Improving outcomes in head and neck cancers [NICE cancer service guideline CSG6]. https://www.nice.org.uk/guidance/csg6.

Oral Cancer Foundation (2020), Osteoradionecrosis. https://oralcancerfoundation.org/complications/osteoradionecrosis (accessed 25 September 2020).

34

Mucus Secretions and Hypersalivation

Lucy Baker

Portsmouth Hospitals University NHS Trust, Portsmouth, UK

Mucus Secretions

A change in the consistency of saliva, developing thicker, stringy, frothy, and sticky mucus, is a common side effect of head and neck radiotherapy. This change in viscosity results in a poor saliva flow that can accumulate in the oral cavity and pharynx.

This alteration in consistency is due to the existence of abnormally high quantities of biological substances in the saliva, which may contribute to nausea, vomiting, loss of taste, smell, halitosis, increased gagging, and dysphagia (Grundmann et al. 2009, 284). Opposite to normal clear, watery, and neutral secretions, this thick mucus is described as viscous, acidic, and semi-opaque. It can also affect nutritional intake and the normal function of talking and breathing.

Thickened mucus is common alongside dysphagia. A study by Pezdirec et al. (2019, 228) discussed that 84.4% of the participates with dysphagia reported thickened mucus in comparison to 54.7% who did not suffer with any swallowing challenges posttreatment. This highlights that thickened mucus can contribute to dysphagia.

Mucus glands are extremely sensitive to radiation, developing acute and chronic reactions to radiotherapy. During head and neck radiotherapy, the salivary glands may be irritated or damaged, affecting the consistency and flow of saliva (Grundmann et al. 2009, 284).

The onset of thickened mucus primarily begins within the first couple of weeks of radiotherapy and may persist for weeks to months. This is very specific to the individual, and the duration can be dependent on age, dose, site, and field of exposure. Saliva function prior to treatment can also have an impact.

Increased mucus production is present following a laryngectomy and stoma placement especially if combined with radiotherapy. Effective care of the stoma and aspiration of mucus plugs is important. A suction machine is available to aspirate the mucus when coughing alone does not dislodge it.

Management of Thickened Mucus

Individuals may find themselves spitting more regularly and coughing partially at night when mucus accumulates. The following tips may be helpful:

- Spit more regularly.
- Increase fluid intake – 8–10 glasses of water a day. Dehydration may contribute to thickened secretions.
- Saline nebuliser – liquid changes to a fine spray that can be breathed through a mask or mouthpiece. This moisture helps to loosen and break up thickened secretions.
- Steam inhalation.
- Humidifier – increases moisture level in the air of a room. Can aid in the reduction of thickened saliva.
- Bicarbonate of soda mouthwash – can be used before and after eating to remove debris. Regular use will help dissolve stickiness and cleanse the oral cavity.

Care of Head and Neck Cancer Patients for Dental Hygienists and Dental Therapists, First Edition. Edited by Jocelyn J. Harding.

- Dissolve one teaspoon of sodium bicarbonate and one teaspoon of salt into 500mls of tap water or cooled boiled water.
- Use a mouthful of the solution to rinse your mouth out before/after meals (with dentures removed), then spit out.
- This mouthwash can be used every one to two hours for maximum effect.
- Discard this mouthwash after 24 hours and make a fresh solution.

Hypersalivation

Hypersalivation (Sialorrhea) is described as overproduction/excessive secretion of saliva or the reduced ability to clear saliva secondary to dysphagia (Paine and Snider 2020, 1333).

Although often a side effect of psychotic pharmaceuticals, in the case of the head and neck cancer patient excess salivation is often associated with anatomical changes of the oral cavity from the obstructing tumour, and following surgery such as mandibulectomy, resection of the lip and injury to the innervation of the head and neck. Sialorrhea is also a manifestation of radiotherapy due dysphagia (Bomeli et al. 2008, 1001).

One of the most challenging aspects of Sialorrhea is from inability to swallow and self-manage secretions, predisposing patients to respiratory issues and infections. Those with the added complication of poor airway control are at risk of aspiration pneumonias. Excess salivation can lead to drooling, especially if the anatomy of the lower lip has changed, with accompanying external skin infections. Both thickened mucus and Sialorrhea can have a psychological impact through depression and social isolation, resulting in diminished quality of life (Paine and Snider 2020, 1333).

Management of Sialorrhea

Where possible a non pharmacological approach is preferred:

- Portable suction device
- Oral rehabilitation with conventional prosthodontics and implant-related treatment
- Functional dysphagia therapy
- Respiratory therapy manoeuvres
- Hyacin patches for corpus amounts of saliva (Paine and Snider 2020, 1336; Bomeli et al. 2008, 1002).

References

Bomeli, S.R., Desia, S.C., Johnson, J.T., and Walvekar, R.R. (2008). Management of salivary flow in head and neck cancer patients – a systemic review. *J. Oral Oncol.* 44 (11): 1000–1008. https://doi.org/10.1016/j.oraloncolgy.2008.02.007.

Grundmann, O., Mitchell, G.C., and Limesand, K.H. (2009). Sensitivity of salivary glands to radiation from animal models to therapies. *J. Dent. Res.* 88 (10): 894–903. https://doi.org/10.1177/0022034509343143.

Paine, C.C. and Snider, J.W. (2020). When saliva becomes a problem: the challenges and palliative care for patients with sialorrhea. *Ann. Palliat. Med.* 9 (3): 1333–1339. http://doi.org/10.21037/apm.2020.02.34.

Pezdirec, M., Strojan, P., and Boltezar, I.H. (2019). Swallowing disorders after treatment for head and neck cancer. *J. Radiol. Oncol.* 53 (2): 225–230. https://doi.org/10.2478/raon-2019-0028.

35

Mouth Care and Quality of Life for Patients Living with Head and Neck Cancer

Jocelyn J. Harding

Gloucestershire Royal Hospitals, Gloucester and
Confident Dental and Implant Clinic, Stroud, UK

FDI World Dental Federation in 2016 defined oral health as '*multi-faceted and includes the ability to speak, smile, smell, taste, touch, chew, swallow, and convey a range of emotions through facial expressions with confidence and without pain, discomfort and disease of the craniofacial complex (head, face, and oral cavity). Oral health means the health of the mouth. No matter what your age, oral health is vital to general health and well-being*' (Glick et al. 2017).

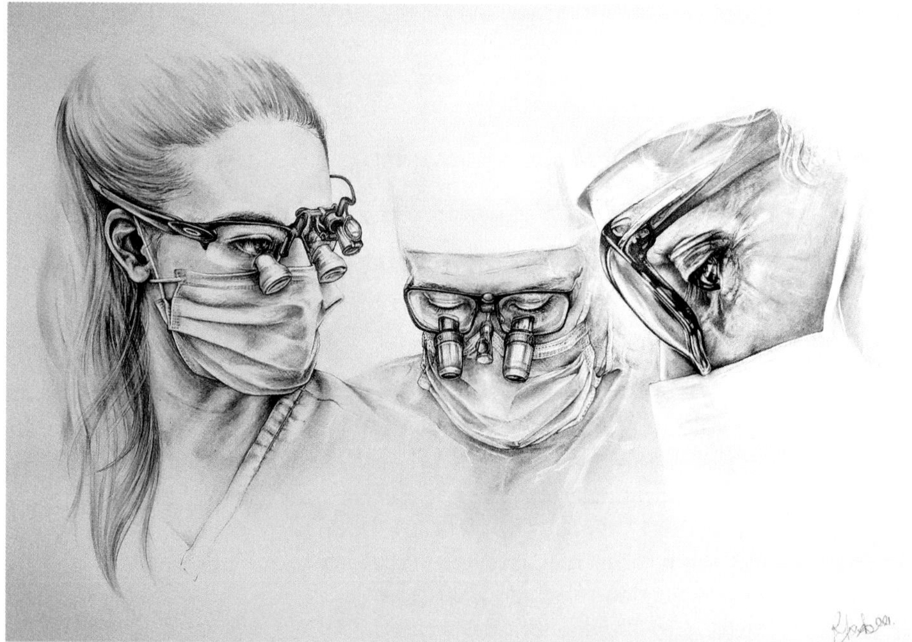

Courtesy of Dr Rachel S Jackson BDS, BSc DTH, BSc Med Ill MIMI, www.medink.co.uk.

Mouth care for this particular patient group in primary and secondary care requires dedication from all involved at the beginning, during, and then onto the important ongoing journey. Is this possible? Good oral hygiene may not always be possible due to many factors, so it is vitally important to build a good rapport with all patients from the first meeting. From patients' initial visits to their discharge, a proactive approach to the mouth care of head and neck cancer patients is truly critical. It is fundamental patient-specific mouth care is provided in the secondary care setting so on discharge this can be maintained by the patient on returning to primary care.

According to Joshi (2010), dental management aims to eliminate or stabilise oral disease to minimise local and systemic infection during and after cancer therapy and help maximise the inevitably reduced quality of life. Cancer treatments are varied and

Care of Head and Neck Cancer Patients for Dental Hygienists and Dental Therapists, First Edition. Edited by Jocelyn J. Harding.

can be complicated; therefore, the process of healing can be complex. Patients will not be aware of the many factors that can complicate continuing oral care when they start their difficult journey. Decisions about which cancer treatment or combinations of treatment or therapies are chosen based on the size of the tumour and location. Due to variations in consequences for individual treatment pathways, balancing patients' expectations before and after diagnosis is challenging and unpredictable.

Optimal mouth care is necessary before commencing cancer treatment; however, according to GP patient survey statistics, fewer than 50% of patients have seen an NHS dentist in the previous two years.

> *Dental questions were originally added to the GP Patient Survey in January to March 2010, as the Department of Health wanted information on NHS dental access and demand for services based on people's reported experience. The GP Patient Survey was chosen to capture this information as a way of accessing the proportion of the population who do not use (or have not recently used) NHS dental services in addition to those that do, to give a fuller picture of people's dental behaviour and experience.*
>
> *(NHS England 2021)*

On commencement of patients' dental treatment, their dental and cancer treatment plans are discussed in detail by the oral maxillofacial and multidisciplinary teams. Many patients often need to come to terms with losing teeth with a poor prognosis. The timing of extractions and other dental procedures is essential to coincide with treatments allowing for healing time. On occasion, the patient may need further confirmation of the treatment plan with other dental colleagues in the team; this is an opportunity to build a professional, supportive relationship.

> *Patients are commonly overwhelmed with their cancer diagnosis and will not take on board the details of the planned journey ahead so shock and denial are to be expected.*
>
> *(Macmillan Cancer Support 2019)*

How can we as dental professionals support this group of patients' lifelong challenge with their oral health? The following sections of this chapter will aim to give practical suggestions for before, during, and after treatment. Many of the considerations covered in this chapter will be discussed in more detail in other chapters. The best advice given to me personally when I began to get more involved with treating cancer patients was to remember to listen to the patient – simple advice but extremely important.

> *Patients diagnosed with head and neck cancer have a life-changing complicated journey, so a clear care pathway before, during, and after treatment can improve, minimise, or prevent complications.*
>
> *(Royal College of Surgeons of England/British Society for Disability and Oral Health 2018)*

Courtesy of Dr Rachel S Jackson BDS, BSc DTH, BSc Med Ill MIMI, www.medink.co.uk.

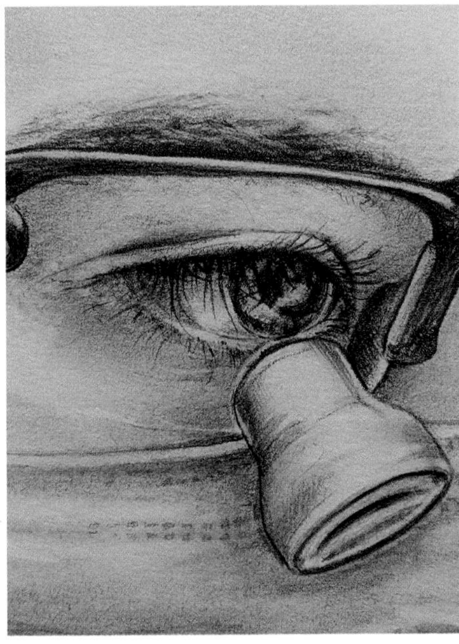

Considerations for the Dental Professional Before Treatment Begins

The following are considerations that should be taken into account by dental professionals before treatment begins.

1) *Booking or cancellation of dental appointments with general dental practices:* After diagnosis, patients will more commonly cancel a routine dental appointment rather than book a dental appointment with their general dental practice. Dental treatments which the general dentist or dental therapist can complete will have been advised in time before commencing cancer treatment, for example, extractions or essential restorations. General dental practices should train all staff to make every contact count (Making Every Contact Count 2021), whether talking to the patient by telephone call or in person, and encourage the patient to attend, time allowing, for oral hygiene instruction or an examination. Despite being overwhelmed with their journey, this can be an opportunity to improve patients' oral hygiene before starting their cancer treatment. However, this may not always be possible due to patient availability, appointments available, anxieties, or financial restraints. It is essential to create a patient-centred approach and not be judgmental of patients if their behaviours adversely affect their health (National Institute for Health and Care Excellence 2015).
2) *Toothpaste:* Patients will generally choose a toothpaste due to cost, taste, and availability; ethical and cultural options are also factors. For patients at high risk of caries, Gov.uk recommends a prescription toothpaste as an option before treatment. As for the appropriate fluoride strength of toothpaste for age, this varies worldwide, alongside importantly advising on the correct amount of toothpaste while reinforcing the recommendation to spit, not rinse, after toothbrushing, a different change in habit for some (Gov.uk 2021). Explaining the benefit of 'spit don't rinse', thereby maximising the fluoride benefit, encourages compliance. (Mouth Care Matters 2019a; Gov.uk 2021).
3) *Toothbrush and toothbrushing:* Patients generally will only change a toothbrush when they perceive it is necessary and in a poor state rather than following professional advice to regularly change the head of their electric toothbrush or manual toothbrush (Rosema et al. 2013; Schmickler et al. 2016) (Figure 35.1). The average patient brushes for 47 seconds rather than the recommended two minutes (Davies et al. 2003). Toothbrushing technique and dexterity vary widely. Consider, is the patient able to clean his/her teeth, or does he/she need support from a professional, partner, or carer?

   Toothbrushing may need to be discussed carefully and sensitively and support offered where necessary. The dental or occupational health team may consider adapting and creating supporting aids to help the patient maintain independence (Mouth Care Matters 2019a). Occupational health colleagues and dental technicians may be contacted for assistance with adapting toothbrushes. Different toothbrush options while in treatment can be mentioned at this stage, as

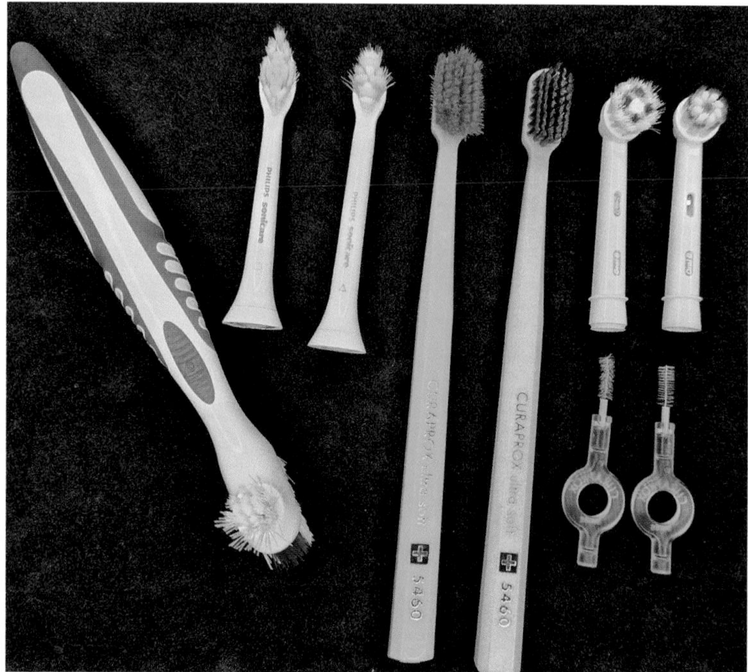

Figure 35.1 Worn toothbrush image. *Source:* http://growingsmiles.co.uk.

the impact of maintaining a basic level of oral health can become extremely difficult due to damage to the oral cavity, for example, oral mucositis. Where the patient cannot use toothbrushes, other options for cleaning tooth surfaces can be considered for the short term (Figure 35.2). When toothbrushing may be limited, waterjets and waterflossers provide an opportunity to keep a percentage of the biofilm under control and freshen the mouth; this can help to improve the patient's overall health and worry of halitosis, that is, quality of life (Figure 35.3).

4) *Mouthwash:* Many patients may have a daily mouth care routine, using mouthwash straight after brushing rather than ideally using at another time of day. Mouthwashes can support patients through treatment if their oral hygiene regime is inadequate. Chlorhexidine mouthwash may be prescribed alongside other prescription mouthwash options to help control biofilm short term, alleviate pain, or manage the symptoms of oral mucositis (UK Oral Management in Cancer

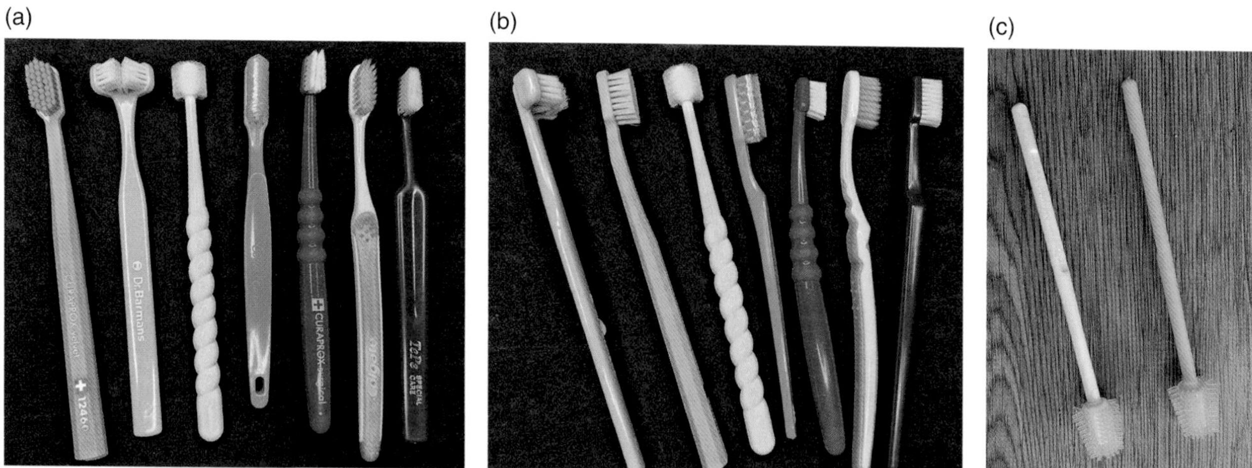

Figure 35.2 (a)–(c) Toothbrush selections – Oralieve 360, Dr Barman, Collis Curve, Tepe special care, Curaprox 12460 and Curaprox surgical toothbrushes, Colgate Slimsoft, and MouthEze oral cleanser. *Source:* http://growingsmiles.co.uk and http://kohc.co.uk.

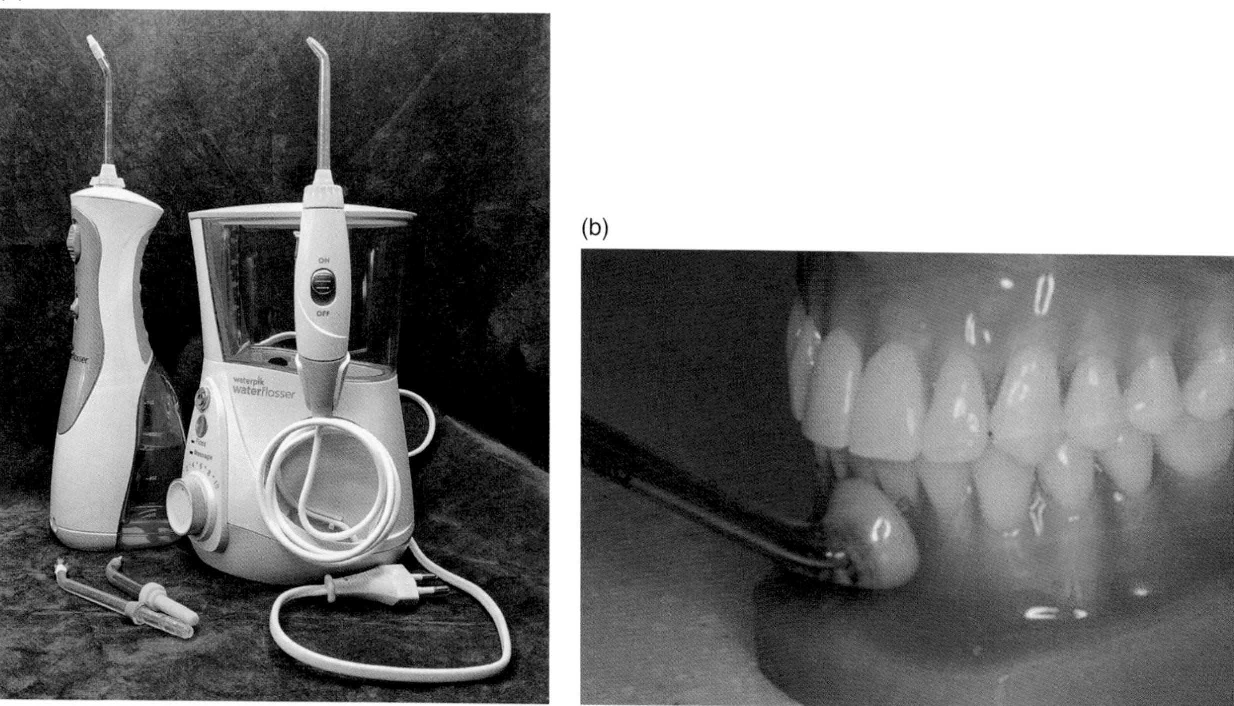

Figure 35.3 (a) and (b) Waterflossers, waterjets, airflossers. *Source:* http://growingsmiles.co.uk.

Group 2019; Elad et al. 2020). A fluoride, alcohol-free mouthwash is recommended to be used at a different time of day to toothbrushing (Burke et al. 2014; Royal College of Surgeons of England/British Society for Disability and Oral Health 2018; Gov.uk 2021).

5) *Gingivitis:* Demonstrating an effective toothbrushing technique before treatment starts is essential while warning patients to persevere with any initial bleeding. Daily interdental cleaning may not be a regular daily routine for the patient, which can be initiated and encouraged. However, specialists may advise cautionary use of interdental cleaning aids during treatment, depending on the type of treatment, the possibility of causing trauma, or clotting disorders (UK Oral Management in Cancer Care Group 2019; Multinational Association of Supportive Care in Cancer 2021).
6) *Periodontal disease:* Patients may or may not be aware of their periodontal disease status before treatment. Teeth with a poor prognosis and/or severe bone loss will be treatment planned for extraction by the hospital team to reduce the risk of osteoradionecrosis after completing radiotherapy treatment. Ongoing periodontal care, maintenance, and oral rehabilitation on a patient's return to practice should be addressed as soon as possible (Royal College of Surgeons of England/British Society for Disability and Oral Health 2018). Loss of teeth affects patient by reduced chewing efficiency, appearance, and trismus (Bhandari et al. 2021).
7) *Xerostomia:* Xerostomia can often be subjective, and many patients will not be aware of the quantity or quality of saliva before treatment due to dehydration/age/comorbidities/polypharmacy (Porter et al. 2004; Epstein et al. 2014). Patients averagely produce 0.5 L or more saliva per day; however, this may be reduced due to the above considerations (Porter et al. 2004).

   Patients will often drink various types of fluids to give variety – caffeinated drinks and squash, or flavoured water as a pleasant alternative – and although these are valuable fluids, they may have a detrimental effect on a patient's teeth (Mouth Care Matters 2019a). Hydration with fluids, ideally water, can be problematic, as patients often mention broken nights of sleep due to increased bathroom visits. Ideally, 6–8 glasses of water per day are recommended (NHS 2021). Sips of water throughout the day and avoiding certain foods may also help (Macmillan Cancer Support 2019).
8) *Angular cheilitis:* This may occur in patients who wear dentures, are immunocompromised, or who have a poor diet. Investigating the cause and helping to resolve a patient's angular cheilitis will improve the patient's health, make toothbrushing easier, and make eating and drinking more pleasant. This complication may improve by applying lip balm or an antifungal prescription (Mouth Care Matters 2019b). Radiotherapy teams will discuss the types of creams, lotions, and soaps allowed during treatment due to some products making the skin more sensitive (Macmillan Cancer Support 2021).
9) *Denture care:* Demonstrating good effective denture-cleaning technique and storage will help remind the patient to leave dentures out at night and reduce the risk of infection (Figure 35.4). Suggest a named denture pot for the patient to take to the hospital to prevent mislaid dentures. If the dentures are a poor fit due to weight loss, this will need to be addressed on completion of cancer treatment.

   Oral Health Foundation denture care summary of guidelines:

   Daily cleaning of the dentures using mechanical action – brushing with a toothbrush or denture brush and an effective, nonabrasive denture cleanser (no dentifrice).

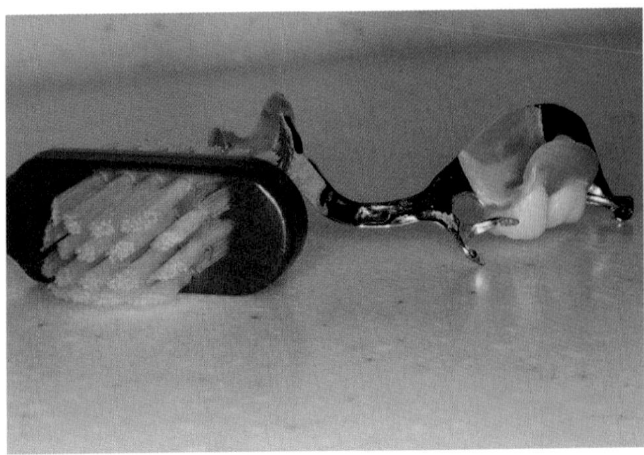

Figure 35.4 A denture brush and denture.

Daily soaking in a denture-cleansing solution – this seems to deliver extra chemical breakdown of the remaining plaque and some level of disinfection of the denture. Denture-cleansing solutions should only be used outside the mouth, and denture wearers should strictly follow the manufacturers' guidelines.

Denture wearers should not keep their dentures in the mouth overnight, unless there are specific reasons for keeping them in. This guideline is even more important for people at a higher risk of developing stomatitis and for frail or institutionalised older people. Soaking in a denture-cleanser solution after mechanical cleaning seems to be beneficial for preventing denture stomatitis and the potential risk of pneumonia events in these groups of people.

All patients who wear removable dentures should be enrolled into a regular recall and maintenance programme with their dental professional. (Oral Health Foundation 2018; Bartlett et al. 2018)

10) *Smoking, alcohol and drugs:* These topics must be discussed sensitively to ascertain patients' status and encourage them to seek support before beginning cancer treatment. Discuss with the patient if they would like signposting to available services and resources (Gov.uk 2021).
11) *Support:* It is good practice to ask about the support network of the patient. Assistance from charities specialising in giving support can be suggested to patients, their families, and friends.
12) *Mood:* Being aware of patients' moods through their journey and beyond is essential, and communicating with their hospital team is critical should patients seem particularly low or possibly suicidal (Osazuwa-Peters et al. 2018).
13) *Empathy:* As dental professionals, life and death conversations are not part of our remit; it is crucial to facilitate the appropriate level of compassion for this group of patients, which can be problematic. What should we say after the diagnosis? Preferring to say, 'Lovely to see you' rather than asking 'How are you?' is an improved way to greet a patient after diagnosis (Fox 2020).

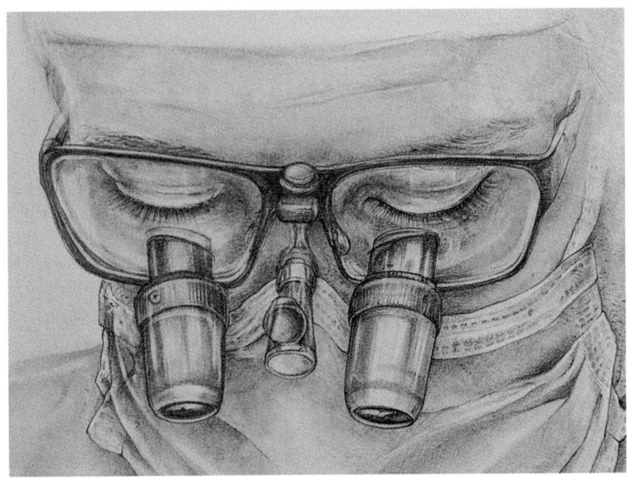

Courtesy of Dr Rachel S Jackson BDS, BSc DTH, BSc Med Ill MIMI, www.medink.co.uk.

During and Beyond Treatment Complications

Some of the challenges during and after treatment may include weight loss related to cancer treatment directly; difficult oral access and ability to clean the mouth due to soreness; consuming high calorific drinks to provide the necessary vitamins and calories; changes to taste sensation (dysgeusia); swallowing difficulties (dysphagia); xerostomia; and fatigue. The patient is vulnerable to tooth decay, periodontal disease, and a high risk of aspirational pneumonia during treatment (Figure 35.5). A patient may have been a motivated regular dental attender before starting treatment, but oral health will become less of a priority due to some or all of the effects of treatment.

1) *Saliva:* The saliva composition for head and neck cancer patients can vary immensely, which cannot be predicted. Xerostomia can be a drastic effect of treatment for many patients. Eating, drinking, speech, swallowing, and intimacy are affected for many patients long term. Hypersalivation can be equally dramatic and frustrating for the patient dealing with a constant flow of saliva. Mucus and thick saliva, described as 'gorilla glue' by one patient, can also be life

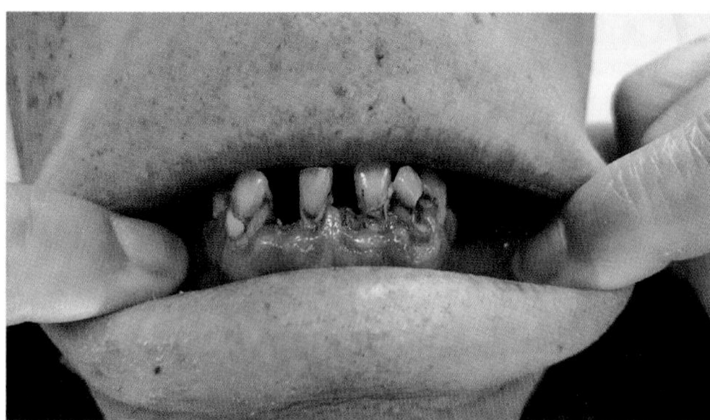

Figure 35.5 Image showing post-treatment oral effects-rampant decay and fractured teeth in a xerostomic patient.

changing. Some effects can improve in the first two months after treatment; however, this can take up to two years to improve or could even be a long-term side effect for many patients (Royal College of Surgeons of England/British Society for Disability and Oral Health 2018).

A nebuliser can be a helpful suggestion providing some relief for mucus, slough, and xerostomia in some patients. This option can be discussed with the patient's medical team.

A lack of saliva will increase some patients' isolation due to not being able to eat with family or friends or taking a long time to eat. This is because the food provided is not the correct consistency for them to manage, or they make noises while eating, or they drool while eating or talking.

Patients' swallowing mechanism can be investigated and subsequently supported, with techniques from speech and language therapists, and, on many occasions, it can be improved. Some patients will notice an improvement. However, it may not return to pretreatment, which must be carefully managed by all teams involved.

Many patients are embarrassed and tend to shy away from social events, negatively affecting their psychological well-being. The control of hypersalivation is equally problematic. Xerostomic patients should be aware of their water intake and remain hydrated. Patients may benefit from medication or saliva substitutes, saliva stimulants, and saliva lubricants available on prescription or over the counter. Advice should be given to check ingredients' pH, contraindications, and animal ingredients. Providing instructions for product application will increase their efficacy, and patients are more likely to comply with helpful recommendations.

2) *Speech:* For many patients, their speech can be affected short term or long term. Partial or total glossectomy, laryngectomy, and xerostomia can all make conversations nonexistent or tiring. Maybe the patient's mouth is still ulcerated or tender from treatment, or perhaps the angles of the mouth are cracked or sore, so be prepared to have a notepad and pen handy for the patient. Keep questions simple and ask one question at a time, because speech problems may go alongside swallowing difficulties. Please discuss this with or refer the patient back to the speech and language therapist.
3) *Hearing:* Patients may notice a difference in their hearing due to radiotherapy treatment. Face the patient and ask questions slowly and clearly and ask one question at a time. Lowering the voice can also help, as these tonal differences can be heard more clearly.
4) *Trismus and shoulder stiffness:* Accessibility to the patient's mouth can vary, depending on the soreness or limited opening of the patient's mouth or restriction due to the effect of the surgery site external to the mouth utilised for reconstruction, for example, shoulder, back, or neck. Oral hygiene will be challenging to perform for the patient and the dental professional. A suction toothbrush may be a helpful option (Figure 35.6). Trismus may be a long-term condition, and referral for exercises by a physiotherapist to reduce the impact may be required. Patients may not be able to lie supine in the dental chair, so this must be considered when examining and treating the patient (Figure 35.7). A dental pillow may help make the patient more comfortable.
5) *Toothbrushing and interdental cleaning:* Oral mucositis and viral and fungal infections can make the mouth sore, so that toothbrushing can become challenging during treatment. Waterflossers, airflossers, or waterjets can be a sensible, gentle option to consider (Figure 35.3b). These options may help remove debris, slough, and thick saliva and allow rinsing the mouth with a fluoride mouthwash if physical cleaning cannot be managed. Soft bristle brushes and other helpful options can be advised; there are many available (Figure 35.2a,b). Pink sponges on sticks are now being discontinued in many Trusts and should not be used. Please check your Trust's recommendations (Elad et al. 2017; UK Oral Management in Cancer Care Group 2019; Mouth Care Matters 2019a).

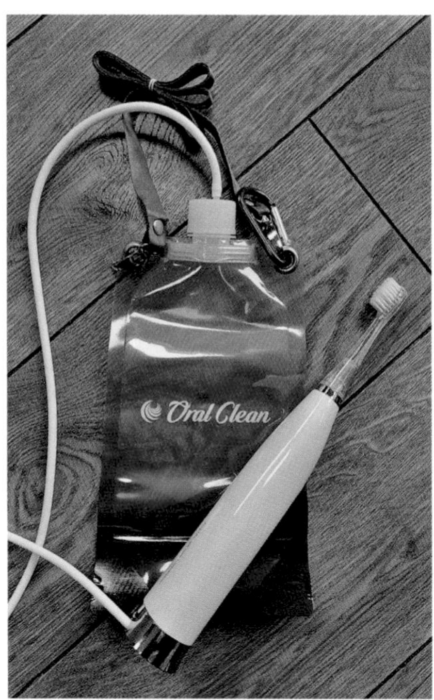

Figure 35.6 Suction toothbrush option helpful for carers or patients not able to perform own mouth care, those lying supine or those with limited opening or trismus to prevent choking. *Source:* http://kohc.co.uk.

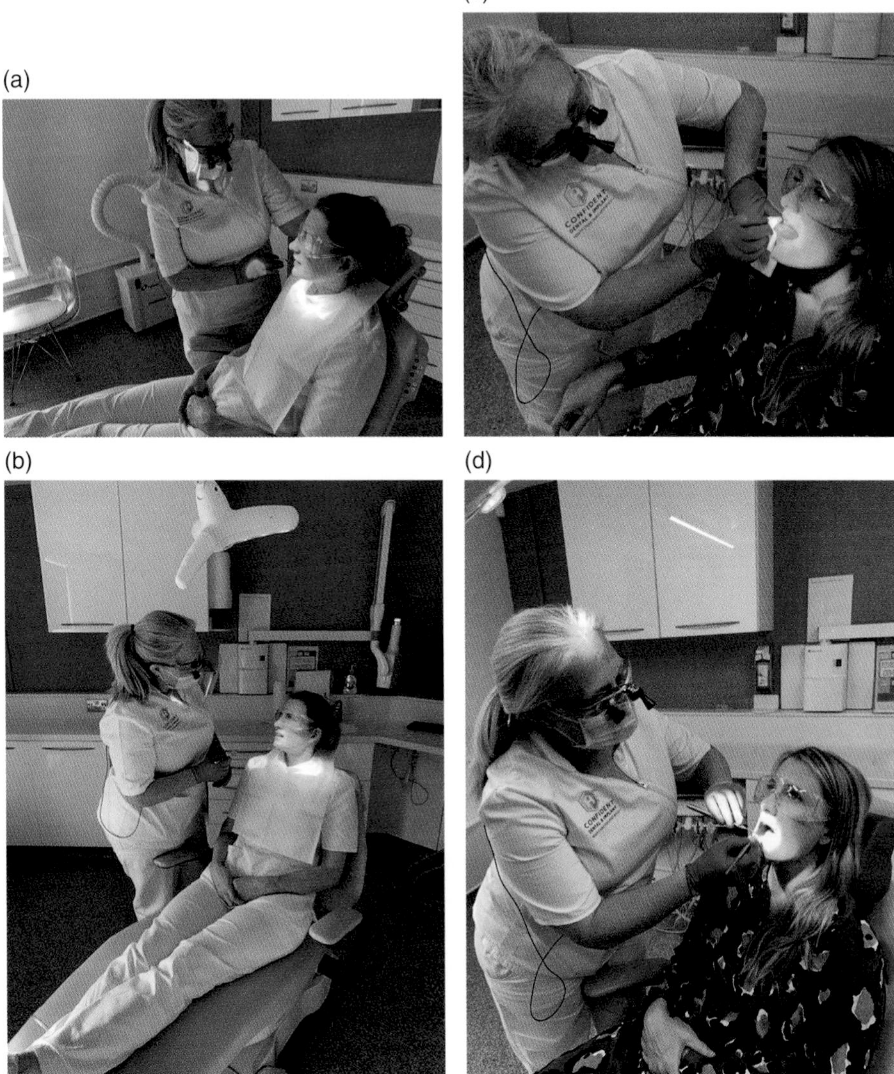

Figure 35.7 (a)–(d) Images showing position of a patient sitting upright for patient comfort and suction when using water, air polishing, or airflow. Face patient to support those with hearing loss and speak slowly and clearly. Provide a head pillow if possible. Check IO, if accessible, and EO. Protect your back position when treating patients upright.

Patients will often have to adapt to a changed, reduced, or complicated dentition. Regular daily interdental cleaning, if possible, is recommended. Demonstrate adaptions and support patients to maintain any change to their dentition. What are they using to clean their teeth and implants or other complex restorative treatment? Do they have the dexterity to use a toothbrush or clean interdentally effectively? Do they need support from their carer or partner? Regular dental visits, and often more frequent PMPR, for monitoring and supporting the patient are vital. Discuss after care maintenance of complicated prostheses and or implants with the restorative specialist if you are concerned.

6) *Toothpaste:* Patients' toothpaste choices will often vary during treatment, mainly due to finding they cannot tolerate mint flavours; other flavoured toothpaste can be suggested, which may be a short-term or long-term change. In some circumstances, many patients may prefer flavour-free toothpaste; OraNurse is one brand available in the UK at present. High-fluoride toothpaste, such as Colgate Duraphat toothpaste, is an evidence-based product recommended by Gov.UK to be used at least two times per day with no rinsing afterwards. Some patients find that not rinsing after toothbrushing during their treatment is difficult due to xerostomia (Gov.uk 2021; UK Oral Management in Cancer Care Group 2019). Check toothpaste ingredients, specifically sodium lauryl sulphate (SLS), a common foaming ingredient. Some patients find this irritating to the mucosa. Selecting an SLS-free toothpaste can improve toothbrushing. Check toothpaste ingredients for contraindications and that products align with patients' ethical choices.
7) *Mouthwash:* Mouthwash is recommended to use at a different time to brushing, so it doesn't reduce the fluoride's benefit in the toothpaste. Alcohol-free fluoride mouthwashes are especially helpful if the patient cannot toothbrush due to mouth soreness (Gov.uk 2021). The hospital team can prescribe different mouthwashes such as antifungals, mucosal protectants, or analgesics to help reduce oral mucositis, ulcerations, and fungal infections (UK Oral Management in Cancer Care Group 2019).
8) *Erosion:* Due to vomiting, acid reflux, the change in appetite, and dysgeusia in treatment, it is common for many patients to deviate from their regular controlled eating habits to either eat more irregularly or consume higher quantities of acidic drinks to help make food and drink more pleasurable. This can lead to tooth surface loss and can be detrimental in some cases, depending on tooth surface loss present before treatment or the length of treatment. Advice from the hospital team to control acid reflux and vomiting will help manage this, as will advice to avoid toothbrushing for 30 minutes after vomiting (Mouth Care Matters 2019a). An alcohol-free fluoride mouthwash can help freshen the mouth and support the patient.
9) *Tooth decay and root caries:* Patients, hospital teams, and carers may not be aware of the raised caries risk during treatment caused by the combination of high calorific foods and drinks, an erratic eating regime, or grazing that may occur. High-fluoride toothpaste is recommended to help reduce the effects of foods and drinks that cause tooth decay (Gov.uk 2021).

   Susceptible teeth will, in many cases, have been extracted before treatment, and not all patients will elect for this; however, this is with the ultimate aim to reduce the possibility of chronic infections becoming acute and monitoring patients' oral health and overall health (Royal College of Surgeons of England/British Society for Disability and Oral Health 2018). The management of rampant tooth decay is an ongoing treatment dilemma for both the patient and the clinician, especially those patients treated with radiotherapy. 'Radiation caries (RC) is a rampant form of dental decay affecting cusp tips, incisal edges, and cervical area of the teeth and the lingual surface of mandibular teeth, which are usually resistant to dental caries in non-irradiated patients' (Kielbassa et al. 2006; Bhandari et al. 2021).

   Exposed root surfaces are at high risk for root caries, which can be challenging to treat, especially during treatment and beyond. Patients should attend their dental practice as soon as possible after concluding treatment to assess any damage and set up a treatment plan for continuing care. When possible, there should be minimally invasive care in the future.

   The dental team can prescribe and routinely apply fluoride varnish to root surfaces to help prevent root caries (Gov.uk 2021). Consider the use of daily alcohol-free fluoride mouthwash and casein phosphopeptide-amorphous calcium phosphate (CPP-ACP) products applied alongside high-fluoride toothpaste as an added preventative measure (Royal College of Surgeons of England/British Society for Disability and Oral Health 2018).

   Xylitol can be considered as a simple recommendation for patients with a dry mouth and an increased risk of tooth decay, one way to support patients with a minimal invasive approach. Xylitol is a natural sweetener that can be purchased in a granular form and added to drinks, sprinkled on cereals, and used in cooking or as a mint or chewing gum. Dr Heff's Remarkable Mints is one brand available and has been developed to help to reduce acidity levels and plaque growth, increase collagen scaffold, and remineralise the teeth with increased calcium phosphate. Different flavours of mints and chewing gums are available and patients can seek out which they prefer (Dentistry.co.uk 2021).

10) *Periodontal disease:* Periodontal disease can be a complication of treatment due to xerostomia, poor accessibility, soreness due to mucosal damage, and suboptimal oral hygiene allowing a more mature biofilm to form and exacerbate periodontal disease progression. Patients will need to have the level of periodontal disease assessed and a future treatment plan discussed on return to their dental practice. Damage from radiotherapy and the risk of osteoradionecrosis will influence the treatment plan to maintain teeth or teeth roots as far as possible. Refer to the oral maxillofacial team for support or possible extractions.
11) *Fatigue:* Tiredness and fatigue are a common complaint from patients during and beyond treatment. Please understand and discuss this with patients to help them keep active as far as possible and to recognise when to stop and relax (Heathline 2019). "The Spoons Theory" is a visual representation of the management of someones energy or fatigue.
12) *Spasm and referred pain:* These are complications of treatment and may occur at any time. Refer to a patient's general practitioner or hospital team for further investigation and support.

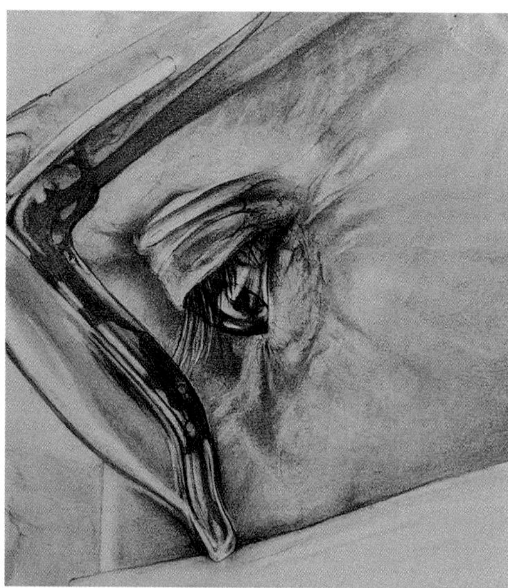

Courtesy of Dr Rachel S Jackson BDS, BSc DTH, BSc Med Ill MIMI, www.medink.co.uk.

Practicalities of Treating Head and Neck Cancer Patients

Some of these suggestions will apply only to patients while in hospital care, some in general practice, and some in both locations.

1) Observe patients as they arrive in the surgery. Take note of any stoop, angle of neck, limp, or neck scarf. These visual differences may give a hint to after-treatment effects related to the patient's head and neck cancer treatment.
2) Please discuss with patients their previous dental history and head and neck cancer treatment journey.
3) A good light source is essential due to restricted opening for many patients.
4) Provide a comfortable headrest for the patient.
5) Have patients lie supine if possible; however, this may, on many occasions, not always be possible.
6) Allow short breaks throughout the appointment when checking soft tissues and treating. Patients may often attend with a bottle of water and take frequent sips.
7) Take short breaks to allow for coughing. Patients will often apologise as they feel this is disturbing the flow of the appointment.
8) Make mouth care applicable to each patient (personal, practical, and positive); demonstrate specific oral hygiene care and give time for patients to copy. Are patients able to perform mouth care themselves? Are they confident? Is their dexterity good/fair/poor?

9) Be aware of restricted access and modify mouth care to the patient. If the mouth opening limits access for preferred oral hygiene aids, consider waterjets, waterflossers, or airflossers as options. Suction toothbrushes are an option if the patient needs more intensive supportive care or end-of-life mouth care.
10) Suggest alternative toothpaste if the patient cannot manage certain ingredients; mint, sodium lauryl sulphate, or prefer flavour-free. Be aware some patients may choose a toothpaste for ethical or other reasons.
11) Give good mouth care advice if the patient is eating orally.
12) Give good mouth care advice if the patient is fed by a feeding tube. In some patients, this may be lifelong.
13) Discuss ongoing dental care while in hospital care before discharge. Is the patient registered with a dental practice? Encourage patients in hospital care to plan their return to general dental practice even if this was not a routine before their diagnosis. Patients sometimes find that returning to hospital for dental hygienist recalls is upsetting because they are returning to the department where they were initially diagnosed. Scanxiety is common (Ennis-O'Connor 2018).
14) Refer to the patient's general medical practitioner if the patient has been discharged from hospital care and needs further psychological support, has swallowing difficulties, or requires nutritional support.
15) Ask patients about their support network and how they are coping with the diagnosis and treatment. Does the patient have children, a partner, parents who also need support?
16) Recurrence – some patients examining their mouths will become 'hyper-aware' of any differences they feel. Recurrence is not uncommon (Mehanna et al. 2016).

> *It is estimated that between 20% and 40% of head and neck cancers will return after treatment and, in England, between 28% and 67% survive their disease for five years or more.*
>
> *(Royal Marsden NHS Foundation Trust 2021).*

17) Look into medical emergency courses for the CPR of tracheotomy and laryngectomy patients.
18) Most importantly, listen to patients. They may discuss their relationship and intimacy complications, financial problems, logistics of attending appointments; in short, many different kinds of worries.
19) Remember to seek help yourself if you feel anxious for a particular patient or procedure, and talk to your colleagues. To have patients tell me personally that they don't sit at the dining table with their loved ones anymore as they are frightened of making noises or they are not able to enjoy a meal with them due to being PEG fed for the rest of their lives, or to have a total glossectomy patient write the word 'miserable' on a pad when communicating, it hits home, hard.

Holistic Care and Ongoing Financial Burden for the Patient Long Term

Patients will have many financial considerations in their lives when diagnosed. The patient may or may not have been a regular dental attender prior to diagnosis. The best patient journey post-treatment would be regular visits to their dental team to check their dental health and general health. However, as there is no financial support presently for head and neck cancer patients for ongoing dental care, this is not always possible and, for some, not important.

Mouth care for all patients is about the care of the mouth; however, if mouth care is not addressed, there may be a detrimental impact to overall health, and mouth care should always be considered an integrated part of care – that is, holistic care.

References

Bartlett, D., Carter, N., de Baat, C., et al. (2018) White paper on optimal care and maintenance of full dentures for oral and general health, https://www.dentalhealth.org/Handlers/Download.ashx?IDMF=8a8a723a-20c5-4064-8f37-1947ab94481a.

Bhandari, S., Soni, B.W., and Ghoshal, S. (2021). Impact of non-compliance with oral care on radiation caries in head and neck cancer survivors. *Support. Care Cancer* 29 (8): 4783–4790. https://doi.org/10.1007/s00520-021-06033-y.

Burke, S., Kwasnicki, A.J., and Kaura, L. (2014). Dental management of patients post head and neck cancer. *Dental. Nurs.* 10 (5): 258–265. https://doi.org/10.12968/denn.2014.10.5.258.

Macmillan Cancer Support (2019). Cancer and your emotions. www.macmillan.org.uk/cancer-information-and-support/treatment/coping-with-treatment/cancer-and-your-emotions.

Davies, R.M., Davies, G.M., and Ellwood, R.P. (2003). Prevention. Part 4: toothbrushing: what advice should be given to patients? *Brit. Dent. J.* 195 (3): 135–141. https://doi.org/10.1038/sj.bdj.4810396.

Gov.uk (2021). Delivering better oral health: an evidence-based toolkit for prevention. https://www.gov.uk/government/publications/delivering-better-oral-health-an-evidence-based-toolkit-for-prevention (Accessed: 27 September 2021).

Dentistry.co.uk (2021). Dr Heff's – the science behind the mint. https://dentistry.co.uk/2021/03/09/dr-heffs-the-science-behind-the-mint/.

Oral Health Foundation (2018). Denture care guidelines. https://www.dentalhealth.org/denturecareguidelines.

Elad, S., Ranna, V., Ariyawardana, A. et al. (2017). A systematic review of oral herpetic viral infections in cancer patients: commonly used outcome measures and interventions. *Support. Care Cancer* 25 (2): 687–700. https://doi.org/10.1007/s00520-016-3477-7.

Elad, S., Cheng, K.K.F., Lalla, R.V. et al. (2020). MASCC/ISOO clinical practice guidelines for the management of mucositis secondary to cancer therapy. *Cancer* 126 (19): 4423–4431. https://doi.org/10.1002/cncr.33100.

Ennis-O'Connor, M. (2018). Coping with scanxiety: practical tips from cancer patients. https://powerfulpatients.org/2018/07/24/coping-with-scanxiety-practical-tips-from-cancer-patients.

Epstein, J.B., Güneri, P., and Barasch, A. (2014). Appropriate and necessary oral care for people with cancer: guidance to obtain the right oral and dental care at the right time. *Support. Care Cancer* 22 (7): 1981–1988. https://doi.org/10.1007/s00520-014-2228-x.

Fox, I. (2020). Compassionate empathetic care: let's talk about the c-word. *Dental Health* 59 (4): 28–31.

Glick, M., Williams, D.M., Kleinman, D.V. et al. (2017). Reprint of: A new definition for oral health supported by FDI opens the door to a universal definition of oral health. *J. Dentist.* 57: 1–3. https://doi.org/10.1016/j.jdent.2016.12.005.

NHS England (2021). Summary of the dental results from the GP Patient Survey – January to March 2021. https://www.england.nhs.uk/statistics/wp-content/uploads/sites/2/2021/07/GP-Survey-Dental-Results-Summary-January-to-March-2021.pdf.

Harding, J. (2017). Dental care of cancer patients before, during and after treatment. *BDJ Team* 4 (1): 10–12. https://doi.org/10.1038/bdjteam.2017.8.

Harding, J. (2018). Oral care in cancer: helping patients with tooth, gum and mouth problems. *Bri. J. Nur.* 27 (19): 1106–1107. https://doi.org/10.12968/bjon.2018.27.19.1106.

Mouth Care Matters (2019a). Improving oral health of older persons initiative. https://mouthcarematters.hee.nhs.uk/e-learning/.

Joshi, V.K. (2010). Dental treatment planning and management for the mouth cancer patient. *Oral Oncol.* 46 (6): 475–479. https://doi.org/10.1016/j.oraloncology.2010.03.010.

Kielbassa, A.M., Hinkelbein, W., Hellwig, E. et al. (2006). Radiation-related damage to dentition. *Lancet Oncol.* 7 (4): 326–335. https://doi.org/10.1016/S1470-2045(06)70658-1.

Making Every Contact Count (2021). Home. www.makingeverycontactcount.co.uk.

Mehanna, H., Kong, A., and Ahmed, S.K. (2016). Recurrent head and neck cancer: United Kingdom National Multidisciplinary Guidelines. *J. Laryngol. Otol.* 130 (S2): S181–S190. https://doi.org/10.1017/S002221511600061X.

Mouth Care Matters (2019b). Mouth Care Matters resources. https://mouthcarematters.hee.nhs.uk/links-resources/mouth-care-matters-resources-2.

National Institute for Health and Care Excellence (2015). Oral health promotion: general dental practice [NICE guideline NG30]. www.nice.org.uk/guidance/ng30.

Multinational Association of Supportive Care in Cancer (2021). Oral care education. https://www.mascc.org/oral-care-education.

Osazuwa-Peters, N., Simpson, M.C., Zhao, L. et al. (2018). Suicide risk among cancer survivors: head and neck versus other cancers. *Cancer* 124 (20): 4072–4079. https://doi.org/10.1002/cncr.31675.

Porter, S.R., Scully, C., and Hegarty, A.M. (2004). An update of the etiology and management of xerostomia. *Oral Surg., Oral Med., Oral Pathol., Oral Radiol., Endodontol.* 97 (1): 28–46. https://doi.org/10.1016/j.tripleo.2003.07.010.

Macmillan Cancer Support (2021). Side effects of radiotherapy for head and neck cancer. www.macmillan.org.uk/cancer-information-and-support/head-and-neck-cancer/side-effects-of-radiotherapy-for-head-and-neck-cancer.

Rosema, N.A.M., Hennequin-Hoenderdos, N.L., Versteeg, P.A. et al. (2013). Plaque-removing efficacy of new and used manual toothbrushes – -a professional brushing study. *Int. J. Dent. Hyg.* 11 (4): 237–243. https://doi.org/10.1111/idh.12021.

Royal College of Surgeons of England/British Society for Disability and Oral Health (2018). The oral management of oncology patients requiring radiotherapy, chemotherapy and/or bone marrow transplantation. https://www.rcseng.ac.uk/dental-faculties/fds/publications-guidelines/clinical-guidelines/.

Schmickler, J., Wurbs, S., Wurbs, S. et al. (2016). The influence of the utilization time of brush heads from different types of power toothbrushes on oral hygiene assessed over a 6-month observation period: a randomized clinical trial. *Am. J. Dentist.* 29 (6): 307–314.

UK Oral Management in Cancer Care Group (2019). Welcome to UK Oral Management in Cancer Care Group. www.ukomic.co.uk.

NHS (2021). Water, drinks and your health. https://www.nhs.uk/live-well/eat-well/water-drinks-nutrition.

Healthline (2019). I'm a 'Spoonie.' Here's what I wish more people knew about chronic illness. https://www.healthline.com/health/spoon-theory-chronic-illness-explained-like-never-before.

Royal Marsden NHS Foundation Trust (2021). World's first research centre for recurrent head and neck cancer launched. https://www.royalmarsden.nhs.uk/worlds-first-research-centre-recurrent-head-and-neck-cancer-launched.

36

Obturators

Rhiannon Jones

Cardiff University, Cardiff, UK

An obturator is "a maxillofacial prosthesis used to close a congenital or acquired tissue opening, primarily of the hard palate and/or contiguous alveolar/soft tissue structures. . .[The word describes the] component of a prosthesis that fits into and closes a defect within the oral cavity. . .[and maintains] the integrity of the oral and nasal compartments resulting from a congenital, acquired, or developmental disease process" (Journal of Prosthetic Dentistry 2017).

The primary function of an obturator is to facilitate speech, mastication, swallowing and, in some cases, improve aesthetics. They can be life changing for wearers, allowing them to communicate effectively, eat a varied diet, and restore their self-confidence. Their ability to make the wearer more confident in everyday activities must not be underestimated by clinicians providing their care.

Obturators are often required for maxillary cancer defects that are not amenable or suitable for surgical reconstruction or where reconstruction has been unsuccessful.

Defects Without Obturation

A defect without obturation could result in the following:

- Speech issues and reduced ability to communicate
- Food impaction or oronasal regurgitation of solid or liquid foods depending on the location and size of the defect
- Poor nutrition/hydration and subsequent weight loss and malnutrition
- Reduced quality of life.

Developmental Defects

Patients with developmental defects such as clefts of their hard and/or soft palate may require obturation. Clefts may result from disturbances of any of the processes involved during palatogenesis (Berkovitz et al. 2018). Babies born with a cleft would be expected to have surgical repair in their first year, allowing them to feed and babble effectively. It is rare for a baby to require an obturator due to effective feeding techniques and timely surgery. However, people born in the first half of the twentieth century may not have received a definitive palate repair and therefore may require obturation of their defect. It is not uncommon for them to have missing maxillary teeth, and they may present with a partial or full denture with an obturator to occlude the defect. The obturators may also contain components for attachment to dental implants (see Figures 36.1–36.3) to aid retention where the alveolar ridge is insufficient. It is possible that younger patients may present with an obturator if they were born in a country where palate repair was not available or successful or to help with speech difficulties.

Care of Head and Neck Cancer Patients for Dental Hygienists and Dental Therapists, First Edition. Edited by Jocelyn J. Harding.

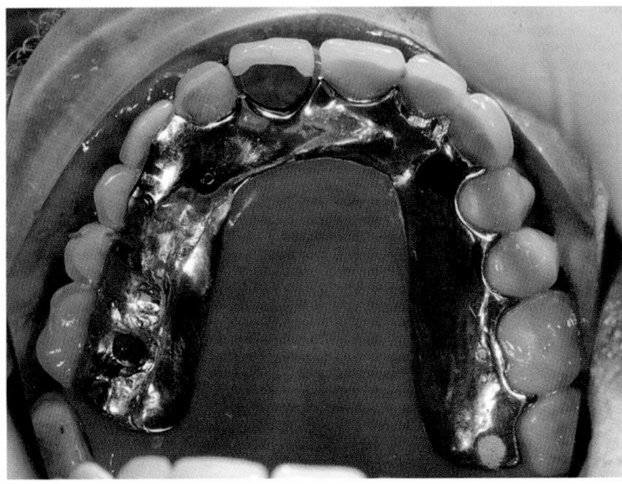

Figure 36.1 Overdenture in situ containing obturator component. *Source:* Image courtesy of Rhiannon Jones, Bristol Dental Hospital and grateful patients of the South West Cleft Team.

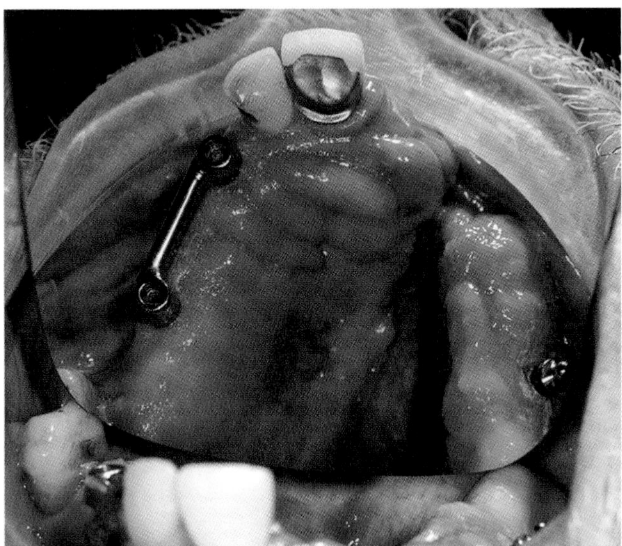

Figure 36.2 Unrepaired cleft with intraosseous implants to aid retention of partial denture with obturator (same case as Figure 36.1). *Source:* Image courtesy of Rhiannon Jones, Bristol Dental Hospital and grateful patients of the South West Cleft Team.

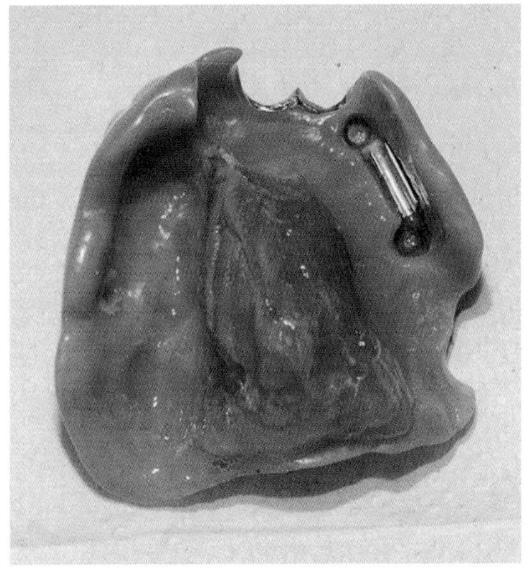

Figure 36.3 Implant-retained partial upper denture with solid acrylic obturator (same as Figures 36.1 and 36.2). *Source:* Image courtesy of Rhiannon Jones, Bristol Dental Hospital and grateful patients of the South West Cleft Team.

Head and Neck Cancer

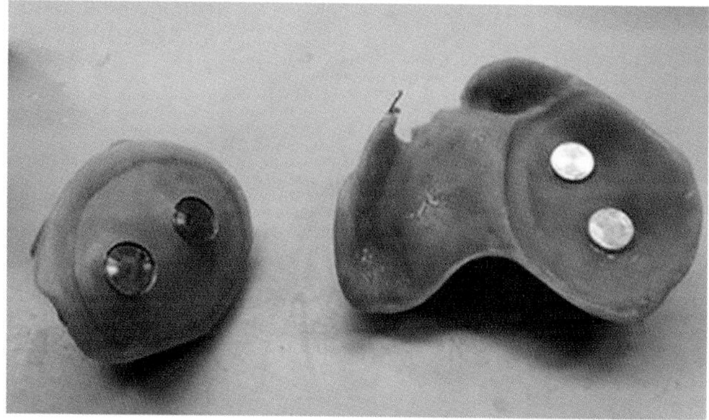

Figure 36.4 Two-part prosthesis using magnets to retain the obturator component. *Source:* Image courtesy of Lucy Tsiopani, Bristol Dental Hospital.

Surgical excision of cancer affecting the maxillary ridge or sinuses can result in a significant defect that requires obturation. Surgical obturators are often required immediately following surgery to prevent nasal regurgitation and to allow the patient to speak, eat, and regain confidence. A multi-disciplinary team (MDT), including speech and language therapists helps patients learn to cope with their new prothesis, and Macmillan nurses provide invaluable care and support to the patient and their family (National Institute for Health and Care Excellence 2018).

Once healing has occurred, an interim obturator is often needed, especially if the patient receives postoperative radiotherapy. A definitive obturator can be provided later and normally no sooner than six months following completion of radiotherapy to allow for tissue remodelling. Recent developments in this area have included immediate zygomatic implants, reconstruction flaps, and early placement of a fixed prosthesis. This requires a specialist team of experienced dental technicians and restorative consultants to plan and create a suitable device and follow-up care (Butterworth et al. 2016). Once fitted, it is critical that the wearer is shown how to care for the obturator to preserve the device and prevent dental diseases such as caries and periodontal disease.

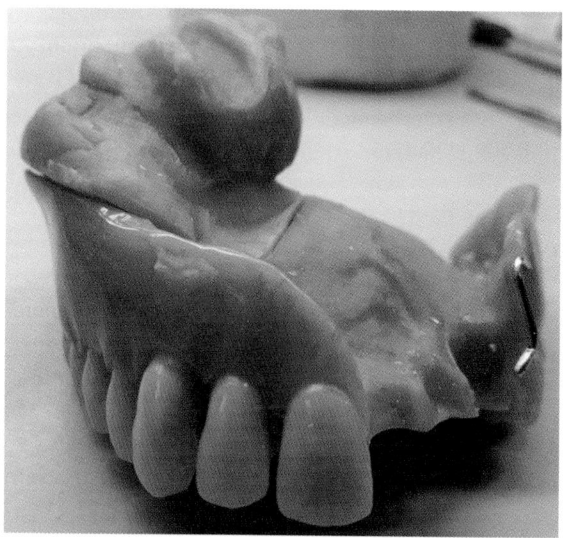

Figure 36.5 Assembled components of an obturator made of a soft material (in Figure 36.4). *Source:* Image courtesy of Lucy Tsiopani, Bristol Dental Hospital.

Obturators for cancer defects are constructed by experienced dental technicians following suitable impressions taken by a restorative consultant. The denture base is normally constructed in acrylic with the obturator being made in acrylic or silicone. Some obturators are hollow, offering a degree of flexibility and closer fit to prevent food impaction and speech issues. Most obturators are designed in one piece but can be made in multiple pieces that use magnets to hold the separate pieces together in situ (Figure 36.4). Some can be designed to attach to intraosseous implants (Figure 36.3). Challenging defects or limited mouth opening may require hollow obturators or soft materials to be used. These materials are more flexible and can obturate the defect more effectively due their ability to be compressed as they pass into the defect and return to their original state (see Figure 36.5).

Mouth Care for Patients with Obturators

Prevention of dental diseases is vitally important to avoid complications and loss of vital structures. The patient should be risk assessed and a tailored oral health plan should be developed following the latest guidance. Regular appointments are required to monitor and maintain health and should include the following as a minimum:

- Detailed history to include medical history, previous surgeries/therapies, and current oral care routine
- Extra and intraoral examination (consider asking your patients to hold a mirror and teach them how to carry out a screening exam at home)
- Use medical illustration to monitor conditions or take an image with the patient's own device

- Full dental examination to include charting, BPE/6ppd chart, tooth surface loss, and indices such as bleeding and plaque
- Radiographs if appropriate and following guidelines
- Tailored treatment plan considering which team member is most appropriate for each item
- Explain the treatment plan to patients and warn them of any risks – for example, obturator no longer fitting well after treatment
- Demonstrate any oral care products and allow patients to try them, especially around implants, and ensure maximum dose of fluoride is used daily
- Make recommendations regarding suitable products for cleaning the prostheses and care of dry mouths
- It can be useful to dampen a gauze square with chlorhexidine or saline and wipe any accretions from the obturator
- Refer back to MDT as appropriate
- Set a recall appointment.

Most prostheses can be cleaned with warm water and soap using a normal toothbrush. Natural teeth should be brushed at least twice a day for two minutes and using an appropriate fluoride toothpaste (Public Health England 2021). There are many pastes available that are flavour and sodium lauryl sulfate free, therefore less irritating to the mucosa. It is important that they contain sodium fluoride for caries prevention. Single tufted toothbrushes can be useful, especially around implants and for cleaning smaller areas of the obturator. Implant care can be challenging when placed high in the palate or other difficult-to-reach areas. It is very important that implant care is stressed to the patient, as loss of the implant may result in a person no longer being able to wear a prosthesis. Advice should be sought from the restorative team as to whether the obturator should be removed at night or for a significant period during the day to prevent stomatitis. It will depend on the prosthetic materials used as to whether a soak is appropriate, so the clinician should keep abreast of current product recommendations. It is often possible for a copy to be made so that the patient will have a spare prosthesis if function would be impossible without it.

Quality of Life (QoL)

Obturators almost always improve the QoL of wearers, but there are some points to be remembered by clinicians providing care (Kornblith et al. 1996). In the case of cleft lip and palate, patients who have had an obturator since childhood have never known life without prostheses and are likely to be very attached to them. In the case of oncology patients who require an obturator suddenly, it can take some time to adapt and may require psychological support from the wider cancer MDT. Many patients have sadly had negative experiences that led to unnecessary upset and embarrassment. A few moments of forethought or asking patients how they prefer the clinician to handle their obturator can prevent poor experiences and demonstrate care for this group of patients.

The following are quotes from patients:

> 'People seem to forget that it's a part of my body. I don't like it being out of my sight'.
> 'Dentists and hygienists have asked me to take it out as soon as I get in the chair. It's such an intimate thing to me, as embarrassing as being asked to take my knickers off'.
> 'I cannot eat or speak without it and fear it breaking or being lost'.
> 'I am always anxious that it will break as thought of the impressions needed for a new one are so awful'.
> 'My partner has never even seen it so removing it in front of strangers is difficult for me. I would rather do it without someone holding a bowl or cup under my chin and I would rather hold it myself and know where it is while I receive care'.
> 'I know that no one is judging me, but I do feel like people are staring and I wonder if they think it is dirty'.

Summary

The following points summarise this chapter:

- Take time to speak to your patients to gain an understanding of their relationship with their obturator. Remember that some patients find it especially difficult with new clinicians.

- Allow them to wear it to communicate with you during the appointment whenever possible.
- Learn about the designs available in your department/laboratory and introduce yourself to the technicians. They love to hear about their successes when you have treated the patient for whom they spent hours designing and creating an obturator.
- Keep up to date with denture care products.
- Ensure excellent preventive care is provided and check for adequate fluoride concentration. Consider the patient as 'high risk' and follow the guidelines in 'Delivering Better Oral Health: An Evidenced-Based Toolkit for Prevention' (Public Health England 2021).

References

Berkovitz, B.K.B., Holland, G.R., and Moxham, B.J. (2018). *Oral Anatomy, Histology and Embryology*, 5e. Elsevier.

Butterworth, C., McCaul, L., and Barclay, C. (2016). Restorative dentistry and oral rehabilitation: United Kingdom National Multidisciplinary Guidelines. *J. Laryngol. Otol.* 130 (Suppl. S2): S41–S44.

Journal of Prosthetic Dentistry (2017). The glossary of prosthodontic terms 9e. https://www.academyofprosthodontics.org/lib_docs/GPT9.pdf (accessed 27 September 2021).

Kornblith, A.B., Zlotolow, I.M., Gooen, J. et al. (1996). Quality of life of maxillectomy patients using an obturator prosthesis. *Head & Neck* 18 (4): 323–334.

National Institute for Health and Care Excellence (2018). Cancer of the upper aerodigestive tract: assessment and management in people aged 16 and over [NICE guideline NG36]. https://www.nice.org.uk/guidance/ng36.

Public Health England (2021). Delivering better oral health: an evidence-based toolkit for prevention. https://www.gov.uk/government/publications/delivering-better-oral-health-an-evidence-based-toolkit-for-prevention (accessed 29 September 2021).

37

Physiotherapy for Head and Neck Cancer Patients: An Overview

Leah Dalby

Leah The Physio, York, UK

It has been a privilege and a joy to be a physiotherapist for more than 30 years, and I am sharing some of what I have learned so far. For clarity, I use the words 'people/person/someone' to refer to the person undergoing treatment and care.

Ideally, you would meet someone before the initial medical treatment, both to explain the role of a physio and explore what the person may want and need. Describe what the person might expect in the way of sensation and function and suggest helpful positionings, exercises, breathing, swallowing, chewing, and communicating techniques. Hopefully, this is done in collaboration with a speech and language therapist (SALT). Explanation around the anatomy involved can be very helpful for some people. Also – and this is important – find out who the person is and what their hopes and needs are, and see how they move before treatment has begun.

After surgery, there is much we can offer as physios, but I understand from the people I work with that they rarely see a physio in hospital, although they often have exercises from the SALT. (Surprisingly, physios are not always a part of the core head and neck MDT.) Even simple things like how to move in and out of bed or negotiate the toilet or staircase with drains can make a difference in those first days. SALT exercises and their useful advice and follow-up are usually described positively and may be continuing after acute intervention (support) has lessened. This can be a great psychological encouragement as well as of practical benefit. Sometimes, people just want to know what's 'normal' after their familiar body, the place where they live, has become an unpredictable stranger.

If your recovery starts on the intensive therapy unit, you are likely to see physios. They may be maintaining airways, optimising respiratory function, and moving people's limbs if they are unconscious or unable to move freely.

In the early postsurgery/radiotherapy days, the correct movements and exercises are important, as are relaxation, nourishing and sustaining breathing and posture (how we rest and function in comfort). Suggestions around pacing, placement of pillows, visualisation, and simple education around anatomy (yes, again! shock and trauma can be fragmenting for concentration) can be helpful. Importantly, we need to ask what someone wants and needs as well as remembering what has helped someone else. Access to surgical notes and local protocols is very helpful.

Some people who have been treated without surgery or with robotic surgery may still need physio even though their scarring and tightness may be unseen.

Significant lymphoedema (swelling caused by the congestion of lymphatic fluid, the flow having been disrupted by surgery and/or radiotherapy) may indicate referral to a specialist lymphoedema therapist or nurse. Treatment options may include manual therapy, use of specialist equipment, compression garments, and advice for skincare and self-care. Some people may find it increasingly difficult to open their mouth or have stiffness, weakness, or altered sensation. As time passes, tightness in scarring may affect facial appearance and function.

There was little undergraduate teaching about head and neck surgery, but I have sought out learning from postgraduate courses and – most importantly, I think – from the people I have been fortunate to work with. Working in independent practice, occasionally I see people before their treatment begins, but more often, several weeks, months, or years later. Sometimes decades later.

Over the last two decades, I have an increasing awareness and understanding of how healing and the fascial system affect functional outcome. This has changed the way I work and greatly enhanced what I can offer people with physiotherapy,

Care of Head and Neck Cancer Patients for Dental Hygienists and Dental Therapists, First Edition. Edited by Jocelyn J. Harding.

with the understanding that however good the exercises and stretches may be and however motivated the person is, they will be hampered by tight, restricted, tethered structures.

The fascia, the connective tissue under the skin that embraces almost everything and enables smooth gliding of one structure over another, can become scarred and stuck after surgery and/or radiotherapy. The light-touch techniques we (and other suitably trained bodyworkers) can use both externally and intraorally can have an enormous impact on function, movement, comfort, and appearance (see Figures 37.1–37.4).

We are integrated beings. Tethering and restriction of one place affects other parts of the body (just as a restriction on a motorway can affect the movement of traffic elsewhere). This may be what brings the person to physio: soreness in the spine or arms due to altered movement or suboptimal mechanics, or changes in arm movements affecting walking patterns. The specialist light touch and vibrational techniques are not a miracle, but the people I work with sometimes describe them that way. Being able to swallow more easily or turn the head without an eye being pulled closed or regaining more subtlety of facial expression can be life changing.

Exercises are important, but they need to be the correct ones for that individual at the right time. With the benefit of 30+ physio years, I realise that one to three exercises done well and attentively are often enough. It is my job to suggest and demonstrate well something that feels enhancing for the person. I need to explain why it matters that they do it. Often it is more about movement than exercise. This is not just semantics; language and intent matter.

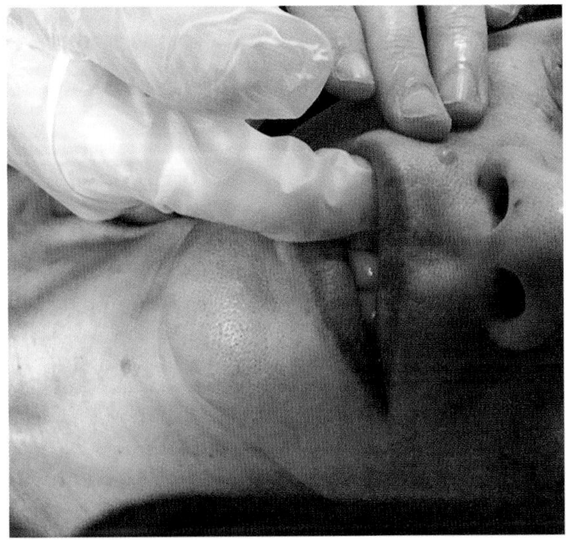

Figure 37.1 Gentle intraoral work can have a profound effect once the area is sufficiently healed.

What we say, how we say it, and why we say it all matter. A person whose life has been in significant peril will be paying great attention. As professionals, we need to be both confident and cautious, checking what is and is not alright for this person trusting us with their precious body. Unless we ask, we have no idea of their previous history or experience – and even if we ask, they may never feel at liberty to say. And they may no longer have a fluent voice!

During an initial assessment, when I ask what someone loves doing, I am often reminded of the person who said, 'sex, eating, and swimming. And I can't do any of those, now'. As part of a team, it is a physio's role to try to facilitate the person's way forward to a fulfilling life, so that the person has not endured significant challenging and life-changing treatment to simply survive.

There may be issues around appearance, intimacy, and sex. Imagine leaning over to whisper in someone's ear when you doubt the smell of your breath, your tongue is stiff and dry, or some paralysis means that saliva may fall out of your mouth as you tilt your head. Or you can no longer speak. Or kissing, with any of the above – with reduced or altered sensation, or your partner is afraid to touch you for fear of any of these or of hurting you.

Communication is essential but not always easy.

And there are those who say to me, 'Who will want me now? Who would look at me?'

The physio's role is seen as primarily physical therapy, and three of our four core elements – respiratory, exercise, and massage – can all make a significant difference to someone who has undergone treatment for head or neck cancer. However, without truly engaging with who the person is as well as their physical body, I believe we may be wasting their time and adding 'insult to injury'.

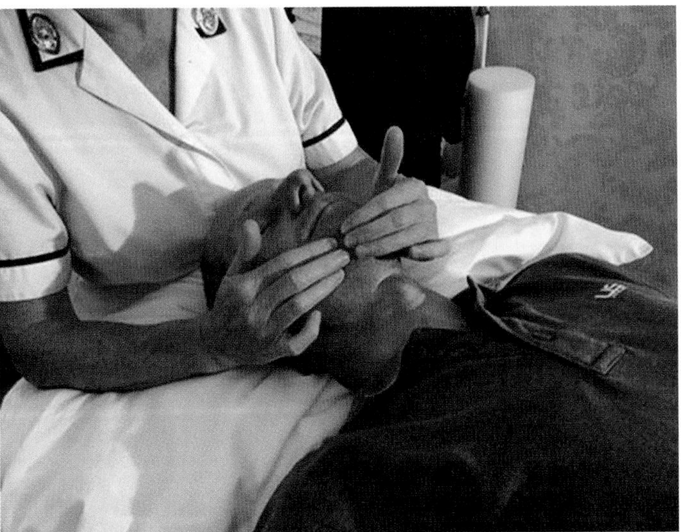

Figure 37.2 Working externally, close to the area treated or in other areas affected, can be relaxing and calming as well as bringing about change in function and decreasing pain.

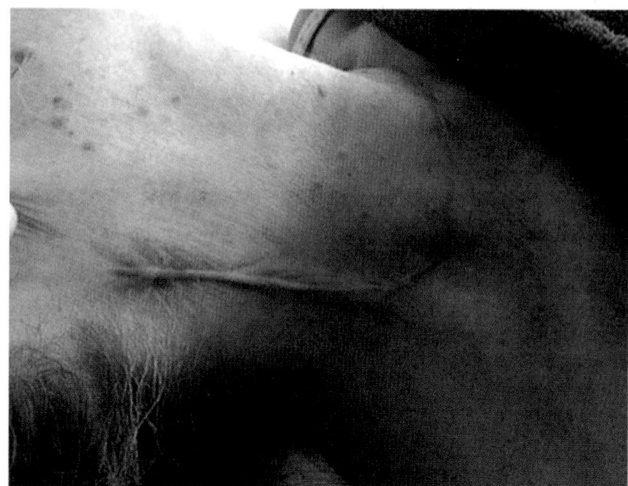

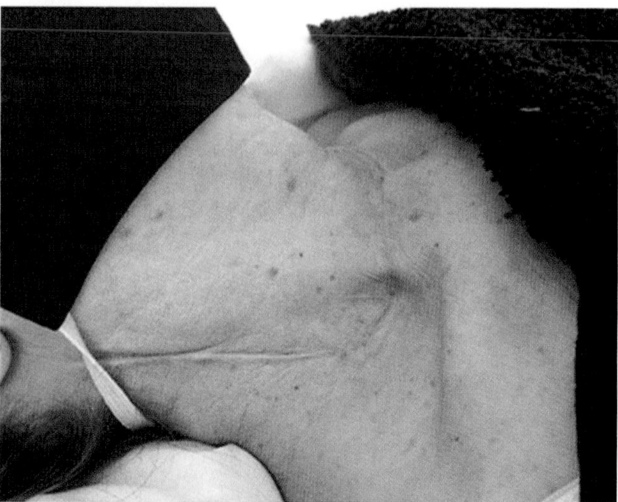

Figure 37.3 Even after working with a scar over several years, with much benefit in movement and comfort, areas of the face can still be pulled by tight scar tissue.

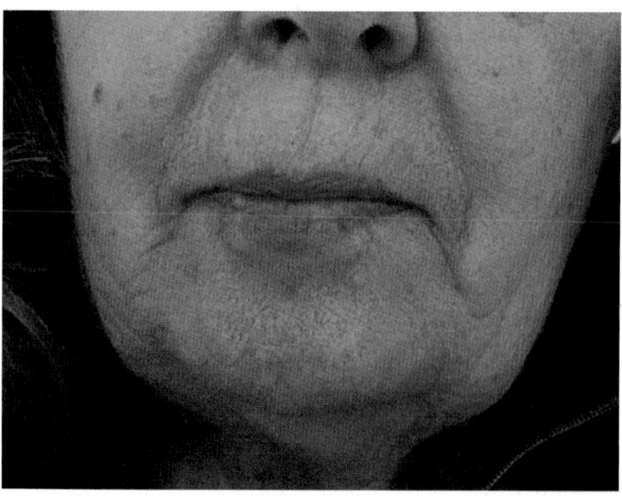

Figure 37.4 Changes in facial expression may happen soon after acute intervention or occur gradually over months or years.

38

Radiotherapy: The Treatment That Keeps on Giving!

Emma Hallam

Nottingham University Hospitals NHS Trust, Nottingham, UK

Radiotherapy is a highly effective treatment for head and neck cancers; however, many patients will experience unintended consequences. It is also well known that multimodality treatments including surgery, chemotherapy, and radiotherapy carry a higher risk of these complex long-term issues.

What Is a Late Effect?

A late effect is a side effect or unintended consequence related to a cancer diagnosis or treatment that can develop months or many years after treatment. It can be an acute side effect that does not settle or gets progressively worse or a new effect that can develop many months, even years post treatment. Late effects are often multifactorial, and patients will frequently have more than one, leading to a reduced quality of life.

Radiotherapy Late Effects

These side effects are directly related to the area of the body that was in the radiotherapy treatment field. The direct damage that the radiotherapy causes to the tissues and organs in that area makes them at risk of radiation induced fibrosis, often resulting in altered function. Patients will also often experience other symptoms such as fatigue and psychological and psychosocial issues as a long-term consequence. These symptoms are often related to changes in quality of life, pain, and nutritional issues that patients experience.

Potential long-term effects of radiotherapy include:

- *Radiation induced fibrosis:* This is scarring of the tissues due to collagen deposition and a build up of a protein substance, fibrin. This effect is progressive and results in reduced tissue elasticity, poor vascularity, scaring and hardening and shrinkage of soft tissue. Patients will experience reduced movement, weakness and loss of function in the area along with pain, muscle and nerve spasms. This can make the tissue less stretchy. Muscles will feel stiff and tough, and patients often experience a loss in movement and any associated function. Muscle spasms, pain, and weakness are also common.
- *Swallowing issues:* Radiation fibrosis and the buildup of scar tissue can, over time, lead to swallowing difficulties.
- *Lymphoedema:* Lymphoedema is the swelling of the head and neck area both externally and internally due to congestion, damage, and fibrosis of the lymphatic system. Lymphoedema contributes to pain and altered swallow function and reduces movement in the head and neck area. Often patients will experience trauma within the oral cavity due to oedema of the tongue and buccal mucosa, leading to recurrent ulcers, pain, and increased anxiety due to the patient thinking this could be a cancer recurrence.
- *Trismus:* Fibrosis and lymphoedema contribute to trismus, a chronic contraction of the temporomandibular joint muscle, resulting in pain and restricted mouth opening, often affecting nutrition and speech.
- *Changes in saliva production:* Damage to the salivary glands can cause a dry mouth and thick secretions, which can be problematic for patients. Lack of saliva or inadequate-quality saliva can have an impact on swallow function and increase

Care of Head and Neck Cancer Patients for Dental Hygienists and Dental Therapists, First Edition. Edited by Jocelyn J. Harding.

dental caries leading to a decline in nutrition and reduced oral hygiene. Patients who experience these effects will often have disturbed sleep that contributes to higher fatigue levels.
- *Burning mouth syndrome:* Chronic burning mouth is often made worse by a dry mouth environment and recurrent oral thrush. Patients experience a burning, scalding sensation along with loss of taste. Intensity and severity can fluctuate over time and throughout the day. Patients may experience anxiety and depression due to pain and isolation, as they often withdraw from social activities.
- *Bone damage:* Radiotherapy can cause small fractures in the bones that were in the treatment field. These can be very painful and worse with trauma. Osteoradionecrosis of the jaw bone is a debilitating and painful complication where the bone is unable to heal after minor trauma such as dental extractions due to damage to the blood supply. This condition needs to be monitored closely by a maxilla facial team.
- *Sinus issues:* If the sinuses and nasal cavity were in the treatment field, patients have a higher risk of developing chronic sinusitis. Problems include postnasal drip, nasal discharge, facial pain, headaches, and dry nasal passages.
- *Skin changes:* Permanent change to the skin includes scarring and fibrosis. This leads to muscle loss and stricture, causing problems with flexibility and reduced movement.
- *Neck and tongue spasms:* Nerve damage can lead to painful and debilitating spasms.
- *Head drop:* Head drop is weakness of the neck extensor muscles that causes an inability for the patient to extend the neck. This results in poor posture and a flexed-forward head. Physiotherapy, along with a specialised collar, can be helpful for some patients.
- *Thyroid problems:* Hypothyroidism is common for many patients after treatment, and thyroid-stimulating hormone levels should be monitored annually. Hyperparathyroidism is less common but can develop.
- *Hearing loss and damage to the ear:* Patients often report tinnitus earache and glue-like ear symptoms due to fluid collection in the middle ear.

The above is just a brief overview of radiotherapy late effects; for patients who have had chemotherapy, peripheral neuropathy is also common, presenting as pins and needles of the hands and feet.

How Can We Help?

- Listening to the patient and acknowledging that this is a long-term problem that cannot be fixed is key, which does not mean that we should take away all hope but that managing realistic expectations is extremely important.
- Ensure that any advice given, including the recommendation of dry mouth products, is maintainable and achievable, as many GPs will not prescribe such products, so often lifestyle tips are more suitable.
- Good oral hygiene advice with plenty of fluids is advisable. Check the patient is not using a mouthwash that is too harsh. Often patients find that a solution of bicarbonate of soda and warm salt water is more beneficial and tolerable.
- Ask if the patient has been given any information on exercises to help maintain and improve mobility and swallow function and encourage the person to do these, indicating that this is a programme for life for long-term mobility and function.
- Hydration of the skin with a suitable moisturiser will also help. Steam inhalation can be beneficial for helping with blocked sinuses and thick secretions.
- Any signs of oedema need to be addressed, as we know that early identification of lymphoedema with appropriate management can be very effective in reducing long-term complications and fibrosis. This can be in the form of simple lymphatic drainage exercises and, again, encouraging exercise and movement.
- Many dedicated late effects services are developing within the UK. Contacting the radiotherapy centre where the patient had treatment or Macmillan Cancer Support would be an excellent place to start for further advice and support.
- As previously mentioned, the area of late effects is multifactorial, and we have addressed the ones commonly seen in this article. Further reading and additional late effects that head and neck patients can experience can be found by accessing Brook (2020) and Purkayastha et al. (2019).

References

Brook, I. (2020). Late side effects of radiation treatment for head and neck cancer. *Radiat. Oncol. J.* 38 (2): 84–92. https://doi.org/10.3857/roj.2020.00213. Epub 2020 Jun 25. PMID: 33012151; PMCID: PMC7533405.

Purkayastha, A., Sharma, N., Sarin, A. et al. (2019). Radiation fibrosis syndrome: the evergreen menace of radiation therapy. *Asia Pac. J. Oncol. Nurs.* 6 (3): 238–245. https://doi.org/10.4103/apjon.apjon_71_18. PMID: 31259219; PMCID: PMC6518980.

39

Management of Intraoral Hair Growth After Flap Reconstruction

Susan Smithies

University of Liverpool, School of Dental Sciences, Liverpool, UK

Patients who have a confirmed diagnosis of a head and neck cancer may be seen either shortly after diagnosis and preoperatively in the dental hygiene therapy clinic or postoperatively, depending on the protocol of a particular hospital. If they are seen preoperatively, the possibility of intraoral hair being an outcome can be introduced to the patient if it has not already been discussed. Those who present postoperatively with intraoral hair may not have realised that this would be an outcome.

> *When it has been decided that surgical excision is the best treatment modality for a particular tumour in an individual patient, one of the main considerations for the surgical team to decide is the site of the donor tissue and its ability to adapt well at the recipient site.* (Wong and Wei 2010, 1236–1245)

The most common sites for harvesting donor flaps are

- Anterolateral thigh and radial forearm; these provide the best harvest of blood vessels, nerve, muscle, fat, and skin (Harris and Bewley 2016, 447–452).
- The donor thigh especially provides volume and bulk, particularly with large defects.
- The pectoral and submental areas are also used.

The disadvantage of all of these donor sites is the presence of hair follicles in the skin (although the radial forearm flap may be predominantly hairless) that continue to produce hair after they have been transplanted into the recipient site. This hair grows, causing discomfort, problems with swallowing, difficulties with maintaining adequate oral hygiene, and trapping food, mucous, and salivary secretions. The hair can be so long and inaccessible that it causes gagging (Figures 39.1–39.3).

The replacement flaps and associated hair growth can be anywhere in the oral cavity: the floor of the mouth, the sublingual area, the hard and soft palate, the pharyngeal area, or the buccal cheek pad. Factors that affect hair growth rate, texture, quality, and quantity in the mouth include

- Site of donor flap.
- Sex – males are more affected than females.
- Skin type – some patients naturally have more body hair than others; ethnicity also has an influence. Caucasian populations have the most density of hair. Asian populations have a faster growth rate than the Caucasian population but less density of hair. African populations have the lowest growth rate and density (Loussouarn et al. 2005).
- Donor site – the submental area is likely to have very coarse and adherent hair in males, as this is 'beard hair'.
- Radiotherapy – if the patient is also to undergo radiotherapy as part of treatment then the hair follicles may be destroyed and growth may be minimal or absent.

Some patients who present in the hygiene clinic with intraoral hair growth find it distressing and uncomfortable and often ask why the hair could not have been removed from the donor site prior to surgery. The simple answer is time. There is no time for the area to be prepared by removing the hair preoperatively. Laser treatments for hair removal from the donor site would take a minimum of five sessions five weeks apart for the hair growth to be reduced or eliminated. Even if time were not of the essence, what if the original donor site is found during harvesting to be unsuitable or fails?

Care of Head and Neck Cancer Patients for Dental Hygienists and Dental Therapists, First Edition. Edited by Jocelyn J. Harding.

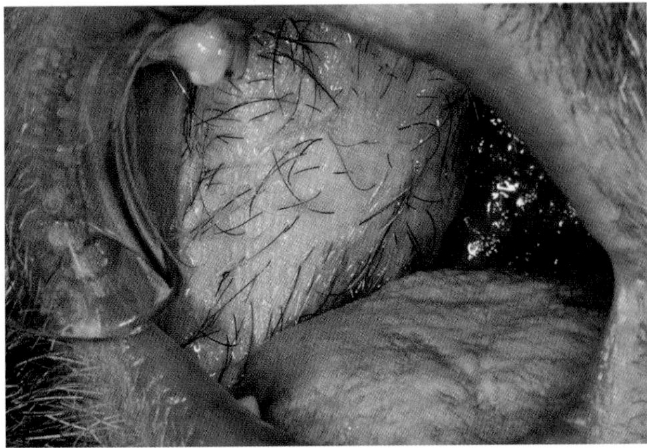

Figure 39.1 Photograph of submental island flap in Patient A, replacing the right pharyngeal area. Hair was growing down into his oropharynx, causing gagging due to an accumulation of mucous attached to the hairs. The patient was PEG-dependent for nutrition.

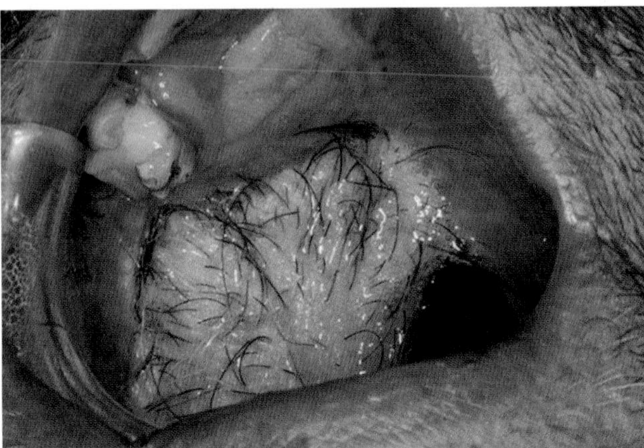

Figure 39.2 Different view of patient A.

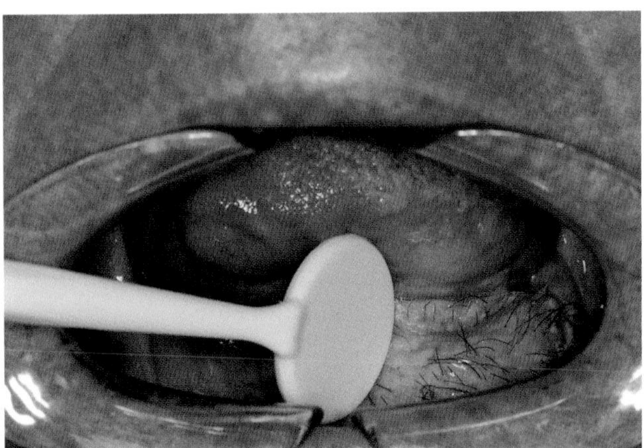

Figure 39.3 Patient B had a replacement of the left floor of mouth. He had very abundant growth and was first seen for hair removal three weeks postsurgery. Photograph of submental flap of patient B.

Postoperative Intraoral Hair Removal

Lasers

Lasers work best on patients with pale skin and dark hair as the light from the laser targets darker pigmentation. Using an Nd:YAG or diode laser for intraoral hair removal postoperatively has been performed with some success (Lumley 2007; Rodrigues et al. 2021), the advantage being that hair removal in some cases may be permanent, although some regrowth can occur.

The disadvantages for using a laser are access, patients may have limited mouth opening, and the head of the laser unit may impede visibility. The graft can be destabilised. There may be postoperative erythema, peri-follicular oedema, pain, and crusting of the site postoperatively (Rodrigues et al. 2021) causing pain and discomfort. The patient may not want to experience any more postoperative pain, having reached to a point where the postsurgery discomfort is manageable and treatment will take multiple appointments four to five weeks apart.

Some patients have sparse hair growth at the flap site and can live with it. It doesn't bother them, and if it gets too long they cut it short.

Electrolysis

This involves an electric current passed into the hair follicle via a fine needle. It is a widely used hair removal treatment in beauty salons. Over time the hair follicle is destroyed.

A search of the literature found no published papers of this form of hair removal being used intraorally.

Cutting

A scalpel or scissors to shorten the hair is the method used by some clinicians and patients, but regrowth is fairly rapid, and what remains will be short hairs that still trap secretions and food.

Plucking

For those patients who wish to have the hair removed or reduced, the least painful or invasive method is to pluck the hair out using haemostatic clips or 'mosquitoes' of the type used in orthodontic clinics to place modules on brackets. The nose of the instrument is slim, which allows access in patients with limited opening and allows the operator to grip the hair near to the root (Figure 39.4).

Removing the hair further up breaks the hair and regrowth is obviously quicker. An alternative instrument is the Adson non-toothed forceps, again gripping the hair near the root (Figure 39.5).

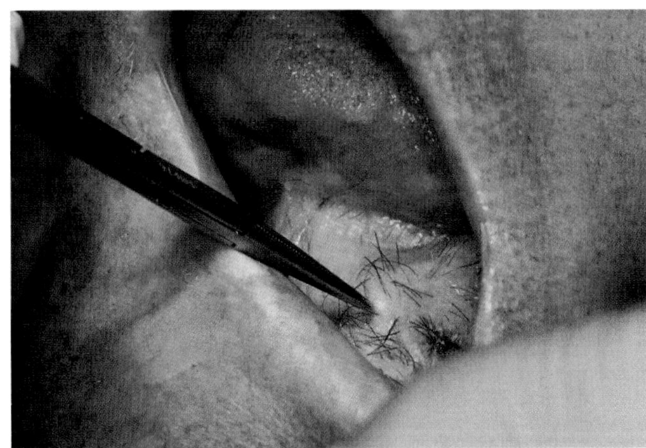

Figure 39.4 Photograph of patient B.

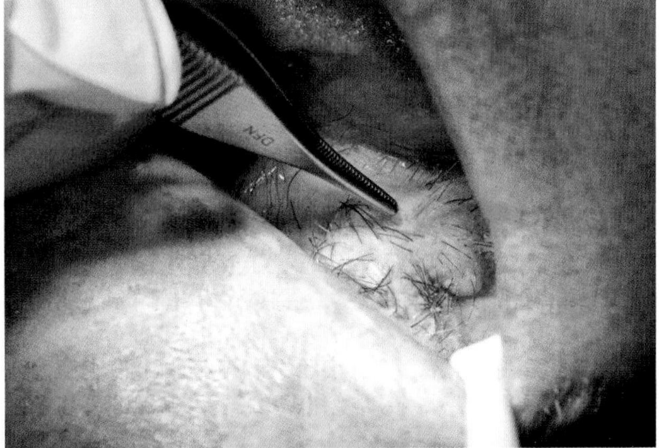

Figure 39.5 Photograph of patient B.

It is useful to use a gauze square to wipe the instrument and the oral mucosa during the procedure, as it removes saliva and stray hairs. A dental nurse who can retract the soft tissues with a mirror is a great help with access. Also, it is helpful to use your nonworking hand to keep the tissue taut as you remove the hair.

Most patients find the procedure painless, but any hairs that grow close to the junction of the flap with mucosa can be uncomfortable to remove, and it is important to remember to support the mandible if working in the floor of the mouth and also be aware that the patient will require frequent rests (Figure 39.6).

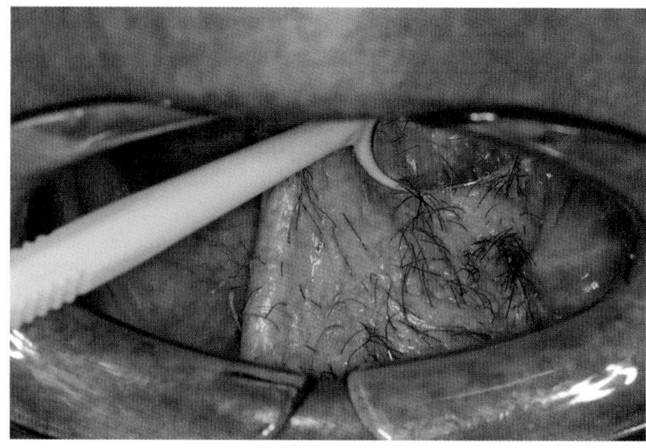

Figure 39.6 Photograph of patient B preremoval.

There are usually no adverse reactions to the treatment and very little discomfort during the procedure, and rate of new growth gradually reduces over time. Initially the patient may need to attend frequently – every two weeks for submental flaps; usually schedule appointments between four and eight weeks apart. The regrowth tends to become less and the hairs finer as time goes on, but this can take a couple of years of regular removal (Figure 39.7).

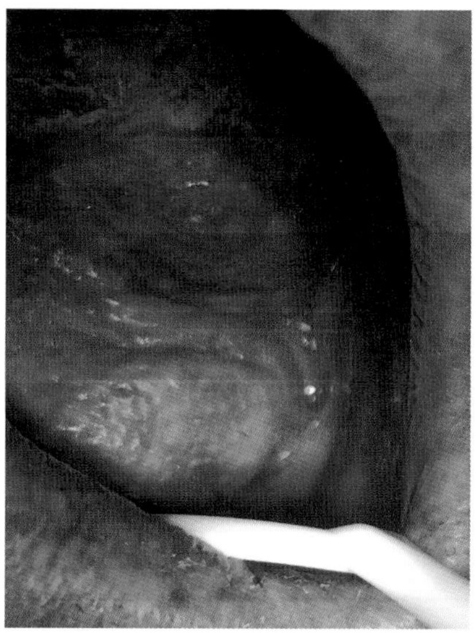

Figure 39.7 Postoperative result for patient B.

The disadvantages of this method of hair removal are that it is time-consuming in some patients – abundant growth can take up to 45 minutes to successfully remove the hair; and some patients may not be able to tolerate keeping their mouth open for this length of time, and fatigue and postoperative muscle ache can be an outcome.

Attending regularly every two to four weeks can reduce the amount of time taken to remove new growth.

Summary

In your clinical practice if you have a patient who presents with intraoral hair, ask the questions: Does it bother you? Would you like me to do something about it? If it doesn't bother patients but is impeding optimal oral health by causing debris and plaque to accumulate, then explanation of why the hair should be removed and that it will be painless can be presented so that they have an informed choice.

References

Harris, B.N. and Bewley, A.F. (2016). Minimizing free flap donor-site morbidity. *Curr. Opin. Otolaryngol. Head Neck Surg.* 24 (5): 447–452. https://doi.org/10.1097/MOO.0000000000000286. PMID: 27455033.

Loussouarn, G., El-Rawadi, C., and Genain, G. (2005). Diversity of hair growth profiles. *Int. J. Dermat.* 44: https://doi.org/10.1111/j.1365-4632.2005.02800.x.

Lumley, C. (2007). Intraoral hair removal on skin graft using Nd:YAG laser. *Br. Dent. J.* 203: 141–142. https://doi.org/10.1038/bdj.2007.683.

Rodrigues, B.T.G., Nunes, L.A.S., Amaral, L.R. et al. (2021). Successful hair removal on intra oral grafts using the diode laser: report of two cases. *Spec. Care Dentist.* 41: 135–139. https://doi.org/10.1111/scd.12541.

Wong, C.H. and Wei, F.C. (2010). Microsurgical free flap in head and neck reconstruction. *Head Neck.* 32 (9): 1236–1245. https://doi.org/10.1002/hed.21284. PMID: 20014446.

40

Lifestyle Factors in Oral Cancer

Mike Nugent

South Tyneside and Sunderland NHS Foundation Trust, Sunderland, UK

> *But all I found was cigarettes and alcohol.*
>
> (Gallagher 1994)

Throughout my time as a dental student in the 1990s, we were taught that the risk factors for oral cancer were smoking and alcohol, smoking being the chief culprit (Mashberg et al. 1993). There was discussion about the incidence of oral cancer being likely to decline, given the decline in smoking (McKean-Cowdin et al. 2000) There was very little discussion of or focus on anything else. More recently, HPV was identified as another risk factor (Elrefaey et al. 2014). Now other modifiable risk factors are gaining the attention of head and neck cancer researchers and clinicians (Kumar et al. 2016). All the while the incidence of oral cancer, touted as declining in the 1990s, has done nothing of the sort and keeps rising (McCarthy et al. 2015).

Why? While the overall incidence of smoking is declining, the incidence in lower socioeconomic groups has not shown the same decrease (Hiscock et al. 2012). Oropharyngeal cancers driven by HPV are also on the increase. But what if it's not all about smoking and drinking? What if there are other modifiable risk factors? Recent studies are showing that the way we sleep, eat, and exercise may influence the risk of getting head and neck cancer (Kumar et al. 2016).

Sleep

Disturbed sleep has been shown to increase the levels of interleukin 6 (IL-6). IL-6 is a protein involved in regulating cell growth and inflammation. High levels of IL-6 are associated with higher stages of cancer, rapid progression, and poorer prognosis (Duffy et al. 2013).

A recent survey in the UK showed that the typical adult gets less than 6.5 hours of sleep per night (Worthington 2018). This is less than the recommended seven to nine hours. Unsurprisingly, in a recent survey those sleeping less felt short-tempered or unable to concentrate as a result. This is bad enough in itself, but this lack of sleep will also reduce the likelihood of having a healthy diet and reduce the chances of us taking regular exercise. Very few would think of their sleep habits as having any of these adverse effects. Getting a good night's sleep needs to be seen as a priority for our patients.

Possible Reasons for Poor Sleep

Our bodies have a natural sleep–wake cycle (aka body clock or circadian rhythm). Many things about modern living and technology disrupt this. Many people will now read on their electronic device in bed or watch TV. Unfortunately, this has two negative effects. Firstly, the content tends to prevent us from relaxing, and secondly, the blue light emitted from the screens inhibits melatonin production, which is necessary for us to sleep properly.

Care of Head and Neck Cancer Patients for Dental Hygienists and Dental Therapists, First Edition. Edited by Jocelyn J. Harding.

What Will Help?

Some suggestions to help with sleep include the following:

- *Routine:* Try to get in sync with your body clock. Have a regular time for going to bed and getting up and stick to it, avoiding lie-ins and daytime napping.
- *Let there be light and dark:* Turn off laptops, tablets, phones, and TVs one to two hours before bedtime. Keep your bedroom dark. This will allow your body to start making melatonin. When you wake up, get as much bright light as possible. Eat breakfast by a window or outside, weather permitting. During the day get as much natural light as possible; get outside for breaks. Exercise outdoors during the day.
- *Exercise (more on this later):* If we exercise regularly, we tend to sleep better at night and feel less tired during the day. Exercise also helps with sleep apnoea and improves both the quality and quantity of sleep. The more vigorously we exercise the better we will sleep, but evidence shows that even a 10-minute walk will make a difference. That said, vigorous exercise should be done at least three hours before bedtime otherwise will tend to interfere with sleep. It's also important to bear in mind that it may take a few months before exercise starts to improve sleep.
- *Eating and drinking (more on this later):* Eating large meals late at night can disturb sleep. Consuming caffeine, nicotine, and alcohol close to bedtime all can have negative impact on sleep too. Although a nightcap can help you get to sleep, alcohol can disturb your sleep cycle. A diet high in sugars or refined carbohydrate can also disrupt sleep, causing wakefulness at night and reducing deep sleep. If a bedtime snack is needed, try a banana, kiwi fruit, milk, or yoghurt (low sugar).
- *Wind down and relax:* Stress, worry, and anger prevent sleep. Our patients who are newly diagnosed or going through cancer treatment will inevitably be feeling some or all of these. Walking can help to relieve stress. Walking in nature will relieve stress better than a walk in an urban environment. Other stress-relieving approaches include breathing exercises, yoga, and mindfulness. Focusing on our breathing or relaxing our muscles one by one can help us to stop the mind racing and help us just to be.

Exercise

Exercise has been recognised as medicine for cancer patients for some time. This is due to a growing body of evidence about the benefits of exercise to our physical and mental health. Recent evidence is showing that higher levels of exercise participation reduce the risk of head and neck cancer (Nicolotti et al. 2011). At the time of writing, this scientific view is unfortunately not yet reflected in day-to-day practice. Exercise interventions do not form part of the standard of care. What is more, there are few guidelines in the UK for promoting exercise in head and neck cancer.

Most head and neck cancer patients will lose muscle during treatment. For the patient this means increased risk of a poor outcome, poor swallowing function, reduced ability to carry out activities of daily living, and low mood. In the longer term there is an increased risk of falls, osteoporosis, and fractures. An exercise programme can counter these issues. The following is a guide to creating a well-rounded exercise programme. Such programmes need to be tailored to fit the ability, needs, goals, and preferences of the individual. If the programme is to be sustainable, then it needs to be enjoyable.

Components of an Exercise Programme

Aerobic Exercise

Ideally 30 minutes of moderate activity three times weekly. This translates to exercising (walking/jogging/cycling/dancing) at a pace where you can talk but not sing. For walking try to build up to around 8000 steps per day.

Resistance Exercise

Twice weekly try to build up strength by either doing body weight exercises or using resistance bands. Start with lighter effort and do 10–15 reps and build up to 2–4 sets of 8–12 reps.

A whole-body workout can be achieved by doing:

- Knee-dominant exercises such as sit to stand, or squats if you are able.
- Hip-dominant exercises such as a deadlift. This can be done with one large or two shopping bags filled with anything to add weight. The bags should be placed next to your toes. Keeping your back straight, bend your hips and knees, reach

down and grab the shopping bag handles, then stand up straight. Ensure you are looking straight ahead the whole time, and focus on pushing your feet into the floor.
- A pushing exercise such as press-ups, which can be done off a kitchen worktop or from the knees to start off with.
- A pulling exercise, such as rowing or pull-ups. A variation of rowing can be done with a weighted shopping bag. Put the bag on the floor in front of a well-secured worktop or bench. Position yourself an arm's length away. Keeping your back flat, bend over, rest one arm on the bench, and grab the bag with the other. Pull the bag off the floor up to your hip and then lower it back down again slowly.

Flexibility

Stretches should ideally be done five days a week. Eight stretches should each be performed for 30 seconds, two times. Yoga, tai chi, and pilates will all also help achieve this.

Neuromuscular Exercises (Balance Exercises)

The simplest exercise here is to try to stand on one leg for 30 seconds at a time. Another exercise requiring no equipment is to go onto knees and hands, then try lifting the left arm straight out in front of you whilst lifting the right leg straight out behind you. Try to build up to holding this for 30 seconds. Repeat this balancing on the left leg and right arm. Again yoga, tai chi, and pilates will all help improve balance and stability.

When Should Cancer Patients Start an Exercise Programme?

Prehab

Improving strength and fitness prior to HNC treatment may reduce the adverse effects physically and psychologically. Prehab also provides an opportunity to empower patients and their carers at a time when they may be struggling to know what, if anything, they can do other than wait for the next visit to the hospital.

Rehab

Most of us will be aware that there is often a low point both physically and psychologically for patients at the completion of their active cancer treatment when they transition into the follow-up phase. This can coincide with less attention from clinicians whose work for that patient is done, as it were. It is conceivable that starting a programme at this point may provide a much-needed lift for the patient and a focus for them.

Diet

A diet higher in fruit and vegetables and low in meat has been shown to reduce the risk of head and neck cancer, and a diet with less fruit and vegetables and higher in meat has been shown to increase the risk. Once patients have head and neck cancer, nutrition does not cease to be important; if anything, it becomes more important (Chuang et al. 2012).

It is well known in the fitness community that your training programme must be supported with good nutrition. The same applies for head and neck cancer patients. Patients undergoing head and neck cancer treatment are often malnourished prior to treatment, and virtually all will lose weight during the treatment. If they're going to make the gains (or minimise the losses during treatment) that are possible through strength and fitness training, most patients will need to significantly increase the amount of protein in their diet. They will also need to maintain a calorie excess. The exact amount of protein patients need in their diet remains controversial. There is a minimum dose of protein that will support the muscle growth pathway, and this is generally felt to be around 1.2–2 g of protein per kilogramme body weight per day. This protein synthesis pathway can only be switched on once every three to four hours, so the timing of meals is also important. In practical terms a patient should be eating a protein-rich meal three or four times daily, with at least three to four hours between each meal. The meal should have 20–30 g of protein. Achieving this for patients with mouth cancers will require some trial and error for the individual patient, given that most of our patients end up eating a soft or liquid food. Many will be tube-fed. In Sunderland, we had a group of six head and neck cancer patients taste test some commercially available protein shakes, and all found them acceptable.

Vicious vs Virtuous Cycles: Sleep, Eat, Rave Repeat vs Sleep, Eat, Train Repeat?

In conclusion, I believe we should view the three modifiable risk factors discussed here as being interdependent. Our patients, and we for that matter, can become trapped in a vicious circle of poor sleep, poor diet, and lack of exercise or a virtuous one where we sleep, exercise, and eat well. These factors will not only impact our patients' quality of life but in all probability the behaviour of their cancer and long-term outcome.

References

Chuang, S.C., Jenab, M., Heck, J.E. et al. (2012). Diet and the risk of head and neck cancer: a pooled analysis in the INHANCE consortium. *Cancer Causes Control* 23 (1): 69–88.

Duffy, S.A., Teknos, T., Taylor, J.M. et al. (2013). Health behaviors predict higher interleukin-6 levels among patients newly diagnosed with head and neck squamous cell carcinoma. *Cancer Epidemiol. Biomark. Prev.* 22 (3): 374–381.

Elrefaey, S., Massaro, M.A., Chiocca, S. et al. (2014). HPV in oropharyngeal cancer: the basics to know in clinical practice. *Acta Otorhinolaryngol. Ital.* 34 (5): 299.

Gallagher, N. (1994). *Cigarettes & Alcohol*. London: Creation Records.

Hiscock, R., Bauld, L., Amos, A., and Platt, S. (2012). Smoking and socioeconomic status in England: the rise of the never smoker and the disadvantaged smoker. *J. Public Health* 34 (3): 390–396.

Kumar, M., Nanavati, R., Modi, T.G., and Dobariya, C. (2016). Oral cancer: etiology and risk factors: a review. *J. Cancer Res. Ther.* 12 (2): 458.

Mashberg, A., Boffetta, P., Winkelman, R., and Garfinkel, L. (1993). Tobacco smoking, alcohol drinking, and cancer of the oral cavity and oropharynx among US veterans. *Cancer* 72 (4): 1369–1375.

McCarthy, C.E., Field, J.K., Rajlawat, B.P. et al. (2015). Trends and regional variation in the incidence of head and neck cancers in England: 2002 to 2011. *Int. J. Oncol.* 47 (1): 204–210.

McKean-Cowdin, R., Feigelson, H.S., Ross, R.K. et al. (2000). Declining cancer rates in the 1990s. *J. Clin. Oncol.* 18 (11): 2258–2268.

Nicolotti, N., Chuang, S.C., Cadoni, G. et al. (2011). Recreational physical activity and risk of head and neck cancer: a pooled analysis within the international head and neck cancer epidemiology (INHANCE) consortium. *Eur. J. Epidemiol.* 26 (8): 619.

Worthington, H. (2018). The Sainsbury's living well index. https://www.about.sainsburys.co.uk/~/media/Files/S/Sainsburys/living-well-index/sainsburys-living-well-index-may-2018.pdf (accessed 30 March 2021).

41

Pain Management for Head and Neck Cancer Patients

Roddy McMillan

Departments of Oral Medicine and Facial Pain, Royal National ENT and Eastman Dental Hospitals, University College London Hospitals NHS Foundation Trust, London, UK

Introduction

Pain is present in the majority of oral cancer patients, with one study suggesting around two-thirds of such patients will be suffering with painful symptoms (Khawaja et al. 2020). The same study found that pain was more common in patients with tongue involvement and more advanced, higher-stage disease. The World Health Organization states that pain management should be integrated within cancer care pathways (WHO 2018). Pain can develop in oral cancer patients through a variety of different and overlapping mechanisms – the tumour can release nociceptive cytokines that sensitise the surrounding tissues, pressure of the expanding tumour against adjacent structures, perineural invasion of the cancer into the sensory nerves, and curative surgery to remove cancers invariably will result in a degree of nerve damage, which can result in a persistent neuropathic pain (Schmidt 2015; Epstein and Miaskowski 2019).

The International Association for the Study of Pain (IASP) defines pain as 'An unpleasant sensory and emotional experience associated with, or resembling that associated with, actual or potential tissue damage' (IASP 2021). A contemporary understanding of the experience of pain is easiest by describing the '3 dimensions of pain'; a collection of three interacting domains: 'sensory-discriminative' (intensity, character, location, and duration of the pain), 'affective-motivational' (unpleasantness and urge to escape the unpleasantness of the pain), and 'cognitive-evaluative' (interplay of cognitions such as past experiences, appraisal, cultural values and distraction) (Melzack and Casey 1968). This elegant hypothesis proposed by Melzack and Casey in 1968 is still regarded as fundamental to the understanding of pain today – in particular, that the experience of pain is subjective and not just determined by the magnitude of the painful stimulus.

Pain Management in Oral Cancer

The WHO previously has published their 'analgesic ladder' as a means to provide guidance for pain medications used for cancer patients; this has since been extended and developed into a more comprehensive guideline for the pharmacological management of cancer pain (WHO 2018). The basic principle of the analgesic ladder is to initiate simple analgesic medications and escalate to stronger analgesics or add different (adjuvant) treatments depending on response (Table 41.1). The aim should be to escalate or de-escalate therapy depending on pain response and potential side effects.

Analgesic Preparations

Paracetamol

Paracetamol is used as an analgesic for mild to moderate pain – it primarily is administered orally but can be provided per rectal or intravenously. The mechanism of action of paracetamol is not fully understood; it is proposed that it inhibits the enzyme cyclooxygenase (COX), in particular COX-2. Metabolism of paracetamol is mainly within the liver and excretion is

Care of Head and Neck Cancer Patients for Dental Hygienists and Dental Therapists, First Edition. Edited by Jocelyn J. Harding.

Table 41.1 Analgesia for oral cancer pain.

Step	Treatment options
1) Mild pain	Paracetamol ± NSAID ± adjuvant
2) Moderate pain	Weak opiate/opioid + paracetamol ± NSAID ± adjuvant
3) Severe pain	Strong opiate/opioid + paracetamol ± NSAID ± adjuvant

Adjuvant – e.g. amitriptyline, gabapentin; NSAID – e.g. ibuprofen, diclofenac; strong opiate/opioid – e.g. morphine sulfate, diamorphine; weak opiate/opioid – e.g. codeine, tramadol.

Source: WHO 2018; Finnerup et al. 2015; NICE 2013.

by the kidneys; the half-life is between one and four hours, hence why four times daily dosing is optimal. Paracetamol is very safe with limited side effects when taking within recommended dosage limits.

Nonsteroidal Anti-Inflammatory Drugs

Nonsteroidal anti-inflammatory drugs (NSAIDs) are a class of analgesic medication that can be used for mild to moderate pain. Examples of NSAIDs include ibuprofen and diclofenac. NSAIDs work as nonselective inhibitors of both the COX-1 and COX-2 enzymes. They are generally well tolerated and safe, although they can be associated with a number of potential side effects – for example, gastroduodenal irritation or ulceration, gastrointestinal bleeds (particularly when prescribed alongside warfarin), exacerbation of asthma (some asthmatics will have exacerbation of their asthma when taking NSAIDs), allergic reactions, and reduced kidney perfusion (should be used with caution in patients with renal impairment).

Opiates and Opioids

Codeine is a naturally occurring opiate (methylated morphine) and is used for mild to moderate pain. Codeine is often compounded with paracetamol (co-codamol). Codeine has a duration of action of around four to six hours and is metabolised by the liver. Tramadol is a synthetic opioid used to treat moderate to severe pain; moreover, it is indicated, as required, for use in breakthrough neuropathic pains (NICE 2013). Codeine binds to the μ-opioid receptor, while tramadol exerts its effect by binding to the μ-opioid receptor and inhibiting the reuptake of serotonin and norepinephrine; both are metabolised by the liver.

Morphine is a naturally occurring opiate and diamorphine is a synthetic opioid – both are used for severe pain via their affiliation with the μ-opioid receptor. Morphine and diamorphine are dangerous in overdose and can cause death by respiratory depression. Metabolism of both preparations is via the liver, and they have a relatively short duration of action of around four hours. Tolerance to the analgesic effects of morphine and diamorphine occurs quickly; hence, patients taking long-term therapy require a gradual increase in dosage over time to maintain the analgesic benefit. Both morphine and diamorphine have the potential for dependence should they be administered over a longer duration.

Adjuvant Medications

Pain management often employs 'adjuvant' treatments that work alongside the conventional analgesic preparations (Table 41.1). Adjuvants are medications that did not originate as analgesics but that are known to have analgesic properties. The most common classes of adjuvant pain medications are the antidepressants and anticonvulsants.

Amitriptyline is a tricyclic antidepressant that was originally marketed in the 1960s for the treatment of depression and anxiety. Amitriptyline is known to interact multiple receptor types within the central nervous system, including serotonin, noradrenaline, dopamine, and muscarinic receptors and transporters. Amitriptyline is taken orally and is metabolized mainly by the liver to the active metabolite nortriptyline – a drug in its own right. Due to the potential for cardiac toxicity, amitriptyline is contraindicated following recent myocardial infarction and in patients with cardiac arrhythmias (particularly heart block). Side effects of amitriptyline include drowsiness (often beneficial for sleep disturbance related to pain), dry mouth, and blurry vision.

Duloxetine is a serotonin, noradrenaline reuptake inhibitor (SNRI) that is used in the management of several conditions that include anxiety, depression, and neuropathic pains. Duloxetine is taken orally and is primarily metabolized by the liver cytochrome system; it should not be issued to patients with liver or kidney impairment. The primary potential side effects of duloxetine are nausea, dyspepsia, constipation, and weight changes.

Gabapentin is an anticonvulsant medication that is also licenced for the management of neuropathic pain conditions – it is thought to work primarily through its effect on voltage-gated calcium channels. Gabapentin is taken orally, is not significantly metabolized, and is excreted through the kidneys; side effects include gut upset and dry mouth.

Pregabalin is an oral anticonvulsant that is also licenced for the management of generalised anxiety disorder and neuropathic pain conditions. Pregabalin works in a similar way to gabapentin through its effect on voltage-gated calcium channels. Pregabalin is minimally metabolized and is excreted by the kidneys; side effects include dry mouth, gut upset, and nausea.

Topical Analgesics

When patient have inflamed oral tissues, or sensitivity of the mouth or face due to neuropathic pain, topical analgesic preparations can be considered alongside the previously mentioned treatments. Benzydamine hydrochloride is a locally active nonsteroidal anti-inflammatory agent that has local anaesthetic and analgesic properties. Benzydamine comes in a 0.15% solution as an oral rinse or spray. Lidocaine can be applied topically to painful oral lesions as either a 5% ointment or as a 10-mg pump spray.

Nonmedical Pain Management

Medications only form one part of chronic pain management, which also includes areas such as patient education, physical exercises/relaxation techniques, physiotherapy, and clinical psychology. When required, oral cancer patients who have persistent neuropathic pain despite successful cancer treatment should have access to nonmedical pain management support in the form of specialist physiotherapy and clinical psychology (British Pain Society 2013).

References

British Pain Society (2013). Guidelines for pain management programs for adults. https://www.britishpainsociety.org/static/uploads/resources/files/pmp2013_main_FINAL_v6.pdfhttps://www.britishpainsociety.org/static/uploads/resources/files/pmp2013_main_FINAL_v6.pdf.

Epstein, J.B. and Miaskowski, C. (2019). Oral pain in the cancer patient. *J. Natl. Cancer Inst. Monogr.* 2019 (53): lgz003. https://doi.org/10.1093/jncimonographs/lgz003.

Finnerup, N.B., Attal, N., Haroutounian, S. et al. (2015). Pharmacotherapy for neuropathic pain in adults: a systematic review and meta-analysis. *Lancet. Neurol.* 14 (2): 162–173. https://doi.org/10.1016/S1474-4422(14)70251-0.

International Association for the Study of Pain (2021). IASP announces revised definition of pain. https://www.iasp-pain.org/publications/iasp-news/iasp-announces-revised-definition-of-pain.

Khawaja, S.N., Jamshed, A., and Hussain, R.T. (2020). Prevalence of pain in oral cancer: a retrospective study. *Oral Dis.* 27 (7): 1806–1812. https://doi.org/10.1111/odi.13701.

Melzack, R. and Casey, K. (1968). *The Skin Senses*, 423–439. Springfield, IL: Charles C. Thomas.

National Institute for Health and Care Excellence (2013). Neuropathic pain in adults: pharmacological management in non-specialist settings [NICE clinical guideline CG173]. https://www.nice.org.uk/guidance/cg173.

Schmidt, B.L. (2015). The neurobiology of cancer pain. *J. Oral Maxillofacial Surg.* 73 (12 Suppl): S132–S135. https://doi.org/10.1016/j.joms.2015.04.045.

World Health Organization (2018). WHO guidelines for the pharmacological and radiotherapeutic management of cancer pain in adults and adolescents. https://apps.who.int/iris/bitstream/handle/10665/279700/9789241550390-eng.pdf.

Section 5

Further Considerations, Patient Experiences and Support

42

Mental Health and Well-Being Post-treatment

Lauren Barry

York and Scarborough Teaching Hospitals NHS Foundation Trust, York, UK

Many patients experience a sense of anti-climax during the immediate period following active treatment. The expectation is that if you are ill you have treatment and then you are better. The reality of cancer treatment is more complex, and many patients feel traumatised as a consequence of the treatment, rather than feeling a sense of recovery. This can make them psychologically vulnerable.

This vulnerable state is often further heightened by the withdrawal of the intense level of support, both from professionals as the active treatment programme ends and from family and friends who rallied around to provide practical and emotional support during treatment and may not realise that support is still needed. People often report feeling alone or abandoned in the period after treatment; they may also feel as though they simply cannot cope now, having used all their toolkit resources during treatment.

The physical impact of treatment may continue to be felt long after the treatment has ceased. There is no clear-cut time frame for recovery from pain, nausea, and eating difficulties. Fatigue and low mood are also common, further adding to feelings of not being able to cope.

Surgery may have had a structural effect on the muscles of the head and neck, and patients may also be experiencing xerostomia and trismus. Individually and combined these can have profound impacts on the patients' capacity to speak and control facial expressions, limiting their ability to communicate with those around them. These challenges to communication can cause some patients to retreat from day-to-day interactions.

Changes to appearance can have a deeply negative effect on self-image and body image. This can lead to a loss of confidence, low self-esteem, and feelings of isolation and loneliness. Loneliness, per se, is linked with low quality of life and can affect those receiving any type of treatment; it is not confined to those patients who have had major interventions as part of their treatment (Dahill et al. 2020).

Intimacy and sex can become difficult for several reasons. Simply being unwell can change the role of the person into one of patient. Body image has an effect on sexual functioning. Cancer treatments can also result in the reduction of sexual desire, changing the relationship dynamics for people with cancer and/or their partner. The mouth itself is a sexual organ, and changes to its health and appearance can have an impact on intimacy and sexuality. Although sexual desire changes through the life course, it is an important part of well-being to consider (Hoole 2020).

Unfortunately, some patients feel worse at this stage than before and during treatment, especially if they were asymptomatic at time of diagnosis. As they try to make sense of what has happened to them up to this point, they can struggle with feelings of 'this is not how I am meant to feel'. Against our typical expectations of a cure following treatment, this experience of the recovery period can be extremely challenging, and some patients find it helpful to see this as a new beginning rather than the end of the dealing with their cancer.

There are no rules about recovery. People are different, and some will move faster than others. Recovery will mean different things to different people. The idea of a return to 'normal' is often desired and discussed. Some patients will not be able to return to the old state they strive for, for reasons outside their control. The loss of their old life can cause great sadness for many patients; for others it highlights further their loss of control of their life, exacerbating their frustration. It can be helpful for these patients to think and plan for what is possible, such as regaining and refreshing old skills rather than

Care of Head and Neck Cancer Patients for Dental Hygienists and Dental Therapists, First Edition. Edited by Jocelyn J. Harding.

focusing on what has been lost. All patients should be able to feel as though they can take the time they need to rebuild their coping strategies and developing a sustainable toolkit.

This huge upheaval, and the changes within the body and the mind, can lead to feelings of distrust of the body. This manifests as a loss of sense of security in one's body, the feeling that the body is no longer known nor its needs understood. Worries about health are common, and there can be a fear that any unfamiliar ache, pain, or change is a return or spread of the cancer. For this reason patients are encouraged to speak to their health care professionals about any worrying symptoms so they can be investigated and the patient reassured. If something abnormal is going on, further investigation can be undertaken in a timely manner.

Other pretreatment anxieties, often suspended during treatment, can also return. These include worries about money, supporting a family, caring for dependents, employment prospects, and many others. The social impacts of cancer cannot be ignored, as they form an integral part of people's lives and well-being.

For some patients the effects of their cancer journey will be long-lived; they may learn to adapt, but there will always be some level of reminder or impairment caused by their illness and treatment. Others seem to move past these events, and there are many examples of patients who have gone on to realise long-held ambitions or made positive changes to their lives as a result of their recovery from the cancer. All experiences are valid and should be given respect and the person treated with kindness and understanding. Some patients may be more guarded about their experience, whereas others will want to talk about it, especially to dental professionals, who would be expected to have a level of insight and awareness of the condition and treatment.

In terms of supporting these patients as a hygienist and therapist, an honest and thoughtful approach is recommended. We are in a privileged position to learn about our patients, and active listening can be one of our biggest contributions. It is important not to feel that we have to provide answers outside the scope of our role.

We are also skilled in communication and thinking creatively to support and motivate our patients. Oral hygiene support and instruction is essential, but it is as important that it is realistic for each individual. Patients who have been through the experience of head and neck cancer and its treatment require some extra time and thought. As has been said in all of these chapters, kindness, rethinking what might be an achievable standard, and time and listening will be of use to these patients.

References

Dahill, A., Al-Nakishbandi, H., Cunningham, K.B. et al. (2020). Loneliness and quality of life after head and neck cancer. *Br. J. Oral. Maxill. Surg.* 58 (8): 959–965.

Hoole, J. (2020). Getting started: assessment. https://maxfacts.uk/help/intimacy/assessment (accessed 18 March 2021).

Further Reading and Resources

Changing Faces: www.changingfaces.org.uk/adviceandsupport. A charity that provides a range of support and information services to patients, carers, and professionals. Supporting those with something that changes their facial appearance.

Look Good Feel Better: https://lookgoodfeelbetter.co.uk/about-us/. National charity that supports patients experiencing any type of cancer. Provides online and face-to-face workshops aimed at trying to improve physical and emotional well-being.

43

Intimacy: Advice for the Patient from a Psychologist

Jo Hemmings

Behavioural Psychologist, London, UK

There are many aspects of having cancer of the mouth that your surgeon or oral hygienist will talk through with you, but the impact it may have on intimacy with your partner is rarely one of them. And yet up to 50% of patients treated for mouth cancers will experience issues with sex and intimacy during and after treatment.

While much of this is down to physiological symptoms, such as dry mouth, our lips and mouth are so inextricably linked with our self-esteem in sexual terms that psychologically, treatment will also have a major impact on our levels of arousal and desire or the sense that we are less desirable ourselves. Decreased libido and arousal, fatigue, and poor self-image can all contribute to a significant decrease in physical intimacy between a couple.

Nearly all relationships start with a kiss. Perhaps a gentle brush of the lips at first, but followed quickly by full mouth to mouth, deep kissing. When relationships begin to go wrong, kissing is also the first element of a sexual relationship to disappear – couples may still be having sexual intercourse, but they may not be experiencing the high intimacy of a deep kiss. And of course oral sex, when you have had mouth cancer, might make you feel self-conscious or feeling that the experience is less pleasurable, even painful, due to discomfort or dry mouth.

Our lips are not only completely unique to us – in the way that a fingerprint is – they also have more than a million different nerve endings, making them one of the most sensitive and sensual areas of our bodies. A hundred times more sensitive than our fingertips, they are also incredibly thin. Just three to six layers of cells, diminishing as we age, compared to the 16 layers elsewhere on our bodies.

If you have had treatment for mouth cancer, it is inevitable that your lips or the inner parts of your mouth will be affected in some way.

So, how can we protect our mouth and lips, postsurgery, to maintain intimacy with our partner?

Talk to your surgeon or hygienist. Intimacy is key to any successful relationship, and they may be able to recommend special gels or other medications to help with dry mouth, taste issues, and production of saliva. All good health professionals should be able to advise, and if they can't they may refer you to a specialist who can. Please do not feel embarrassed about talking about this with them; they will have most certainly heard it before.

Talk to each other. Don't shy away from discussing how you are feeling. Your partner is much more likely to be sensitive and supportive if you are candid about how are feeling rather than withdraw from the person altogether.

Keep hydrated, drink plenty of water, and use a mouthwash regularly to keep your breath as fresh as possible.

Exfoliate, moisturize, and generally protect the lip area to encourage regrowth of the skin there and to keep them from drying out.

There are many alternatives that you can do to maintain intimacy in your relationship, even without using your mouth or lips. Use your fingertips – not as sensitive as the mouth but a pretty good substitute – or use other tactile and sensory playthings like feathers or silk scarves.

Be reassured that once your treatment has started, progress and healing will be relatively swift. With such few layers of skin on our lips, they are designed to replenish themselves quickly, so diminished sensation or discomfort will pass in due course.

Care of Head and Neck Cancer Patients for Dental Hygienists and Dental Therapists, First Edition. Edited by Jocelyn J. Harding.

44

What Is Palliative Care?

Emma Husbands

Gloucestershire Hospitals NHS Foundation Trust, Gloucester, UK

Palliative care (PC), sometimes also referred to as 'supportive care', describes the approach of active holistic care for individuals with serious health-related suffering due to severe illness. It aims to improve the quality of life of patients, their families, and their caregivers (Radbruch et al. 2020). Traditionally associated with care of the dying, the principles of PC are recognised to provide benefit earlier in the course of cancer treatments: helping to improve quality of life, possibly lengthening survival, and reducing the need for aggressive treatments near the end of life (Temel et al. 2010). HNC treatments mean that many people receive anticancer therapies over many years, more are living beyond cancer, 'off treatment', and either in remission or cured, and others are living with progressive disease (National Cancer Survivorship Initiative 2013; NHS 2016).

All health care professionals can provide PC; many of them do not have specialist training but their own skill sets will enable relief of symptoms, optimization of comfort/function, and an enhancement of quality of life. Interdisciplinary care is crucial to optimising palliation, with allied health care professionals playing a key role in supporting rehabilitation and adjustment to life after cancer treatment, be that curative or noncurative. For people with HNC, the role of the dental hygienist is vital, providing initially preventative care before cancer treatment, moving through to restorative care and education around maintaining oral health, as well as interventions for complications as they arise – all are integral to the care of a person with HNC.

Of course, specialists in PC can also be needed where someone's needs are more complex and not responding to standard measures. Specialist PC teams are present in most hospitals across the UK, as well as working in community settings and hospices. Teams consist of a range of professionals who have undertaken additional training, most often including doctors, nurses, occupational therapists/physiotherapists, and psychologists. They work with a person's usual team to support symptom control and optimise care.

What Symptoms are Seen with Head and Neck Cancers?

The following are symptoms commonly seen with HNCs.

Swelling/ulcer/sore in mouth	One of the commonest symptoms/signs. These may be initially identified at a routine dental check-up and people may be unaware that they are present. If identified, it is important to explain the findings to them honestly but avoid unnecessary alarm.
Hoarseness or change in voice	This may be noticed by friends/family rather than the person.
Pain – tongue/throat or ear pain	Pain may be a persistent sore throat, pain in the tongue/jaw, or painful lumps in the neck. Pain can be referred and felt in the ear or shoulders/arms, depending on the location and impact of tumour. Pain is very individual and people will describe it differently. It can be helpful to explore what people mean when they say they have pain, its impact on them, and anything they might have tried to help it, as well as things that can make it worse.

Care of Head and Neck Cancer Patients for Dental Hygienists and Dental Therapists, First Edition. Edited by Jocelyn J. Harding.

Difficulty swallowing (dysphagia)	Can relate to certain foods/fluids and can cause choking episodes that can be quite frightening.
Ill-fitting dentures/ loose teeth.	May be the prompt for a review with the hygienist, and the fact it can be a sign of a cancer may well be unexpected for many people.
Foul mouth odour not explained by hygiene	Again, this may be a trigger for someone attending for a dental review. This can be a particularly embarrassing symptom.
Lump, bump, or mass in the head or neck area, with or without pain	It is a misconception that cancers are always associated with pain; they can be entirely painless. Any unusual 'lumps' that are not resolving should be reviewed.
Coughing up blood in saliva or phlegm.	Sometimes an intermittent problem and may be more likely to be discussed with a doctor than the dental team.
Nonspecific symptoms	These can include shortness of breath, poor appetite, weight loss, and/or fatigue.

It is likely that the initial approach to symptoms will be referral for investigations to confirm the cause. The identification of disease and approach to any treatment often has a role in treating symptoms, and anticancer treatments such as surgery/chemotherapy/radiotherapy or immunotherapy can all reduce tumour size and hence improve things.

You may be able to offer some general advice on oral hygiene and simple pain relief initially. Any suspected cancer is treated as an urgent referral under what is known as the 'two-week wait', and the NHS remains committed to any such person being seen within that time frame, often sooner. It is unusual for someone to present with very severe symptoms, but if this were to happen, a more urgent referral may be required to your local head and neck team.

What are the Effects of HNC Treatment?

The treatment of any cancer has long-lasting effects, but there is no doubt that the nature of treatments for head and neck cancers can impact not only because of the potential for symptoms such as pain but also the effects that may be had on very basic human functions such as eating/drinking, communication, and appearance. Figure 44.1 is an illustration of the impact of pain for a person following curative treatment for tonsil cancer. It shows very clearly that the pain can be incredibly debilitating, and it is important to ask people about symptoms when considering their needs/preassessing or treating them. For some people, the long-term effects can be significant enough that they regret undergoing treatment in the first place; cure is not always associated with acceptable quality of life, and a decision to decline radical treatment is an important choice for people to be allowed to consider, even accepting their life will likely be shortened.

Disease can also be small/superficial and respond to much more simple treatment.

Common Post-treatment Symptoms

Common post-treatment symptoms include the following:

1) *Dry mouth or xerostomia* can be an almost inevitable consequence of HNC treatment. Many treatment regimens include radiotherapy or surgery that can affect the function of salivary glands. People may report a more mucoid consistency to their saliva – it can feel sticky and difficult to clear.
   Dental/oral hygiene is particularly important where saliva production is reduced or consistency altered. Saliva is a hugely important substance in maintaining oral health and aiding mastication/digestion. Sipping water regularly or using a water spray or artificial saliva can be beneficial. There may be a role for medications to try and stimulate saliva and also medications to try and thin more viscous mucus.
2) *Pain after treatment* is common. The principles of assessment and management are fairly standard, and tools such as 'SOCRATES' are useful aide-mémoires to undertaking a pain assessment (see below). It is unlikely you will need to discuss pain in such detail, but a pain history is key to helping to manage pain.

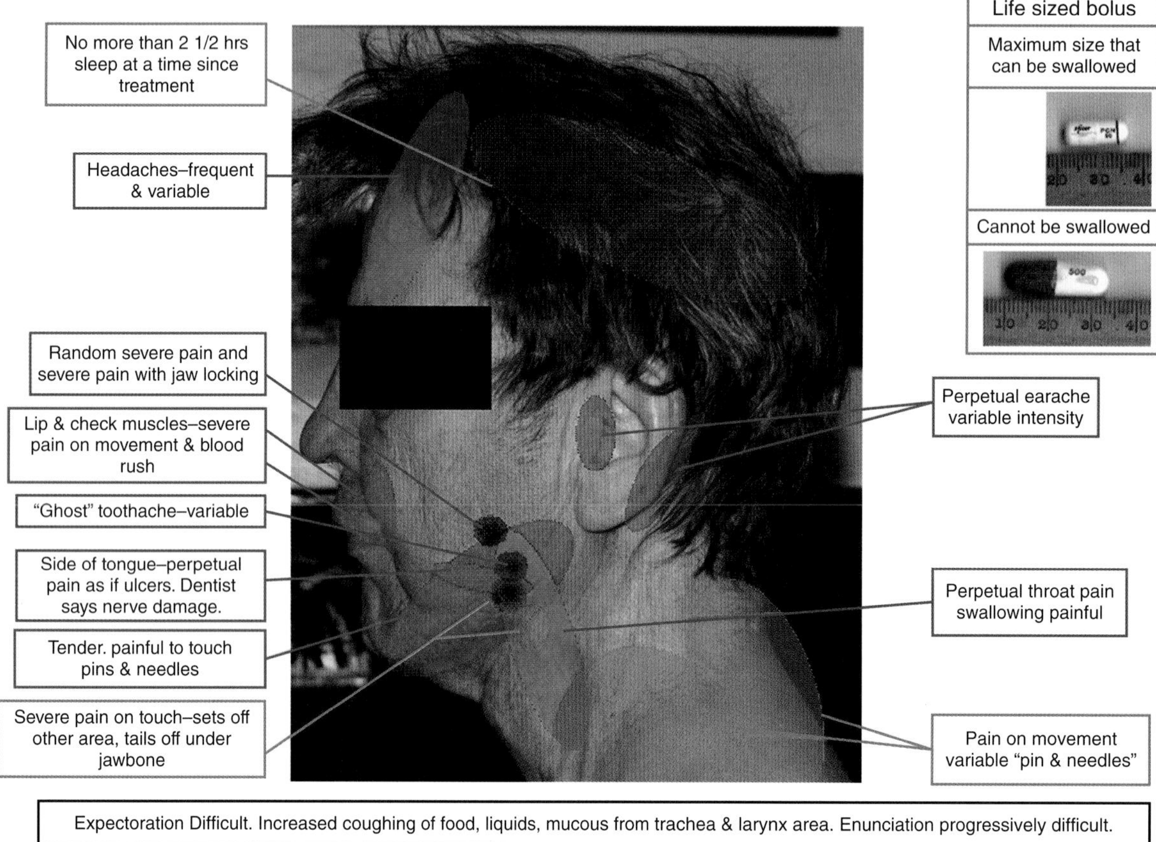
No more than 2 1/2 hrs sleep at a time since treatment
Headaches–frequent & variable
Random severe pain and severe pain with jaw locking
Lip & check muscles–severe pain on movement & blood rush
"Ghost" toothache–variable
Side of tongue–perpetual pain as if ulcers. Dentist says nerve damage.
Tender. painful to touch pins & needles
Severe pain on touch–sets off other area, tails off under jawbone
Life sized bolus
Maximum size that can be swallowed
Cannot be swallowed
Perpetual earache variable intensity
Perpetual throat pain swallowing painful
Pain on movement variable "pin & needles"
Expectoration Difficult. Increased coughing of food, liquids, mucous from trachea & larynx area. Enunciation progressively difficult.

Figure 44.1 Impacts of pain.

Letter	Aspect	Example questions
S	Site	Where is the pain? Or the maximal site of the pain.
O	Onset	When did the pain start, and was it sudden or gradual? Include also whether it is progressive or regressive.
C	Character	What is the pain like? An ache? Stabbing?
R	Radiation	Does the pain radiate anywhere?
A	Associations	Any other signs or symptoms associated with the pain?
T	Time course	Does the pain follow any pattern?
E	Exacerbating/relieving factors	Does anything change the pain?
S	Severity	How bad is the pain?

Following extensive treatment, a period of recovery over many months may be needed with physiotherapy/occupational therapy as well as oral care all playing a part in the rehabilitation of people living beyond cancer. The mouth may feel sensitive due to the effects of treatment, so do bear this in mind when examining/undertaking treatment. The approach to pain is influenced by the state of people's HNC. If they have ongoing disease, the use of medications such as morphine regularly may be really important, and this is often supported by their medical teams. If pain isn't controlled with standard measures and they aren't already known to a palliative/supportive care team, they may be referred on for pain assessment. When people have completed curative treatment or for those in remission, the management of pain may be slightly different. When present for more than three months, pain is classed as chronic, and it can be less responsive to some of the standard pain medications; there may also be greater risk to them staying on some medications over many years. In the absence of disease recurrence, the pain is effectively indirectly caused by the cancer, and there is often greater importance in nonpharmacological approaches to pain management and optimizing techniques of living with pain. This might include a pain management programme as well as psychological interventions. That said, medications can certainly have a role, and either the HNC team/supportive care or chronic pain team may be asked to advise.

3) *Stiff jaw/trismus* is particularly common after radiotherapy treatment and can contribute to pain but also impact on ability to speak and eat/drink if very severe. For dental treatments, this may mean that adaptations need to be made or more time allowed.
4) *Dysphagia or difficulty swallowing* may or may not be associated with pain. The knock-on impact of dysphagia can be weight loss and sometimes increased risk of aspiration of food/fluids leading to episodes of choking and even chest infection. Speech and language therapists can support people in trying to improve their ability to swallow and can guide on textures and techniques. Dieticians also have a role in optimizing nutrition, but it is often important to remember that diet may be altered and include supplement drinks, which can be quite sugary or acidic. This will be important for oral hygiene and protection of remaining dentition.
5) *Difficulty speaking/dysphasia*: surgery and other treatments can have a real impact on speech; some people will have loss of muscle function and difficulty making their speech understood and others may, as part of their treatment, lose their voice box and find themselves either having to communicate through a speech valve or by artificial means such as a paper and pen or electronic device. This is important to understand before your consultations, to ensure that you can give people adequate time and support to enable them to have their 'voice' heard.

There are many other symptoms reported after treatments for HNC, such as depression and challenges with body image and self-esteem. So many really basic aspects of life can be affected and people can feel like a different person and may feel incredibly vulnerable. They may feel very aware of their appearance and be embarrassed by it.

Communicating with People Who Have Experienced HNC

Introduce yourself and explain your role, in plain language without using 'dental jargon'! Try to build a rapport and be open and friendly. Remember that patients may have had their cancer diagnosed in a dental setting and so it may cause them anxiety, and it will be important to tell them what is happening.

Allow people to set the scene and ask them if there is anything they want you to know in order for you to support them – this might include their communication needs or advising you of any pain/restricted movement or impact of their experiences during treatment.

Listen proactively and be present with people; demonstrate you are interested and connecting to their words and feelings. Using some open questions can give people permission to say things and express their concerns. Whilst there isn't an endless amount of time, try not to make people feel rushed.

Ensure that any advice given is understood; don't assume it has been heard as you said it. For advice around oral hygiene, it is important to ask people if they feel it is possible – if for some reason they don't feel that it is, then adjusting the advice to something that they think they can do will be far more beneficial than encouraging a gold standard approach that may not get done.

Finally, remember to communicate with any relevant members of people's care teams if needed and, of course, with their permission. Teamwork is always the key.

References

National Cancer Survivorship Initiative (2013). Living with and beyond cancer: taking action to improve outcomes. https://www.gov.uk/government/publications/living-with-and-beyond-cancer-taking-action-to-improve-outcomes.

NHS England (2016). Enhanced supportive care: integrating supportive care in oncology. https://www.england.nhs.uk/wp-content/uploads/2016/03/ca1-enhncd-supprtv-care-guid.pdf.

Radbruch, L., De Lima, L., Knaul, F. et al. (2020). Redefining palliative care – a new consensus-based definition. *J. Pain Symptom Manag.* 60: 754–764. https://doi.org/10.1016/j.jpainsymman.2020.04.027.

Temel, J.S., Greer, J.A., Muzikansky, A. et al. (2010). Early palliative care for patients with metastatic non-small-cell lung cancer. *N. Engl. J. Med.* 363 (8): 733–742. https://doi.org/10.1056/NEJMoa1000678.

45

My Cancer, My Journey

Roy Anthony

Retired Dental Hygienist, Stockton on Tees, UK

In March 2015 when a human papillomavirus squamous cell carcinoma of the right tonsillar region was confirmed, it seemed death had knocked on my door. Life changed for me and my family as events accelerated in a way that our wonderful National Health Service achieves when urgency is required.

This account of my personal journey is, well, very personal. It's a narrative, not a science paper. I had a foot in both camps as I was a dental hygienist and a patient, and so I hope by writing this it will give colleagues a perspective and an insight into what our cancer patients may go through.

I found a tiny asymptomatic swelling immediately below the right-side angle of my mandible. I found it when I subconsciously went to scratch an itch whilst driving.

That moment will stay with me for the rest of my days.

There was nothing to see, no redness or pain, no discernible change to my breathing or voice; nothing. I felt curious. Cancer was the furthest thing from my mind; it was more likely a blocked subcutaneous or salivary gland. When it persisted for a couple of weeks, the consensus at work was a blocked salivary gland, and my GP even showed me Google images of a blocked salivary gland. However, blocked salivary glands are supposedly episodic, and this one was persistent.

A referral to the oral surgery department followed. Other than the extraoral, same-sized lump, there was nothing to be seen or felt intraorally, any sign or symptom lying tantalisingly beyond the reach of the longest fingers. There followed an ultrasound scan of the site and a fine needle biopsy, neither of which proved conclusive.

As there seemed little urgency involved, it was late March 2015 before I saw the consultant oral surgeon. Alarm bells must have been ringing as he sent me straight away for a CT scan and kindly waited beyond office hours to discuss the findings with me. The scan showed what appeared to be an enormous pear-shaped tumour with the 'top of the pear' pointing outwards and allowing me to feel it beneath my skin. A follow up appointment was hastily arranged for Monday, 30 March 2015, and two days later on the Wednesday, 1 April, I was one of the first on the list for a biopsy/resection.

At the review appointment two weeks later and with blissful naivety, I attended by myself as I was certain that whatever it was it would be nothing sinister.

I was wrong. The diagnosis was a T2 N2b HPV SCC.

It is a body blow knocking all the wind from you being told you have cancer. I left the department reeling, and I remember little of what was said to me beyond those few words. I found myself reeling, completely overwhelmed. I pulled myself together and went and broke the news to my wife, who was at work. Together we went and cried with my two teenage boys before my usual stubborn spirit kicked in and I proclaimed to the family that I was not going to die from this.

The next few weeks were a whirlwind of appointments, many of which were a blur but, in many cases, although I was nodding and smiling, the enormity of the various discussions was largely lost on me. All staff, all departments were excellent and in a well-rehearsed process took time and effort to talk me through the treatment pathway.

I still wonder if, through the whole time, I was still mentally in denial.

My wife and I attended a multidiscipline team meeting to hear the full treatment proposal. This was quite daunting and humbling, as there must have been at least 15 team members surrounding us, all of whom were dedicated to my well-being.

Care of Head and Neck Cancer Patients for Dental Hygienists and Dental Therapists, First Edition. Edited by Jocelyn J. Harding.

My treatment started at oral surgery, where my oral hygiene and the possible need for a molar clearance were assessed. A second appointment with the resident dental therapist was attended, where a full mouth ultrasonic scaling was completed. A molar clearance was not indicated.

I was sent for a PET scan, which thankfully showed that there was one primary lesion and no secondary lesions. I had to attend with a full bladder, and the scanning team had to escort me to the toilet while clearing public and staff from my path as I had been injected with a radiotracer. This substance, normally fluorodeoxyglucose (FDG), emits a radiation that is picked up during the scan and shows where the cancer is located.

I visited the chemotherapy and radiotherapy departments, had impressions taken for my radiotherapy mask and had it fitted and marked up, and had a targeting tattoo inked on to my chest before having my feeding tube placed. This PEG tube was a necessary evil and was to prove problematic. I also convinced myself that I would only use it as a last resort. The Fortisip food product that was to be used with the PEG was supplied by a private company, and the nurse came to the house and talked us through the tube's maintenance and use. She also scared us with talk of it falling out and reassured us that the food would arrive shortly.

So much Fortisip food arrived I was afraid I would be living with the PEG for several years.

Chemotherapy was to take place every Monday for six weeks and would take all day. At some stage during the day, I would be taken for my radiotherapy. We arrived early morning and my general health was checked: no temperature or cold-like symptoms. I was cannulated and placed on a drip for approximately two hours, ensuring full hydration. I was also given a steroid injection and an antiemetic. Towards lunchtime I was given a diuretic and the chemotherapy began. Cisplatin was the therapy of choice and was also delivered over two hours. Each therapy is specific to the individual, and as cisplatin deteriorates in daylight, it was always delivered via drip and covered in a black plastic bag.

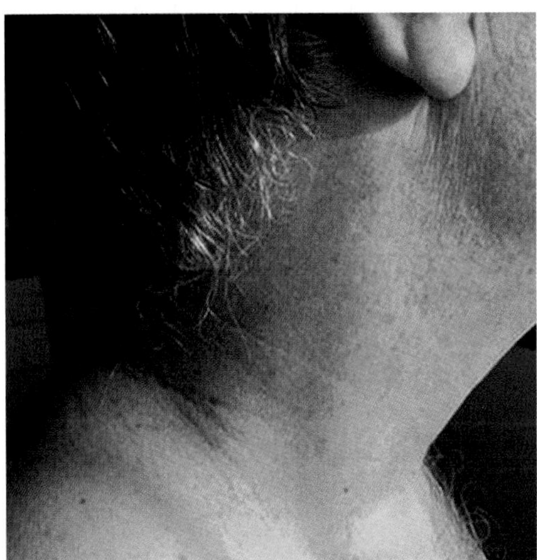

Figure 45.1 Two weeks into radiotherapy.

The diuretic prompted regular visits to the toilet. Following the cisplatin a further two hours of rehydration followed, and I was normally free to leave at about 4 o'clock.

IMRT began the Thursday prior to my first Monday of chemotherapy and then every morning, except weekends, for six weeks. Each appointment was about a half hour. I would lie on a surprisingly comfortable wooden bench and was positioned by staff after I had put on my 'swim cap', into my radiotherapy mask. I used a breathing tube, and as the mask was so closely fitted, I lay with my eyes closed. Treatment followed the same format daily as I entered the machine initially for about 5–10 minutes, removed for a further 5 minutes as, I presume, settings were checked prior to treatment. I would then re-enter for the further 10 minutes or so of treatment.

My worries were understandable, even though staff constantly reassured and supported. On reflection, though, I believe my cheerful, 'manly' approach hid the fact that information was not sinking in. I am so grateful to my wife for being there at every step as she was able to organise information for me.

My first chemotherapy session over, I wondered what all the fuss was about. I felt cheerful and full of energy for a couple of days until the effects of the steroid wore off, and I then felt tired and down. For the first couple of sessions this cycle was repeated, but as therapy went on, I became more tired and, eventually, exhausted. It became increasingly difficult to motivate myself to do the most simple and mundane of tasks, for example brushing my teeth. It took a monumental effort to have a shower every day.

Two weeks into radiotherapy, it followed a similar pattern. Initially I was pleased that treatment seemed so straightforward with seemingly little effect. However, while signs extraorally began looking like localised sunburn (Figures 45.1–45.3), by the end of radiotherapy the skin was a marked burn with tissue sloughing off (Figures 45.4 and 45.5).

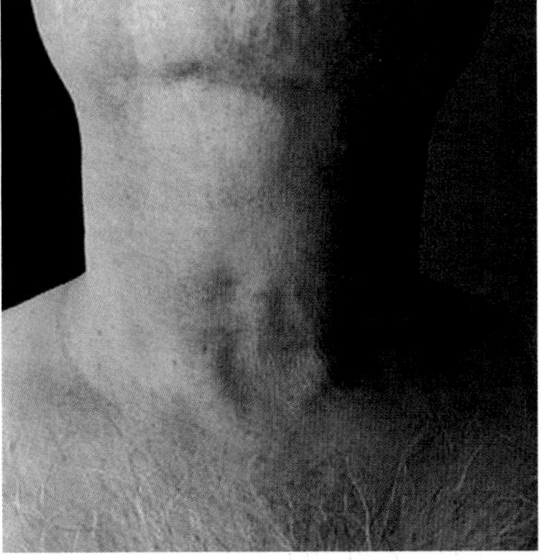

Figure 45.2 Two weeks into radiotherapy.

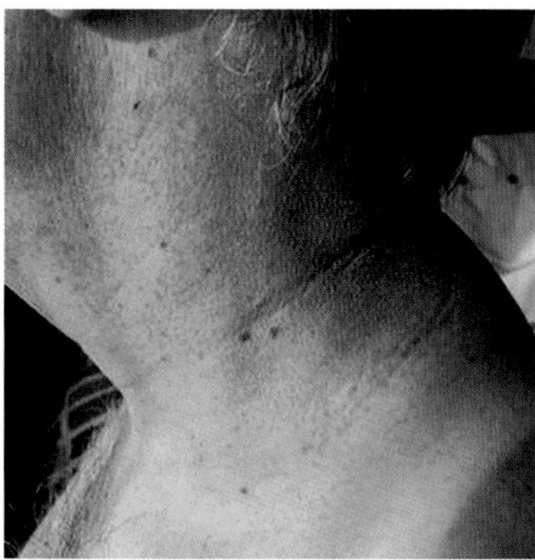

Figure 45.3 Two weeks into radiotherapy.

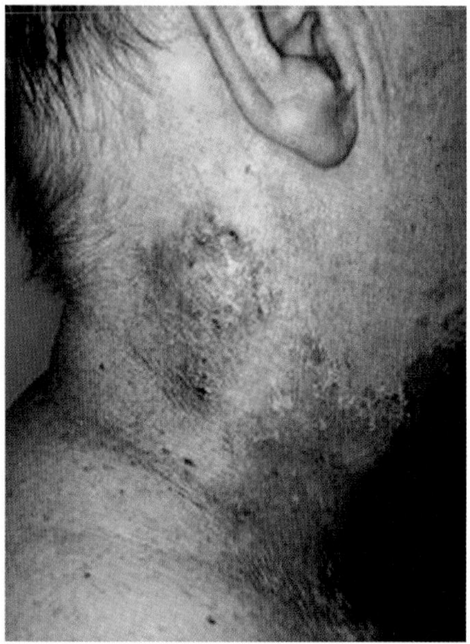

Figure 45.4 The end of radiotherapy.

Radiation burns at the end of six weeks of radiotherapy were treated by the pain management team with Flamazine cream and a Polymem cover (Figures 45.6 and 45.7), which managed to calm the area. The Polymem was worn every day for two weeks and gave off an unfortunate odour.

Intraorally the soft tissues rapidly broke down, resulting in a very painful and two-month presence of oral mucositis. Initially presenting as an ulcer along the right border of the tongue, this rapidly developed into an ulceration covering most soft tissues in the oropharyngeal region. The only area largely untouched by the radiotherapy was the anterior region. The gingivae took on a chronic inflammation and bled spontaneously. Acts of cleaning and eating were becoming progressively more difficult and were further complicated as I developed a severe, spontaneous gag reflex. I continued to clean my teeth throughout, despite the prolific bleeding and pain. Oncology had prescribed a mouthwash tablet, Telladont, which I was sceptical about using, doubting its efficacy. However, late on in treatment I tried it and was surprised at how fresh it made my mouth feel. I diluted one tablet into a litre of water as anything less was far too intense a flavour.

Eating became unbearable. After two weeks of treatment, I used the PEG full time for food and medication. I should have used the PEG from the outset as my stubbornness could have jeopardised my ongoing treatment – maintaining my body weight was crucial as the radiotherapy mask had been fitted to my pretreatment size, and any weight reduction could have halted treatment (Figures 45.8 and 45.9).

The combination of tiredness and exhaustion from the chemotherapy and the mounting pain from the radiotherapy began to take their toll. I felt as if I was always asleep. The pain was controlled, initially and well, by paracetamol, but as

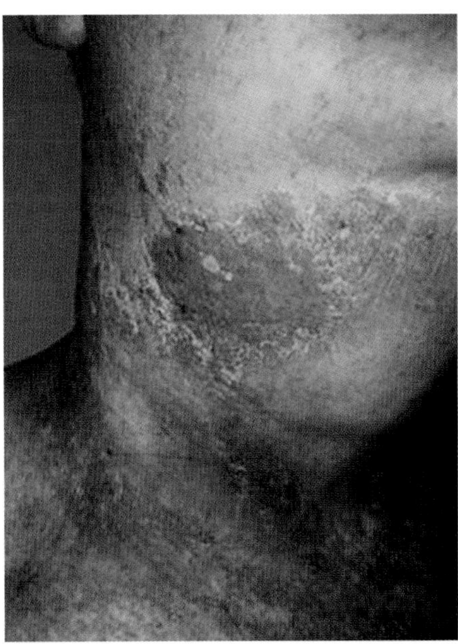

Figure 45.5 The end of radiotherapy.

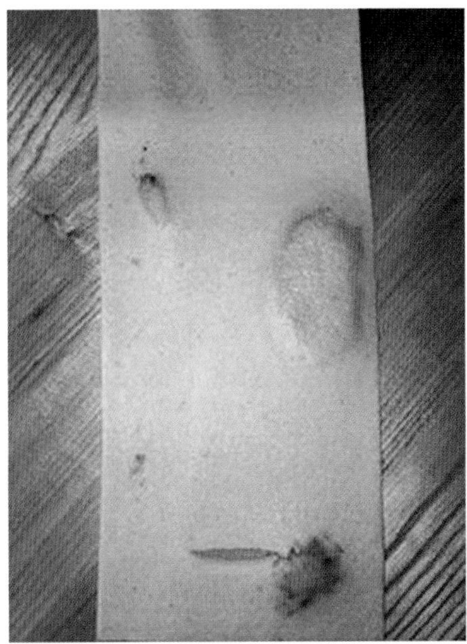

Figure 45.6 Treatment for radiation burns.

treatment progressed and the pain mounted, then pain relief became stronger until Oramorph was consistently used. This had the added side effect of making me more tired. I was also taking daily antiemetics, iron tablets, and lansoprazole. A laxative was also added to the list.

To ease the intraoral pain and to help with the healing process of the soft tissues I was prescribed Caphosol. I describe this as a supersaturated salt/mineral mouthwash that has a similar pH to saliva and is designed to help maintain the moisture level of the mucosa and aid healing. It also acted as a very mild topical anaesthetic for me. I had to mix vial A with vial B and rinse to a maximum of 10 times per day. Although Caphosol proved very useful, it did cause me to gag. As treatment progressed this involuntary reflex became more painful and so I had to pick my time carefully as to when to use it.

The PEG was also becoming a problem. During its placement a small blood vessel at the stoma site had failed to heal. This resulted in both external and internal bleeding: externally it showed as a substantial bleed but internally resulted in the projectile vomiting of about 2 pints of blood and many trips to A&E culminating in a few hours in resuscitation as my wife tried valiantly to help by catching everything in an oversized kidney dish.

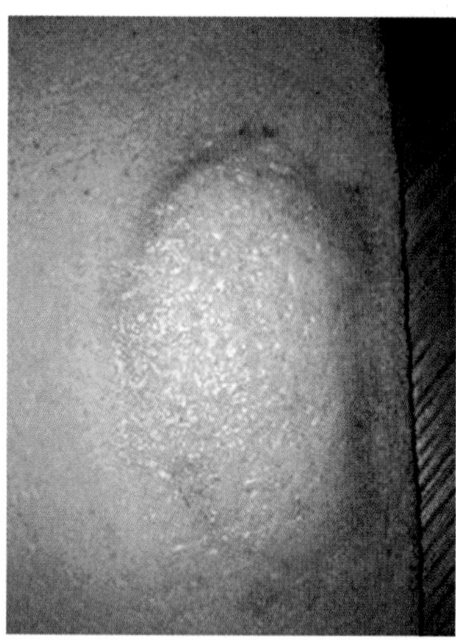

Figure 45.7 Treatment for radiation burns.

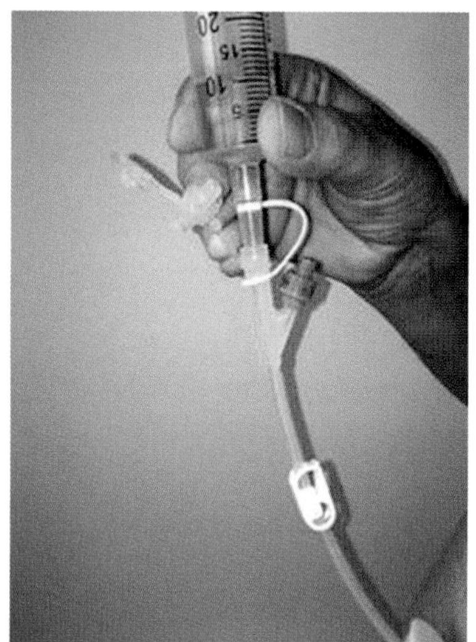

Figure 45.8 The PEG.

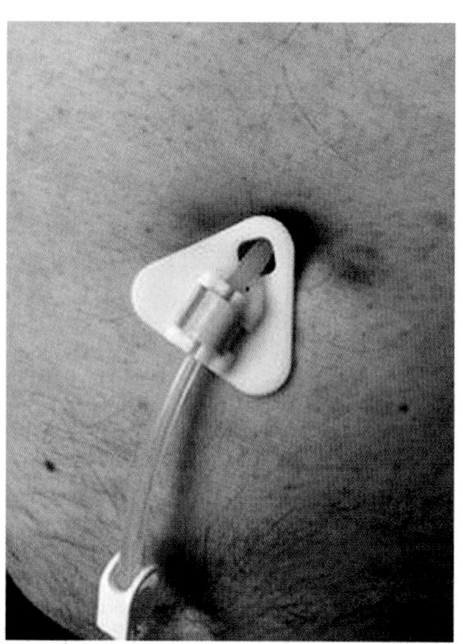

Figure 45.9 Using the PEG.

It also resulted in needing about 10 units of blood to be transfused over five visits. I am so, so grateful to all those unknown people who kindly and generously donated their blood for me.

The PEG was replaced by an NG tube as soon as practical when chemoradiotherapy was finished. The first tube was held in place with a sticking plaster (Figure 45.10) that body oil caused to loosen, and when I realised in the middle of the night that it had become dislodged, I just pulled it out. This did mean needing a second tube placed, which was held in place with the bridle system, tying it in place behind the nasal septum.

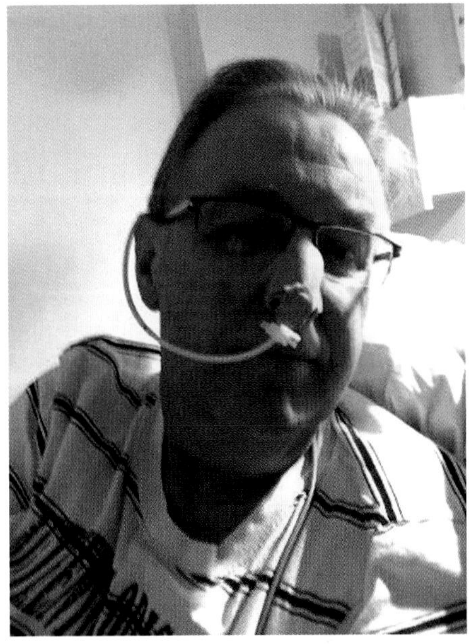

Figure 45.10 Using a nasogastric tube.

There were two parts to recovery, the physical healing and the exhaustion. Physically I could do little to speed the healing process. My diet for several weeks after treatment completed was still supplied artificially by Fortisip, and when my NG tube was fitted, pumped into my stomach, leaving me feeling bloated. If I remember correctly, it was the soft palate that healed the quickest, although during the healing process there would often be setbacks as the tissue seemed to stretch and split. There was also a nasty ulceration on my uvula that required a further biopsy under general anaesthetic, which proved innocent.

One of the first things I noticed as healing took place was an increase in salivary production. This was a poor-quality saliva and I carried tissues continually to wipe away embarrassing excess. I was prescribed hyoscine patches, which were placed behind my ears, and they seemed to help reduce the flow.

An unusual creeping sensation appeared in my scalp during the first and second month of healing. I could feel something crawling in my hair behind my ear. There was, of course, nothing there, but this part of the healing process is known as formication and only lasted a couple of weeks.

It was shortly before my three-month review that the first ulcer that had appeared on the border of my tongue eventually healed. It was also at about the same time that I was able to stop using analgesics. The radiation burns on my neck had healed quickly with the use of the Flamazine/Polymem combination, although it has left me with no hair follicles below my jaw line. During healing there was also a marked increase in lymph drainage, leading to a dewlap swelling around my throat. Although now receded, it has left me with stretched skin in the area.

Throughout treatment and recovery my weight had been carefully monitored, and I had spent some time with the dietician, who continually monitored my calorie intake. As recovery progressed and I was considering returning to a solid diet, the speech therapist joined us and examined me as I drank water, ensuring that I hadn't lost any capability to swallow.

My stubbornness continued to confound my family as, when my NG tube was removed, I took it upon myself to increase my exercise level and went cross country running with friends.

Needless to say, exhaustion overwhelmed me, and I probably put back my own recovery by a month at least.

My first review was at three months. Prior to the appointment I had a second PET scan, results showing that there were no further lesions present and that treatment was successful. Visually, intraorally, and a check of all lymph nodes in the head and neck region was completed. The team were again supportive and took time to explain the ongoing process. Reviews would continue at three monthly intervals for the first year, as this period has the highest potential of recurrence. It was noted that my salivary production had decreased, and reviews for the second year would also remain at three-month intervals.

Each review that I attended and that proved uneventful was met emotionally, and I freely admit to crying at my second year all clear.

Reviews followed the same pattern for the remaining three years, although the interval between reviews was extended to four months and, arbitrarily, six months. Each review followed the same pattern, a check on my well-being and my weight and a full exam of my oral mucosa and associated lymph nodes.

At the time of writing, I was given my five years all clear about six months ago.

It was emotionally overwhelming. I am so lucky.

There are so many lessons to share with colleagues that I am sure that I forget some.

But I do always know where to start, and that is detection.

Unless we actively look for lesions, intra- and extraorally, at every appointment opportunity and then act on anything suspicious at the earliest possible moment, then we run the risk of doing a great disservice to the patient. To all colleagues, I urge you to routinely check all relevant intra- and extraoral tissues, including lymph nodes. If confidence is an issue when checking nodes, then I suggest practicing on partners and your children. I used to talk my patients through this examination, which helped involve them in their care and may help them become more self-aware and check for anything suspicious themselves. It also acted as an aide-mémoire for myself as I developed a rhythm to the process.

I do think that patient information can become more effective. Verbal information didn't sink in or left us confused, and written information wasn't read.

Is it possible to condense and simplify everything into three A4 sheets of paper: one to describe treatment progress, another to list contacts as well as listing any additional reading, and a third to list medications and a daily timetable for them?

I would recommend that whenever possible, a patient attends appointments with a second person. This would help all parties with the information given and the emotional support required.

My reluctance to use the PEG tube leads me to suggest that patients are encouraged to use their PEG from the outset and to be helped and watched by staff, even prior to treatment commencing. This would help reduce any mental barriers a patient may have and help prevent any withdrawal of treatment due to weight loss.

Dentally, I would encourage patients, prior to treatment commencing, to improve their oral hygiene. This would help reduce the need for a molar clearance. As treatment progresses and the possibility of oral mucositis increases, toothbrushing will become more difficult and may even be impossible. Any time spent improving dental hygiene will be time well spent. I would also suggest that it offers the patient another shoulder to lean on as all support offered will help the patient both mentally and dentally.

Many patients will also see a reduction in salivary production following treatment, which can lead to the risk of a higher caries rate. A high-level fluoride toothpaste, for example Duraphat 5000 ppm, may be prescribed prior to treatment commencing and may be required for future use. However, I found that the sodium lauryl sulphate (SLS) found in many toothpastes made the paste unbearable to use. An SLS-free paste, for example Curaprox Enzycal, may be more tolerable. Similarly, I found my powered toothbrush too aggressive, quickly resorting to a manual, soft bristle toothbrush.

Issues still present are still a reduced saliva level making it difficult to chew and swallow certain foods, for example apples and rice. Chilli I now find unbearable, but each patient will be different.

The last few years have been an emotional and physical rollercoaster for me and my family. We have been incredibly lucky and are so grateful to everyone involved for their care, skills, support, and passion. Every day will be lived to the full; no day will be taken for granted, and if by writing this chapter just one person is helped in any way, then it will have all been worth the effort and the experience.

A colleague, Debbie Hemington, told me that a patient of hers undergoing similar treatment to myself described the treatment as a 'cutting, burning, and poisoning' process. I cannot find much to disagree with there. . .but it works.

46

Life 2.0: How My Life Has Changed Since My Cancer Diagnosis

Shrenik Shah

25-Year Stage IV Vocal Cord Cancer Survivor, Ahmedabad, India

I would like to share my life journey in two parts: Life 1.0 – before cancer – and Life 2.0 – during and after cancer.

Life 1.0

After graduating with a degree in organic chemistry in 1972, I joined a family business producing colours for applications for dyeing on textile, leather, paper, and so forth, and worked as a key administrator for 13 years. In 1985, I entered the colour export business and traveled the world as a marketeer, visiting 37 countries and making more than 200 overseas trips from 1986 to 1996 alone.

Life 2.0

Until the first half of 1997, I was speaking normally; then my voice started changing from normal to hoarse to whispering. A clinical examination was done twice, but nothing remarkable was diagnosed. Gradually, I started losing weight, developed acute breathlessness, and was unable to lie flat on my back and had to sleep in a slanted position.

During mid-August 1997, at age 44, I started coughing blood, which was very alarming. I visited my family physician, and he suspected something most unusual and advised me to visit a head and neck cancer surgeon. During the preliminary examination, the surgeon suspected cancer of the vocal cord, explained the necessary outcomes, and advised a laryngoscopy on an urgent basis. The next day, laryngoscopy was done and a tumor was found over the vocal cord, blocking the opening of the trachea. The surgeon performed a tracheostomy and a biopsy was done and sent for pathological analysis.

The biopsy report came stating stage T4aNOMO, IV. A and massive wide-field total laryngectomy was performed along with partial removal of the thyroid gland and 56 nodes. The surgery lasted nearly nine hours. A week later, I was discharged with rice pipe. After one week of recovery, 30 rounds of radiotherapy were advised. As the first step, I bravely accepted the diagnosis and result – a resounding victory over advanced-stage cancer.

The molding technology of the radiotherapy mask was not as advanced as at present. It was made from ABS plastic and used on a five days/week schedule. The skin around my neck and throat burnt out completely but slowly recovered to normal colour.

I began trying to return Life 2.0 to normalcy by using pen and paper in place of my natural voice. In December 1997, I started practicing speaking with an electrolarynx. In those days, the services of a speech and language pathologist/therapist were not available, and I had to learn on my own to speak with this new device. It took about a week to locate a sweet spot under my chin from where audible sound could be generated. While speaking in public with my differently enabled voice, many surprising incidents occurred – people were running away from me because they were scared of the sound.

I was the only wage-earning member of my family, and as export marketing was my key job function, I had to accept this midlife crisis and the challenge of rejection of my voice. I continued speaking with my newly developed voice with full courage and confidence and without any fear. Needless to say, there was full-time, unparalleled support from my wife, Nilam, sons, Maulik and Ankit, and from my cancer surgeon. Caregivers are the backbone, and without them, the journey is incomplete.

Care of Head and Neck Cancer Patients for Dental Hygienists and Dental Therapists, First Edition. Edited by Jocelyn J. Harding.

For the first five years after surgery, I stayed away from closed public places like theaters, auditoriums, and restaurants because of passive smoking, and I visited my surgeon regularly for follow-ups. I started my international business travel alone, meeting customers and speaking with them over the phone, and I continued managing my business the same as before.

The best advantage of my differently enabled voice is that the moment I start speaking over the phone, I am not required to announce my name – people recognise my voice immediately. Seeing me speaking with my distinct voice is inspiring and gives hope to those with similar problems.

Another 10 years passed, and beginning in 2011, I started counseling head and neck cancer patients in private hospitals three days a week. With word-of-mouth publicity, patients and caregivers started reaching out through various social media platforms. I have counseled more than **50000** patients to date.

My journey was featured as chapter 1 of the coffee table book *10/10: Immersive Narratives of 10 Cancer Winners* (Bharadia 2017), with the chapter title 'I Am Here to Stay'. During the book launch event, I was invited to address a huge audience (500+) in an auditorium, especially medical professionals and super specialists. Since then, I have had the privilege of adding momentum to my in-person and online talk shows.

I have given numerous professional live presentations with slides in India and abroad as a global patient leader and motivational speaker emphasising quality of life after cancer. I have delivered extensive live talk shows at hospitals, universities, and conferences in India, the UK, the US, and elsewhere to global participants. It is my relentless pursuit to touch the lives and hearts of millions through my motivational talks (see, e.g. Figure 46.1).

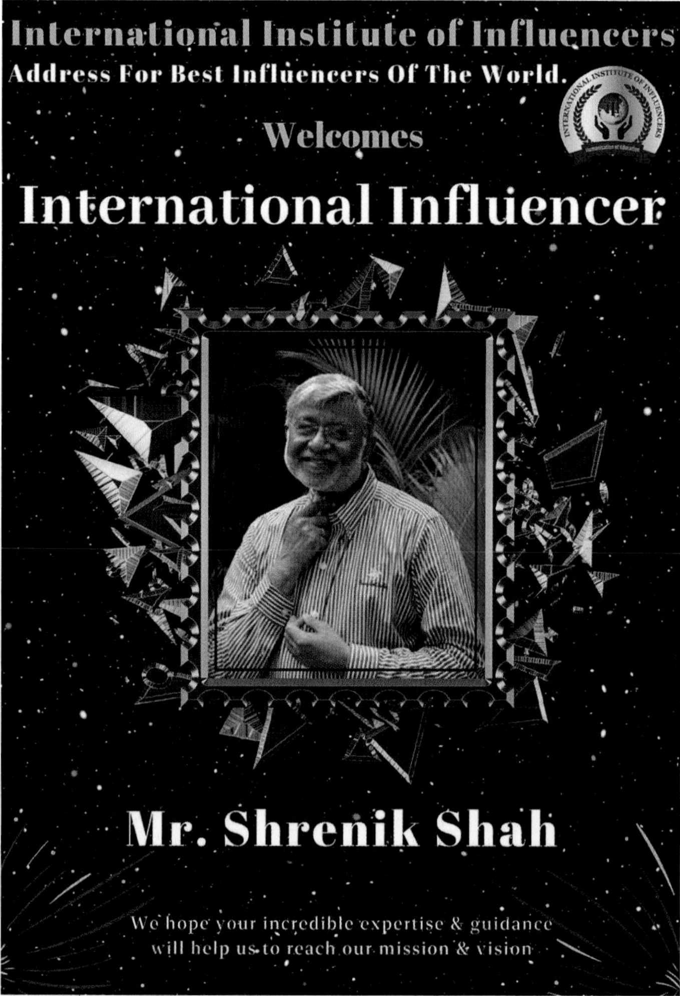

Figure 46.1 Poster for a motivational speaking appearance. *Source:* Shrenik Shah.

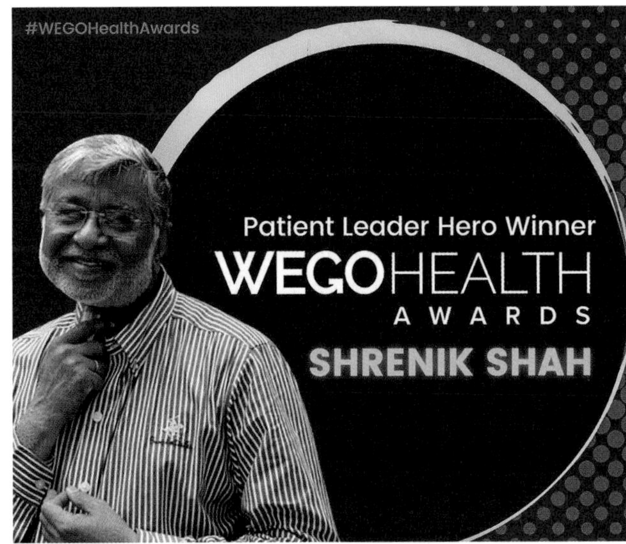

Figure 46.2 Poster for the WEGO Health awards. *Source:* Shrenik Shah.

I delivered **several hundred in-person and online talk shows** and interviews during the coronavirus pandemic, and a story on my cancer-winning journey was published by the prominent newspaper *Divyabhaskar*, which has close to a million daily circulation in the state of Gujarat, India

I have received various awards in India and elsewhere, including the Patient Leader Hero Award from WEGO Health in the US (see Figure 46.2). My biography, **SHAHEN SHAH:** *Story of Shrenik Shah, the Cancer Conqueror*, was published in 2020 (Dangi 2020).

In October 2020, I conceptualised and launched a one-to-one interview and talk show e-health series on Facebook, inviting distinguished medical professionals to bridge the gap between patients and doctors for early diagnosis, timely treatments, and saving precious lives. As of December 2021, I have completed 18 episodes, and more are scheduled.

I survived my cancer diagnosis thanks to my 'will to win' approach coupled with a dedicated team of doctors who left no stone unturned to aid me in my fight. Post-cancer I have learned so much from the university of experience and living, especially acceptance, courage, confidence, and troubleshooting, and I learned to live in the moment.

I express deep gratitude to one and all who were, are, and will be part of my cancer journey. I am grateful to God for giving me a bonus Life 2.0. I spend every moment of life without any regret and without seeking sympathy.

Please see my website, https://shrenik-shah.com for more information.

References

Bharadia, R. (2017). *10/10: Immersive Narratives of 10 Cancer Winners*. Ahmedabad, India: Ahmedabad Cancer Foundation.

Dangi, J.S. (2020). *Shahen Shah: Story of Shrenik Shah, the Cancer Conqueror*. Chhattisgarh, India: Evincepub Publishing.

47

Steve's Story

Steve Baker

Head and Neck Cancer Survivor, Blackpool, UK

2017 hadn't been the best year; my relationship was fast breaking down, work was hell, and I was feeling fatigued. Could things get any worse?

There was only a couple of weeks to a long-awaited holiday and then 'boom!' one morning I awoke with a slightly sore throat and swollen glands in the left side of my neck, couldn't believe that this was happening just before going away, and no time to get a doctor's appointment before leaving – I took myself to the chemist and got some over-the-counter remedies. The soreness in my throat disappeared after a couple of days, but the glands were still swollen; this bothered me as I have never suffered from this type of inflammation, but I decided it must be because I was feeling a bit run down.

So three weeks passed. Back from holiday but still sporting the swelling in my neck, I booked a doctor's appointment and went in and explained my misfortune. She said, 'it's a reactionary gland, they can take a couple of weeks to go down', but in her opinion, there was nothing wrong with me and I should leave it to go away naturally. I felt uneasy about this as the swelling had been present for over a month now and expressed my concern to her that perhaps there was an underlying infection that may be causing the issue. She then gave me the option of having a five-day antibiotic course, if it would make me feel better about the situation, explaining that even with the antibiotics it could still take a couple of weeks for the glands to settle down, but if no change after that to make another appointment. On leaving the surgery I stopped at the reception desk and booked another consultation with a different GP at the practice for two weeks' time; something was telling me all was not well.

Round two! And what a difference. I once again sat down and explained my predicament, the doctor looked over the notes from my previous visit – 'ah, you were diagnosed with sinusitis', he said; 'news to me'! I replied. . .that had never been mentioned at all; he then checked me over and sat back down to deliver his opinion: he thought I looked very well, no other issues, but I was over 45 with a swelling in the neck, which would qualify me for a fast-track appointment to see an ENT consultant. If I would like to take this route he would make the necessary arrangements. I agreed straight away as I knew something wasn't right.

Fast track was spot on! Five days later, I was at the hospital. I was seen by the consultant's associate – I had a superficial examination, glands were still swollen, she looked inside my mouth and also had a nasoendoscopy. She said everything looked okay, but she would extract some fluid from the gland area to send to pathology, but as these tests could be inconclusive, I would be referred for a biopsy of the gland in a day surgery operation – wasn't expecting that! But still thinking it was some kind of infection.

The next day the letter with my appointment for day surgery arrived; it was within the week. I really couldn't believe how quickly things were moving, but I truly thought it was positive as I could get 'it' sorted and get back to sorting the rest of my crumbling life out! So I presented at the hospital on the day of the operation at 6 a.m. and booked in; I was quite calm about the whole thing really, but my partner had come with me, who had no patience at all; he then proceeded to just wind me up over the next three hours of waiting by complaining about anything and everything, so eventually I asked him to leave, there was nothing he could do, and I just needed to calm down. Within 10 minutes of him leaving the show was on the road! I was called through to have initial blood pressure checks and so forth, then I was to see the surgeon and anaesthetist, calm was restored, everyone was putting me at ease. I felt comfortable about everything. I spoke to the surgeon, who explained what seemed to be a fairly simple procedure, and then on to the anaesthetist. Within about two minutes of being

Care of Head and Neck Cancer Patients for Dental Hygienists and Dental Therapists, First Edition. Edited by Jocelyn J. Harding.

in with him there was a knock on the door, and the surgeon came in and asked to speak to the anaesthetist. He excused himself and left the room. Totally unaware, I sat there for about 15 minutes before the two men returned; little did I know it then but the next 5 minutes would change my life.

The surgeon sat down and explained that the operation was to be cancelled – my heart sank a little at the thought of delay but also there was a spark of joy at the reprieve! He then went on to explain that the results of the fluid extraction from the week before were literally just back from the lab, and they meant the biopsy was no longer appropriate; he explained that the biopsy would have been looking for evidence of lymphoma and that I didn't have; this was my first jolt, as I didn't think that was what they were looking for! He continued then to apologise because this was not the usual scene for a diagnosis, but the fluid test was conclusive. . .a very high cancer cell count but not lymphoma. You have cancer, but we don't know where exactly, but it is in your head or neck. I was to be contacted later that day by someone from the hospital to arrange my 'next steps'; I was dumbfounded! In no way, shape, or form was I prepared for that; shell-shocked, I left. I wandered, totally dazed, through the hospital. . .wondering why everyone was just going about their business while my head was imploding. I called my partner, who was surprised to be hearing from me so soon, and I just couldn't bring myself to say the words 'I have cancer'. . .so simple but so irrevocably life-altering. Even then I knew that I had to overcome my internal meltdown and face this demon head-on. I had the perfect example of resolve shown to me in my formative years when my father went through hell facing bowel cancer treatment in 1980; at this point standing outside in the November rain my mind wandered immediately to him. I just cried and wished I had that perfect parental love around me now, Mam and Dad were long gone physically, but how on earth they had dealt with it all in such a dignified way I will never know, but I had to go home and find my own strength.

Still in a state of disbelief, I took a call a couple of hours later from Jo, my Macmillan nurse; she was fantastic, calm, sympathetic, informative, and friendly. She was to be my port of call for anything from now on. I was to return to the hospital the next day for a CT scan, and within the next 10 days had a PET scan with a radioactive tracer and an MRI scan before returning to the consultant for the verdict. The PET scan was full body, so he took me coldly frame by frame either pronouncing no cancer or cancer; it was cancer of the left oropharynx near and tonsillar pole/base of tongue (squamous cell carcinoma) with lymph node involvement but had not migrated any farther at this stage (T3 N2 M0). The race was on to get rid of this nemesis, and a date was arranged to remove the tonsils and some tissue from the tongue and throat.

I then saw the oncologist, who explained they were to tackle my problem with a belt and braces solution designed to irradicate the cancer, 6 rounds of chemotherapy and 30 radiotherapy sessions; I was to see a dental consultant to make sure all was in order with my teeth, She looked over my x-rays and told me I would need nine teeth removed before I could start my treatments, and she explained why each tooth was compromised either by location or previous treatments that could cause complications in the future after the chemoradiation. Devastated again, I was to wait to see the surgical team to book the extractions; she asked if I would prefer to have a general anaesthetic and I said yes, the prospect of this was terrifying! So I waited to see the surgical team, who informed me that if I wanted a general anaesthetic, I would be waiting weeks, and that would delay the further treatments, so a hospital appointment was booked for extraction under local anaesthetic. I was booked for the 27th December (dread of this appointment totally finished off any prospect of enjoying my potential last Christmas!). I arrived at the hospital, and the maxillofacial surgeon was 1 hour 45 minutes late on the day of the surgery; he went through the whole thing again with me and declared it would be too much to put me through under a local anaesthetic, and I was to return one week later to have a general anaesthetic, and he would do the deed in one go. I was relieved, returned a week later at 6 a.m. just to watch everyone be called up and then leave the surgical unit; the NHS was overwhelmed due to seasonal flu, and all nonessential surgery was cancelled. The ward sister cried when I told her my surgery was cancer-related and that without having the operation that day my treatments would be put back, but she said there was no way any operation would go ahead unless I was admitted through A&E, so off home I went and called my Macmillan nurse, Jo.

Two hours after returning home and speaking to Jo, I was called by another hospital and was added to their trauma list for a couple of days' time; I went, waited all day, and got my surgery in the evening as no emergencies had come in! Ironically it was done by the surgeon who said I couldn't have the general anaesthetic! I was bundled out of the hospital very quickly, about 6 p.m., only to return at 1 a.m. the next morning as the bleeding wouldn't stop; the surgeon was called back in to deal with me.

In the next week, I attended the specialist cancer centre to be measured for the radiotherapy mask that was to keep me pinned down to the table during treatments and chat and meet the team who were to care for me. I was also booked for day surgery to have a feeding tube put through my stomach; this too I was dreading – my throat, mouth, and gums were still sore, and healing from the previous operations and the prospect of having this done while awake was not a good one. Lying on the table having a hose pushed down my throat watching my insides reveal themselves on the overhead monitor and feeling totally violated, I was surprised after a few minutes of jiggling around when everything was pulled out. Wheeled out to recovery, I started to run my fingers tentatively over my stomach. . .no PEG! I felt confused; it was then explained to me that my stomach was too high and the tube couldn't be passed out safely because of my rib cage, potentially a massive problem as the majority of radiotherapy patients are rendered unable to swallow; I had to keep eating!

My treatments started on time at the end of January, chemotherapy every Monday taking approximately seven hours per session followed by a dose of radiotherapy, which was about five minutes, and back again Tuesday to Friday for the subsequent radiotherapy sessions.

I used to quite look forward to chemo day! It was a perfect time for myself once the cannula was fitted; there was nothing else to do. I was given a dose of steroids and antisickness drugs (more of those to take at home for three days after), and I would just rest up and visualise a happy and healthy me. I remained upbeat to the best of my ability throughout my treatments, and I believe this was a massive part of my recovery – never underestimate the power of positivity!

For the first three weeks of treatment, I kept on working; my throat was getting progressively more uncomfortable after each radiotherapy session, but I could still manage to eat and swallow soft foods, and my pain medication regime of paracetamol, ibuprofen, and liquid codeine was working well. I had been given the parameters of where I could dose myself up to and could fluctuate the dosages accordingly; morphine was to be the next step if I needed it. Sundays turned into my day of hell. I'd finished the steroids from the chemotherapy session by Friday, leaving me to totally 'crash' by the weekend. I felt totally wiped out and sick (I did have extra antisickness drugs for such occasions), but the worst part was total constipation; it was absolutely agonizing – I could spend hours in the bathroom in tears. I mentioned this to my oncologist in our weekly meeting and was prescribed Movicol, which helped a lot, but as the weeks passed this too was becoming more difficult to ingest as my throat worsened, so to a certain extent the problem returned. Also, there were weekly meetings with the dietician; she advised me to lace my food with cream and sugar (even though I'd been advised never to touch sugar again by the dental consultant). Keeping my body fed with calories was the priority no matter where it came from as long as I could manage to swallow; I couldn't taste anything after the first 2 weeks, so porridge with 10 dessert spoons of sugar was the norm! I was also prescribed Ensure Plus drinks to replace meals, but even those were becoming more difficult to get down; sometimes I could have one a couple of hours in front of me before I could pluck up the courage to take a sip. Everything now was like swallowing broken glass, except the liquid codeine, which was now at the maximum dose. My oncologist kept suggesting morphine, but I didn't want to go there unless I really had to.

I really tried to remain upbeat throughout the weeks. Every day I got up, took my medication, went back to bed for about an hour until the codeine 'trip' wore off, and then I would shower and put on fresh clothes. one morning about two weeks into treatment I was standing in front of the mirror, wondering what was different; after about five minutes I realised that the stubble on the left-hand side of my face had washed off in the shower. I shouldn't have been surprised, really – a clump of hair had come out in my hands a couple of days earlier. This disease and treatment were taking everything one piece at a time, although I was very lucky with my skin; I had been told not to wet shave and to keep my skin drenched in oil-free moisturiser, and it worked as my skin remained intact. Quite a few of the other patients had nasty wounds opening up on their necks, and it wasn't until the last week of my treatment that my mouth started to ulcerate, so some things were going really well. The oncologist and team at the cancer centre said it was remarkable how my body was handling the whole thing. I must admit it didn't always feel like that, but seeing other patients' journeys week by week, I realised truly how lucky I had been.

I was elated when the six weeks were over and my last session was complete. I had two days feeling fabulous, then woke up one morning feeling a bit off; my temperature was 38.5. I'd been advised all the way through the treatments that if I had a temperature over 38 °C, I was to be hospitalised, so I phoned the cancer unit, and they arranged for me to be admitted to the hospital straight away. I had developed a sepsis infection and spent two weeks in isolation on intravenous antibiotics day and night before my blood returned to normal. This indeed was the lowest point for me; once home, I rested for a few weeks, and eventually, things got better.

I'm now almost four years down the line and have made a very good recovery; although my personal life had been the last casualty of the whole thing. My relationship had totally broken down by the end of my treatment, so I moved on with my life, six-weekly check-ups have now been extended to every three months, and generally, I feel pretty normal. I do suffer from daily facial cramps, and energy levels are definitely not what they used to be. Dryness in the mouth can be an issue sometimes, but I have good movement in the jaw, so eating isn't a problem. Taste began to return after a few months, and I'm now living a pretty normal life, happy and hopefully healthy!

48

Living with the Legacy

Debbie Hemington

Dental Therapist, London, UK

> *They cut you, they poison you and then they burn you.*
> *—Mark Batchelor, QC, European Association of Oral Medicine, London 2010*

My experience differs from Roy Anthony's in that it was a long time ago now and not an oral cancer; however, the long-term side effects have now made me an interesting dental patient.

My story begins in September 1985 aged 24, when on holiday in France with my husband of one year and friends, I woke up to find a large lump had appeared on my neck overnight. It was on the left-hand side just above my collar bone and approximately 4 × 3 cms firm and moveable.

I felt fine, hadn't been bitten, no other symptoms at all so decided as we were due home in two days' time, I would wait and go and see my own GP rather than navigate the French health system in the rural Dordogne with my phrase book.

Once home, I went to my prebooked osteopath appointment and showed him the lump, thinking it might be a pulled or torn muscle, and he said straight away that I ought to see the GP.

At the GP the next day, it was pronounced a mystery, and I went for an ultrasound scan that showed it was a diffuse area that looked like a haematoma. The lump was measured, and it had reduced in size a little. It was decided to keep an eye on it; best guess was a cyst on the thyroid that had burst and bled overnight. Blood tests showed nothing unusual other than a raised ESR (erythrocyte sedimentation rate), which can occur for lots of reasons.

I felt tired and run down but we had been through a very stressful year, so it didn't seem out of place.

Over the next five weeks, the lump got smaller then suddenly bigger again, once again overnight, and then carried on increasing in size slowly. Scanning again showed the same picture, so no further forward with a definitive diagnosis. The lump was then big enough to mean I couldn't do up the top button of a shirt, and if I rolled over on that side in my sleep I would wake up because it was impinging on my airway.

My GP was flummoxed, so were both of his partners, and everyone came to have a look at the mystery lump! I was asked if I was happy to go and see a surgeon at Guys, a friend of my GP, because it was felt it needed another set of eyes and probably a biopsy. Off I trotted and saw a charming surgeon who was also puzzled but felt it had been going on long enough and it needed sampling at the very least to find out what it was.

Consenting to the surgery for the biopsy, I asked the surgeon to go ahead and remove it all if he was able once he had seen what it was; he agreed and said he would be sending it for a frozen section while I was in theatre to get a definitive diagnosis.

I woke up in recovery to hear someone saying 'no, don't let Debbie go back to the ward, she's got to go back into theatre again at the end of the list, they need more tissue', so that's what they did!

That evening back on the ward, feeling very sore, someone appeared to take some blood, and then twice the next day the same thing happened too. . .I wondered why?

On day three after the surgery, after a sleepless night with two elderly dementia patients who were climbing out of bed and shouting all night, a young and very confident surgical senior house officer (SHO) came to see me, sat on the chair in

Care of Head and Neck Cancer Patients for Dental Hygienists and Dental Therapists, First Edition. Edited by Jocelyn J. Harding.

my bay on an open ward, and told me they knew what it was. . . Hodgkin's lymphoma and had I heard of it, which I hadn't. He said it was a cancer of the lymph system and I needed to get hold of my family as the doctors would need to speak to them. He asked if I had any questions, and the only thing I could think of was whether I was going to die. He said he hoped not but couldn't say and walked off! I was utterly stunned.

I went to the payphone on the landing and rang my parents (I couldn't get hold of my husband as he was a sales rep and it was before mobile phones) and as soon as I heard my dad's voice I broke down. I could hear his voice breaking too. Dad said they would be up as soon as possible, and I put the phone down.

I went back to the ward and the consultant was doing his ward round; I saw him say he wanted to see me last. When he got to me, he pulled the curtains round and sat next to me on the bed (you were allowed to do that back then!) and asked me what I had been told as he could see I was upset. I repeated the conversation with the SHO and he rolled his eyes and took my hand and told me that Hodgkin's lymphoma treatment had come on in leaps and bounds in the previous five years, and it now had a good prognosis, especially if caught early. He then said something that changed my whole outlook and lifted my day beyond words: 'Debbie, I would be far more upset to have to tell you you were diabetic, because you would never get rid of that and it would likely cause you more problems as you got older, but this can be cured, it will be tough but you will be cured'. He said he would arrange for one of the oncologists to come and speak to me, and he wanted me to go home that day as it was such a noisy busy ward, he thought I would probably have got more sleep at London Bridge station than I had got in there!

I went back to the payphone to ring my parents again and told my dad I wasn't going to die after all! He said he would still come up and meet me but I said I'd be ok to get the train home on my own if he could pick me up at the station. He couldn't believe the change in my mood, and neither could I, but I knew I was determined to prove the SHO wrong, and I would do this!

The oncologist came to see me a bit later and asked me why I was looking a bit upset. . .I thought 'oh here we go!' so relayed the SHO conversation again, and she was furious! She stayed with me for over half an hour explaining everything about the disease, its history, and the groundbreaking treatment that was now available. Thomas Hodgkin, who discovered the disease, was a Guys physician, and they were one of the leading centres for treatment.

She told me to go home and get some rest and come back to her clinic the next day with anyone I wanted to bring with me, and she would start arranging scans and so forth. She told me to keep a pad and pen with me and jot down anything at all that came into my head that I wanted to know and bring it with me. She said I would probably be awake all night and would probably have lots of thoughts. . .she was right!

The next day my husband and I went back to see her and I was given a list of dates for scans and bloods and so on, and she asked for my list and went through every single point as if she had all the time in the world. She made sure my husband understood and was comfortable with everything.

So, the rollercoaster of tests began, some of which were deeply unpleasant, and the crucial point was how far it had spread; if it was confined to the nodes above my stomach then I would be having radiotherapy, and if it was in my stomach or further it would be chemotherapy, which was very much a blunderbuss approach back then, and infertility would be guaranteed. I was praying for radiotherapy!

My prayers were answered and I was grade 2 A (two sets of nodes involved, cervical and mediastinum, and 'A' as no symptoms. . .usually weight loss, night sweats, tiredness (yep, had that but had other reasons for it I thought), and pain in the lump on drinking alcohol (well I tested that one extensively and it was a no!). Radiotherapy would start the following week, so I had to go the radiotherapy department the following day to be 'planned'. I met with a lovely radiotherapy oncologist who explained everything again and made sure I understood; she also arranged for one of the radiographers to come and talk to me as she had been treated the year before for Hodgkin's! It was great to talk to her and see someone who had come out the other side. The visit involved measuring my torso in various different ways and using the scans so they could work out where they needed to deliver the radiotherapy. To ensure I was lined up correctly each day, I had to have two dots tattooed on my front and back, they looked like big blackheads! It was surprisingly painful, so I decided I probably wasn't cut out for a big heart-shaped design at any point!

A frame was laid on top of me (like a small coffee table) and a sheet of acetate sellotaped on to it lined up with my blackheads that had tracings of my vital organs on (heart, thyroid, lungs), and small lead shields were laid on the tracings to protect the organs. They would irradiate one set of nodes above and below the affected ones just in case there were any cells not detected in the diagnostics, so I would be treated from my earlobes to my armpits every Monday to Friday for six weeks alternating lying on my front and back. I was gunning to get started and had a massively positive attitude about it all. My dad was convinced I was so cross at the SHO that it spurred me on; I think he was right!

Monday arrived at last and I was raring to go! The radiotherapy department was in the bowels of the hospital next to the boiler plant and boiling hot! There were a mixture of people there but mainly middle-aged ladies with breast cancer. I was called in, got on the table, and was zapped for about two minutes, and that was it. . .bit of anticlimax! Off home I went with a 'see you tomorrow', and my routine for the next six weeks had started. That evening I felt very sick and told myself I was overreacting, but the next day the staff asked if I had had any problems so told them and they arranged for antiemetics for me as apparently some people do feel sick very quickly, usually if the treatment area is large, which mine was.

My life then revolved around getting the train every day to get there on time, weekly blood tests, and consultations with the radiologist, who remained hugely supportive and approachable throughout.

By week two my saliva was drying up (my submandibular glands were in the line of fire; unfortunately so were my lower 8s, so more problems later when they needed extracting!). Eating became more difficult and I turned to soft foods washed down with glasses of water. I was advised to suck lemon drops to stimulate my saliva. . .luckily I couldn't tolerate the flavouring so I didn't do that! My skin looked like I had been on holiday and sat in the sun a bit too long, and I was getting more tired.

At four weeks I couldn't eat solids at all so bought Complan soups and Build-Up milkshakes (no Fortisip etc. in those days), but after a short time I couldn't tolerate the flavourings. My right Eustachian tube had ulcerated due to the treatment; I had horrendous earache whenever I swallowed, and my throat felt like glass shards. I could see the lump in my neck shrinking each day, and that kept me going.

My sixth and final week of treatment was so hard, I could only drink lukewarm water and had been prescribed morphine for the earache. I needed someone with me to travel by now, I was exhausted and only got out of bed to go to the hospital, I had lost more than nearly two stone in weight, my earlobes were splitting from the side of my face and my armpits were also splitting, and my entire torso was like a really bad case of sunburn; wearing a bra or anything with seams was too painful to manage. My hair had fallen out where it was in the field of the beam. I still think radiotherapy was the easier option back then, but oh my goodness it was hard.

My final treatment was on my 25th birthday, and when I walked into the treatment room, the staff all sang 'Happy Birthday' to me! It was so touching.

I then had a week of no appointments, which I spent in bed just sleeping, and then I started the round of scans and reviews that would last for the next 15 years. I was over the moon when I was told the treatment had been successful and concentrated on recovering and building my strength up again.

I felt so grateful to have had such groundbreaking treatment and to live within easy access of a major centre for care. To this day my mouth remains quite dry, my skin burns easily in the sun, I have marked muscle fibrosis in my neck and shoulders, and my oral mucosa can't tolerate any strong flavours – a small price to pay, I feel.

The years ticked by and the interval between reviews increased with each visit and scan, still with the same consultants, which made such a difference. I had my two children and they sent congratulations cards each time.

After about 10 years of reviews, the consultant told me that they were discovering some people developing an underactive thyroid due to the treatment, so I was tested and yes, it had happened so was put on thyroxine. Then a couple of years after that they discovered a high incidence of breast cancer in these patients (this was all over the papers at the time; skin cancer and lung cancer risks were also found to be increased too), so I was put on a programme for a yearly appointment at the breast clinic and mammogram.

I developed high blood pressure and saw a cardiologist because of my history, and he had done a lot of research with his colleagues in America before my appointment and told me that not enough was known about people like me yet as we were the first long-term survivors.

Fast forward to 2015, so 29 years later, and I went to the doctor (same GP after all these years!) after coughing up some blood during a mild but persistent chest infection. He suggested a chest x-ray as I hadn't had one for a while and with my history felt it was sensible, so off I trotted. The x-ray showed some areas of calcification, probably consistent with a chronic infection, but I was referred to the chest clinic as a precaution, again because of my history. At the chest clinic, my chest was clear but I had to have an electrocardiogram immediately as my heart rate was 142 and I was in fast atrial fibrillation (AF). I had no idea at all and didn't feel any different to normal. I was escorted straight round to resus and given beta blockers and monitored; the consultant said it can happen for many reasons, thyroid and menopause the usual causes, but 'because of your history' he wanted some cardiac investigations. I ended up staying in overnight as the heart rate was slow to reduce and sent home the next day and told to get the rate checked at the GP three days later. Did as I was told, and my GP was alarmed that the rate was 156 that day, so I was sent straight back to resus and once again in overnight to get stabilised, and this time discharged on beta blockers and also warfarin for stroke prevention due to the AF.

I started another huge round of investigations, again some of them very unpleasant although very clever, such as a transoesophageal echocardiogram (TOE), where the echo is done from inside the stomach to get a better view of the heart. Topical anaesthetic is sprayed down your throat, which is horrible – you feel like your throat is closing up and have to breathe through your nose. A plastic 'letterbox' is taped into your mouth so they can get the scopes down easily, and then thankfully some amazing sedation is given so the rest is a blur.

It is now known that radiotherapy affects the coronary blood vessels and causes calcification of heart valves; even though they were shielded by the lead on the 'coffee table' the scatter is huge, and this damage is now becoming apparent as long-term survivors emerge.

I was passed on to a cardiologist, who told me I needed to make sure I had excellent oral hygiene before she asked my occupation. I was impressed! She had all my results, and my aortic valve was severely calcified, causing marked stenosis. She remarked it looked like the valve of an 85-year-old, not a 55-year-old. The mitral valve wasn't performing well either, and I had paroxysmal AF (this is where episodes of AF come and go, as opposed to persistent AF). Her gut feeling was that I would need valve surgery but because of the radiation scar tissue in my chest and heart it was very high-risk surgery. Life had suddenly become a bit daunting again.

I went up to Kings to see a cardiovascular surgeon (who was a friend of a friend and had looked at my test results and felt I needed seeing urgently). He said the aortic valve was beyond repair, it definitely needed replacing. A new technique exists now for minimally invasive valve replacement, transcatheter aortic valve implantation (TAVI), but I was not a candidate for this because of the scarring in my chest. We discussed the choice of valve, whether animal or mechanical; he favoured animal as that doesn't require anticoagulation – he felt lifelong warfarin was very restrictive. I said I would leave it to him to decide what was best when he was 'in there' and that I trusted his judgement. He said I also needed a repair to the mitral valve, closure of a small hole in the heart that I never knew about, and ablation to tackle the AF. . .quite a shopping list!

Hindsight is a wonderful thing, but I had been complaining about breathlessness for a while so had tried more exercise, losing weight, and an inhaler and nothing made much difference. I was in fact exhibiting classic aortic stenosis but at completely the wrong age, so it was missed.

The surgery was planned and I was on the waiting list. It was decided I ought to have an angiogram as belt and braces as I had thrown up so many surprises, and guess what, I didn't disappoint them! I had an 85% blockage in my main coronary artery, wasn't allowed to go home, and was taken straight to the coronary care unit for rest and constant monitoring. Surgery would now be urgent and planned for two days' time. The blockage was too severe for a stent; even though I didn't have high cholesterol, radiotherapy roughens up in the arterial lining, making it more prone to atherosclerosis. Before I left home for the angiogram in the morning, I had pulled the full wheelie bin down the drive as it was bin day. . .I was a heart attack waiting to happen!

Thirty years and one week after I had my final radiotherapy session, I was taken into a cardiac theatre for major open heart surgery. It was daunting. Six hours later I was in the intensive care unit, having had a mechanical aortic valve placed, an aortic resection to allow the valve to be placed as the calcification was so bad, and a double bypass. There was no time to do the ablation or close the small hole as I had been on bypass for long enough by that time. My lovely surgeon came to see me and told me it was exceptionally challenging surgery, my chest was so full of scar tissue and the damage to the valve had been very extensive. He opted for the mechanical valve because he didn't want to have to go back in ever again! On the plus side, the mitral valve was better than expected so he left that alone – one good thing at least!

Recovery was long and slow and not the immediate improvement I had hoped for. I was still very breathless, my leg wounds from the vein donor sites got infected and needed dressing regularly, the AF came straight back, and my international normalised ratio (INR) needed stabilising (different makes of valves have different thrombogenicities so the INR target range will vary), which involved a hospital trip every couple of days to the anticoagulation team. The mechanical valve is very loud and took a lot of getting used to, and the chest wound made sleeping very difficult as I couldn't lie down.

At my surgical review six weeks post-op, the breathlessness was still very troubling, and it was decided that the beta blockers were causing it, so I was swapped to Verapamil instead (a rate-limiting calcium channel blocker), which improved things enormously. I religiously attended the cardiac rehab classes, and after four months I returned to work.

I am now reviewed annually and will be forever. The mitral valve will need attention at some point in the future, but it is hoped that can be done less invasively. My INR is tested every two to six weeks, and it is important that my diet remains similar each day in terms of eggs, green vegetables, and chickpeas. I also need antibiotic cover for dental treatment as the mechanical valve puts me in the high-risk category, and the amoxycillin for that sends the INR a bit haywire for a couple of weeks.

I have been so lucky and have had excellent care from the NHS; thank you to them for saving my life for a second time. Huge thanks to the wonderful staff at Guys, the Princess Royal University Hospital, and Kings College Hospital and especially to Mr Ranjit Deshpande, a supremely talented surgeon to whom I owe so much.

49

Look Good Feel Better

Lisa Curtis

Look Good Feel Better UK, Epsom, UK

Look Good Feel Better is an independent cancer support charity set up in the UK in 1994 to help women combat the visible and psychological effects of cancer treatment. The initiative is global, starting in the US more than 30 years ago, and is now available in 27 countries across the world.

The charity could not have started in the UK without the support of a number of the leading beauty companies, who provided the time and expertise of their employees as well as donating some fabulous products for the attendee gift bags given to everyone who goes along to a Look Good Feel Better workshop. Initially there were 17 'member' companies who helped set the charity up, and today the charity is supported by more than 50 companies who regularly donate their time, funds, and products. Quite simply, Look Good Feel Better could not operate without their support.

Look Good Feel Better's skincare and makeup workshops provide practical tips such as how to look after your skin during and posttreatment; and how to plot and draw eyebrows back if these have been lost, or how to use eyeliner to give the illusion of lashes. Aside from what can be learned at a workshop, one of the key benefits is meeting other people on a similar journey, sharing experiences, and hopefully making some new connections. It's a wonderfully uplifting couple of hours usually full of fun and laughter.

The workshops are run by expert volunteers who are specially trained to deliver the Look Good Feel Better programme. They very kindly give up their time to share their expertise and make the whole experience very special. The charity is very fortunate to work with more than 2500 of these special people across the UK.

Look Good Feel Better partners with more than 140 hospitals and cancer centres to deliver its services across the UK. Operational as far north as the Shetland Islands, through Scotland, Northern Ireland, the Isle of Man, Wales, England, and the Channel Islands, the charity has good national coverage, which means there should be a Look Good Feel Better service within easy access to most parts of the country.

All workshops are two hours long and completely free of charge. People can attend the one time during their current treatment and up to a year after, receiving a special Look Good Feel Better 'gift bag'. If they want to attend again during this time, they can do so but will need to take their gift bag with them as Look Good Feel Better has a limited number of these and so they need to be shared fairly. If, further down the line, there is a cancer recurrence or new diagnosis and treatment must start again, then people can attend again and get a new gift bag. Look Good Feel Better does not include hair or wig advice in these workshops; they are purely about skincare and makeup. All the charity's expertise is supported by a series of useful tutorials on its website, so if someone who has been to a workshop needs a refresher, these are a useful tool. Alternatively, if a group session is not for you, then the tutorials will be a great alternative.

In 2018, the charity launched a new service for men living with cancer. The skin fitness workshops cover advice on looking after your skin during and posttreatment, safe shaving, grooming, sun protection, and how to deal with scars. These workshops are delivered by volunteer professionals from the male grooming and barbering industry and take place in a number of hospitals and cancer centres across the country. Like the women's service, the men's workshops aim to teach practical tips but also offer that great opportunity to connect with others on a similar journey. The men also receive a fabulous gift bag of full-size skincare, grooming, and sun protection products.

Additionally, Look Good Feel Better provides a series of men's tutorials on its website including all that is covered in the workshops with very useful extra information on image and styling. There is also a comprehensive manual for men

Care of Head and Neck Cancer Patients for Dental Hygienists and Dental Therapists, First Edition. Edited by Jocelyn J. Harding.

available that covers skincare and grooming advice, sun protection, nail care, hair care, oral health care, nutrition, fitness advice, and a great section on image and styling. This can either be downloaded or sent in the post.

Look Good Feel Better runs special teen and young adult workshops for both the women and the men's programmes, following a similar format but working with products and trends suited to the younger market. These workshops are run in collaboration with charities like the Teenage Cancer Trust, CLIC Sargent, and Teens Unite.

When the pandemic hit in March 2020, the charity was able to move all its services online very swiftly, ensuring support was still available at such a crucial time. All workshops are run via Zoom, enabling people to attend in the comfort of their own home. In addition to its existing workshops, Look Good Feel Better has been able to expand the support it offers by launching new services, enabling the charity to help people on their cancer journey more than just the one time.

The charity can now offer a hair loss workshop working in collaboration with the charity Cancer Hair Care. These sessions are run twice a month and cover hair loss; hair regrowth; scalp care; scarves, headwear, and accessories; wigs; scalp cooling; and colouring hair.

The new nail care service was also launched in 2020, running biweekly sessions covering advice on the importance of using nail oil, how to safely file nails, how to hide discolouration and ridges, dealing with sore and split nails, and how to look after your hands and nails during treatment.

Lastly, the charity has launched a new service addressing the challenges faced around body image. For more information on all of the services Look Good Feel Better offers, please visit www.lookgoodfeelbetter.co.uk.

Appendix A

Head and Neck Cancer Charities UK

Mouth Cancer Foundation, info@mouthcancerfoundation.org, www.mouthcancerfoundation.org
2 Larchfield Close, Weybridge KT13 9DD
01924 950950

The Head & Neck Cancer Foundation, info@hncf.org.uk, www.hncf.org.uk
The Coach House, Somborne Park, Little Somborne, Stockbridge SO20 6QT
03301 330 724

The Swallows Head & Neck Cancer Support Charity, info@theswallows.org.uk, www.theswallows.org.uk
The Michael Stenhouse Centre, 68-70 Waterloo Road, South Shore, Blackpool, FY4 1AB
07504 725 059

Saving Faces – The Facial Surgery Research Foundation, https://savingfaces.co.uk/
71 Tonbridge Street, King's Cross, London WC1H 9DZ
020 3417 7757

Heads2gether, www.heads2gether.net
0800 0234 550

Crokus Club, crokusclub@hotmail.co.uk
07704 366705

HNChelp – Laryngectomee and Head and Neck Cancer Support for Chesterfield and the North Midlands, www.hnchelp.org.uk
Text to: 07826 219345

Faceup Cymru, www.Faceupcymru.org.uk; faceupcymru@outlook.com

The John Wilkinson Face Cancer Charitable Trust, www.facecancer.org.uk

Head and Neck Cancer Support Group, Email: astra.hall@nnuh.nhs.uk
01603 288198

Headstart Cancer Support – Head & Neck Cancer Support for Kent & Sussex, Email: headstartnews@gmail.com, www.headstartcancersupport.org.uk/

The Look Ahead Cancer Campaign, Email: enquiries@headandneck.info, www.headandneck.info/
Mrs Pam Cooper | Secretary Telephone: (01642) 531109 Mobile: 07710 449823

About Face, About Face Centre, 111 Longfleet Road, Poole, Dorset BH15 2HP
01202 677340

Oracle Cancer Trust, info@oraclecancertrust.org, www.oraclecancertrust.org/
0203 475 3471

Maggie's, www.maggies.org, Email: enquiries@maggies.org
Maggie's, The Gatehouse, 10 Dumbarton Road, Glasgow, G11 6PA
0300 123 1801

Throat Cancer Foundation www.throatcancerfoundation.org
hello@throatcancerfoundation.org
0203 4754 065

Care of Head and Neck Cancer Patients for Dental Hygienists and Dental Therapists, First Edition. Edited by Jocelyn J. Harding.

Index

NOTE: All index entries refer to head and neck cancer (HNC), unless otherwise described. 'Treatment' refers to HNC treatment, unless otherwise specified. Page numbers in *italics* indicate figures and those in **bold** denote tables.

a

actinic/solar keratosis (AK) 17, *17*
acupuncture, in xerostomia 187, 191–193
  patient assessment 192
  possible mechanisms/theories 191
  treatment regime, needle position 192, *193*
adjuvant treatment 69
  see also chemotherapy (CT); radiotherapy (RT)
airflossers *221*, 224
airways, altered 88
  see also laryngectomy; stoma
alcohol use 223
  dependence on 29, 30
  as risk factor 38, 116
amitriptyline 251
anaemia 104, 174
analgesic ladder 249–250, **250**
analgesic preparations 249–250, **250**
  topical 251
anatomy, head and neck *109*
angular cheilitis 196, *196*, 222
antidepressants 250, 251
antiemetic drugs 211, **212**
anxiety 3, 169–170, 256
aortic valve damage 278
appearance, altered after surgery 91, 95, 237, 255, 261
appetite, reduced **80**
artificial intelligence 48–49, *49*
aspirational pneumonia 223
atrial fibrillation 277, 278
atypical mole syndrome 17
augmented reality (AR) 157, 159

b

bacillus Calmette-Guérin (BCG) vaccine 116
bad news, breaking 63, 98
balance exercises 247
basal cell carcinoma (BCC) 14, **15**, 16, *16*, 98
basal cell naevus 16
benzydamine hydrochloride 251
biofilm, plaque 177, 179, 182, 183, **184**, **186**, **198**
biopsy 44, *45*, *53*, 62, 98
  examination/diagnosis 45, 273
  journey 44, *45*, 272–273, 275
  sentinel node (SEN) 67
  tissue processing 44–45
bio-psycho-social model 51
bisphosphonates 94
blood, coughing up **259**, 269
blood tests, normal results 174–175
body image 255, 261, 280
bolus (gravity) feeding 83
bone damage, radiotherapy late effect 240
  see also osteoradionecrosis (ORN)
bony free flap 68, 69, *71*, *72*, 94
botulinum toxin 188
Bragg peak 124, 125, *125*
Breslow thickness 17
bruxism 30, 31
burning mouth syndrome 240

c

cancer
  dysplasia *vs* 45–46, *46*
  sites/types of HNC 109, *109*
cancer cells, histology 45
Cancer Hair Care 280
cancer resection specimen 48
candidosis 183, **184**
  chronic erythematous 195–196, *196*
  photobiomodulation therapy for 150
  pseudomembranous (thrush) 194, *195*
cannabis 27, 29, 31, 32
carcinogens 31, 63, 96
cardiovascular complications 277, 278
care plans 76
  oral 181, 219
case stories/histories *see under* patient journey
cetuximab, OPSCC 38
Challacombe Scale 179
charities 279–280, 281
cheilitis, angular 196, *196*, 222
chemoradiotherapy (CRT) 63, 69, 103, 116
  case studies/stories 263–267, 273, 274
  oral mucositis due to 205, 208
  see also chemotherapy (CT); radiotherapy (RT)
chemotherapy (CT) 69, 103–106, 116, 173
  adjuvant 104
  administration 104–105
  case studies/stories 263, 274
  concurrent 103
  dental treatment and 103, 105, 106, 173–175
    considerations during/after 105–106, 174, 175
    risk assessment 173, 174, 175
  drug groups/types 104, 173–174
  mechanism of action 103
  neoadjuvant 103
  palliative 104, 116

Care of Head and Neck Cancer Patients for Dental Hygienists and Dental Therapists, First Edition. Edited by Jocelyn J. Harding.

side effects/complications 104, 105, 144, 169, 173, 174
myelosuppression 174
oral mucositis 104, 105, 144, 169, 205
photobiomodulation therapy for 141, 144–146, **147**
xerostomia *see* xerostomia
chewing ability 92
chewing gum, sugar-free 183, **184**, **185**, 186, 192, 212
Chinese flap *see* radial forearm flap
chronic erythematous candidosis (CEC) 195–196, *196*
cigarette smoking *see* smoking
cleft palate 231, *232*
clinical nurse specialists (CNSs) 52, **58**, 63, 64, *75*, 76–77
as integral member of MDT **58**, 76, 77
referral to, initial meeting 63, 76
role 63, 64, 76–77
clinical oral dryness score (CODS) 179
close margin 64
coagulation tests 175
cocaine 29, 31, 32
codeine 250
COM-B model, for behaviour change 176, 181
communication, by dental team
with oncologist/oncology team 105, 106, 173
with patients after HNC 224, 261
with patients before diagnosis 4, 5
communication, by patient 85–86, 92, 224, 255, 261
after laryngectomy 88, 161, 269, 270
see also voice prosthesis
assessment 85–86
nonverbal 86
ongoing rehabilitation for 85, 92
physiotherapists' role 236, 237
tracheostomy impact 88
treatment by SLTs **58**, 64, 85, 86, 88, 261
see also speech, impairment; voice disturbances
complications of HNC treatment 3, 141, 259–261
of chemotherapy *see* chemotherapy (CT)
dental care/oral hygiene in 223–227, *225*, 259
photobiomodulation for *see* photobiomodulation therapy
of radiotherapy *see* radiotherapy (RT)
see also specific complications (e.g. xerostomia)
computed tomography (CT) 62, 157
planning scans for 3-D conformal RT 107, 112
planning surgery 62, 159, *159*
cone-beam computed tomography (CBCT) 98, *100*
coping strategies 51
core biopsy 44, 62
corticosteroids 208
counselling 4–5, 270
COVID-19, halitosis and 202
crack cocaine 31
cryotherapy 208
cyclotron 124, 125
cytochrome c oxidase 142
cytotoxic drugs 103, 104

d

da Vinci robotic surgical system *130*, 130–132, *131*, *132*, *133*
operating room configuration for 133, *134*
patient-side cart *130*, 130–131, *131*, *135*
surgeon's console 132, *132*
vision cart 132, *133*
see also transoral robotic surgery (TORS)
decayed, missing, and filled teeth (DMFT) 30
dental anxiety 32
dental appointments 220
dental assessment, pretreatment
before radiotherapy 110–111, 214
by restorative dentist 93
see also dental treatment
dental caries 30, 31, **185**
during/after HNC treatment 91–92, 223, *224*, 226
home-care and risk reduction 183
see also radiation caries
dental erosion **185**, 211, 226
dental hygienists/therapists **58**, 258
attitudes to substance users 32
lip cancer prevention/detection 20
oral complication management role 141, 151
pretreatment phase role 52, 111, 179, 258
restorative care, role 96
routine examinations 4
skin cancer recognition/management 14, 18
as source of advice for patient 18, 20, 51, 52, 111, 170
support for patient after treatment 141, 256
see also dental professionals
dental implants *see entries beginning* implant
dental nurse 98–100
dental pain, substance users 32
dental professionals 173
challenges relating to chemotherapy 173–175
considerations before HNC treatment 220–223, 268
considerations during/after HNC treatment 223–227
consultation with oncology colleagues 105, 106, 173
empathy 223
examination by *see* examination
halitosis (oral causes) management *200*, 200–201
help for, and seeking help 228
nausea and dental erosion prevention 211–212
practicalities for treating patients 227–228
support for patients 4, 219, 223
see also dental hygienists/therapists
dental surgeons 60
dental treatment 173
after cancer treatment 105, 218–219, 228
after chemotherapy *see under* chemotherapy (CT)
after radiotherapy 111
practical considerations 105–106, 227–228, 259
treatment complications and 223–227, *225*, 259
before cancer treatment 111, 179, 207, 219, 220–223, 268, 273
before radiotherapy 110–111, 214
oral mucositis risk reduction 207
restorative dentist's role 93
emergency 105
medications and challenges of 173
obturator use and 233–234
patient access and funding issues 181, 228
planning 173–175, 219
before radiotherapy 110–111, 214
myelosuppression impact 174, 175
routine, delayed during chemotherapy 105
routine examinations 4, 5, 269
see also tooth extraction
dentine hypersensitivity **185**
dentists, general 220
denture brush 222, *222*
dentures 95, *95*
care in HNC patients 183, 222–223
chronic erythematous candidosis 195–196, *196*
cleaning 222–223
difficulties with, in xerostomia 95, **185**
ill-fitting 20, **259**
implant-supported 95, *95*, 96, *99*, *232*
removable partial 92
replacement 96
depression and anxiety 3, 169–170, 256, 261
developmental defects 231
diagnosis (of HNC) 61–63, 259
early, importance 3–13
emotional response 51, 52, 76, 95, 169, 219, 262, 273
flowchart, patient journey *53*, 61–63, 273
impact on patient 3, 51–52, 273
MDT discussion after 46, 48, *53*, 63
pathologists' role 44–48
diamorphine 250
diet 247
during/after HNC treatment **80**, 183–184, 214, 226, 247, 274
halitosis management 200, 201
healthy 183–184, 214, 247

diet (*cont'd*)
meals, timing 247
nausea and vomiting, advice 212
for oral health in patients 183–184, 222
oral mucositis management 208
palliative care 261
sleep quality and improving 246
dietary requirements 81, 88, 247
dietetic advice 88
barriers to implementing **80**, 80–81
for specific complications **80**, 81
sugar 81
dietetic review pathway *79*
dietitians **58**, 78–84, 261
in home enteral feeding team 83
in MDT **58**, 78, 79, 81
role 78–80, *79*, 81, 111, 214, 274
working with SLTs 85, 88, 261
digital pathology 48–49, *49*
discharge from hospital 69, 228
disclosing agents 182
dressing plates 93
drug abuse *see* substance dependence
drug resistance 173
dry mouth *see* xerostomia
duloxetine 251
dysgeusia **80**, 176, **185**, 223
chemotherapy causing 104
photobiomodulation therapy for **148**, 150
radiotherapy causing 114
dysphagia 86–87, **185**, 223, **259**
assessment 86–87
chemotherapy and 105
consequences 86, 261
management 87, **185**, 224
photobiomodulation therapy **147**, 149
oral-/pharyngeal-stages 86
radiotherapy causing 92, 113, 216, 239, 274
speech and language therapists' role 86–87, 88, 224
transoral robotic surgery and 137
dysphasia 261
dysphonia 5, 85, 176, **185**, **258**, 269
dysplasia (oral epithelial) 45–46, *47*
dysplastic cells, histology 45

e
edentulous patients, rehabilitation 95
EGFR inhibitor 38
electrolarynx 161, 269
electrolysis, intraoral hair removal 243
electronic cigarettes (e-cigarettes, vapes) 24–27
cariogenic potential 27
market size, global industry 25, 26
nicotine in 25, 26, 27
regulation (UK) 26, 27
respiratory damage 27
types 24–25, *25*
emergency dental treatment 105
emotions
after treatment 255–256, 268
response to diagnosis 51, 52, 76, 95, 169, 219, 262, 273
empathy 223
employment 52
EndoWrist instruments 131, *131*, 132, *132*, 133
ENE (extranodal extension) 64
enteral nutrition 83, 87
epithelium, oral, normal *vs* dysplastic 46, *46*, *47*
examination 5–13, *61*, 61–62
describing to patient, counselling *4*, 4–5
intra-oral tissues/structures 10–13, *10*, *11*, *12*
by nasendoscopy *61*, 61–62
palpation of head and neck 5, *6*, 7, *7–9*
recording findings 11
routine, and frequency 4, 5, 268
self-examination 13, *13*
substance users 33
what to look for 13
exercise 246–247
exercise programme, components 246–247
extractions *see* tooth extraction
extravasation, chemotherapy 105

f
facial expression *238*, 255
facial nerve, high-definition MRI 157, *158*
fascia/fascial system 236–237
fatigue 104, 105, 112, 169, 223, 227, 255
case studies/stories 264, 267, 277
feeding routes 81–83, *82*, 87, 111, 169, 228
enteral feeding methods 83
gastrostomy tube *see* gastrostomy tube
jejunal tube 83
nasogastric tube *81*, 81–82, 87, 136, 267, *267*
tracheoesophageal tubes 82, *82*
tube removals 83–84
fibreoptic endoscopic evaluation of swallowing (FEES) 86–87
fibula bone, bony free flap 68, 69, *71*, *72*, 94
financial implications of cancer 3, 52, 228
fine needle aspirate 44, 62
flaps, types 61, 68–69, 94
donor sites, intraoral hair growth 241
free *see* free flaps
local, or pedicled 61, 68
submental island *242*
floor of mouth
cancer 63, 64, *72–75*
intraoral hair growth after *242*, *243*, *244*
examination 11, *11*, *12*
flowchart, and journey *45*, *53*
patient journey *see* patient journey
specimen (biopsy) journey *45*
fluoride varnish 226
fluorodeoxyglucose (FDG), PET scan 63, 263
follow-up 70, 75, 96, 106
after radiotherapy 114–115
case studies/stories 267, 270, 274, 277, 278
frequency/duration 70, 114–115
food and drink *see* diet
formication 267
Fortisip food 263, 267
free flaps 61, 68, 69, *69*, 94
bony (fibula) 68, 69, *71*, *72*, 94
intraoral hair growth and 241
radial forearm 68, *69*, *70*, *71*, *74*
frozen sections 67
full blood count 174
fungal infections *see* candidosis

g
gabapentin 251
gastrointestinal transit, altered **80**
gastrostomy tube 69, 81, *82*, 82–83, 87, 111
PEG *see* percutaneous endoscopic gastrostomy (PEG)
radiologically inserted endoscopic (RIG) 82, 83
gender, risk factor for OPSCC 37–38
gingivitis 201, 222
glutamine, oral 208
Gorlin–Goltz syndrome 16
grafts 61, 68, 69, 94
skin 69, 98
see also flaps, types

h
haemoglobin 175
hair, intraoral *see* intraoral hair
hair loss 114, 274, 277, 280

halitosis **185**, 197–204, **259**
  aetiopathogenesis 198, **198**, 199, 200
  classification 198, **198**
  COVID-19 and 202
  diagnosis *199*, 199–200
  epidemiology 198
  genuine or nongenuine 198, **198**
  management of oral causes *200*, 200–201
    counteractives 201–202
  physiological 198, **198**, 200–201
head and neck cancer (HNC), as 'umbrella' term 109
head drop 240
healing process **184**, 208, 214, 219, 236
  case studies/stories 265, 267
  diet role 78, 81, 88, **183**
  impaired 23, 207, 213, 214
  photobiomodulation 142, 144, *145*, 146, 149, 208
health education 14
healthy diet 183–184, 214, 247
hearing loss 113, 224, *225*, 240
heat moisture exchange (HME) device 163, *166*, *167*
herpes simplex type 1 (HSV-1), recurrent infection 194, *195*
HNSCC *see* squamous cell carcinoma (SCC)
hoarseness 5, 176, **185**, **258**, 269
Hodgkin's lymphoma 275–278
holistic care 228
holistic needs assessment 52, 76
hologram 157–159, *158*
home enteral feeding team 83
home self-care, oral hygiene 181–184, **184–186**
honey 208
human papillomavirus (HPV) 36–43, *39*, 245
  head and neck cancer 36–37, 63, 245
    HPV-negative *vs* HPV-positive 36, 38, 116
    immunohistochemistry 45
    OPSCC *see* oropharyngeal squamous cell carcinoma (OPSCC)
  HPV16 and HPV18 (high-risk types) 36, 39
  oncogenes, viral-human DNA hybrid episome 37
  oral infections 36, 38, *39*, 45
  vaccine/vaccination 36, 39
hyperbaric oxygen therapy 215
hypersalivation 217, 223–224, 267
hyposalivation 176, 179, 192, 239–240
  photobiomodulation therapy for **147**, 148–149
  see also xerostomia
hypothyroidism 169–170
  immunotherapy adverse event **120**
  radiotherapy late effect 169–170, 240, 275

i

imaging 62–63
  3D, hologram 157, *158*
  see also specific modalities
immediate obturator 93–94, *94*, 233
immune checkpoint inhibitors 117, 120
  administration 118–120
  agents used/approved 117–118
  benefits in HNSCC 118
  mechanism of action 117, *118*, 120
immune system 116, 117
  overactivation, by immunotherapy 120
  tumour control by *see* immunotherapy
immunohistochemistry (IHC) 45, *47*
immunotherapy 116–122, 173–174
  adverse events (IrAE) 120, **120**, *121*
    grades 121, 122
    management 121–122
  future use in HNSCC 122
  in OPSCC 38
  principles, and indication 116
  tests before 118–119
  in tongue cancer *119*
  see also immune checkpoint inhibitors
implant, dental 94, *95*, 96
implant bar 95, *95*
implant-supported obturator *94*
implant-supported overdentures 94, 95, *95*, 96, *99*, 231, *232*
incidence of HNC 109, 116
infliximab 122
information for patients 268
integrated care, substance dependent patients 33
intensity-modulated radiotherapy (IMRT) 69, 91, 108, 123
  case study/story 263
  treatment plan 108, *108*
  xerostomia reduction/prevention 177, **178**
interdental cleaning (IDC) 182, 222, 224, 226
interleukin 6 (IL-6) 245
international normalised ratio (INR) 175
intimacy 237, 255, 257
intraoral hair growth 241–244, *242*
  flaps and factors affecting 241
  postoperative removal methods 242–244, *243*, *244*

j

jaw carcinoma *64*
jaw opening, reduced *see* trismus
jejunal tube 83

k

keratinocytes 14
key worker 76
kindness to self 52, 170
kissing 237, 257

l

laryclips *166*
laryngectomy 61, 88, 161, 216
  care 160–168
    baseplates and HMEs *162*, 163–164
    stoma care 161, *161*, 163, 216
    voice prosthesis 161, 163
  case story 269–271
  equipment used after 164, *164*, **165**, *165*
laryngectomy bib *163*, *168*
laryngectomy tube 161, **165**, *165*, *166*
laryngopharyngectomy 61
larynx 61
  cancer, radiotherapy fractions 110
  endoscopic evaluation (EEL) 86
  removal *see* laryngectomy
laser therapy 142, *142*
  cancer excision 67, *68*
  intraoral hair removal 242–243
  low-level (soft laser) *see* photobiomodulation therapy
  terminology 143, **143**, *143*
  training/learning about 151, 152
laser–tissue interaction *142*, 142–143
lidocaine 251
lifestyle factors 245–248
  halitosis management 200
  oral/lip cancer risk 20, 245–248
  see also diet; exercise; sleep
light-matter interactions *142*, 142–143
light-touch techniques 237, *237*
linear accelerator (LINAC) 107, *108*, 123, *124*, 125
lip balm, SPF 21
lip cancer 20–22
  prevention 21–22
  risk factors and aetiology 20, 22
  signs/symptoms 20–21, *21*
  squamous cell carcinoma 20, 21, *21*
lip care 21, 257
lipoma *158*
listening, importance 52, 219, 228, 256, 261
liver function tests 175
local anaesthetics 32
Look Good and Feel better (charity) 279–280

Lugol's iodine 64, *65*
lung injury, e-cigarettes and 27
lymphadenitis 6
lymph nodes
  cervical 7, *7*, 64
  enlarged, infections 6
  examination (microscopic) 48
  groups/chains 7, *7*
  involvement in cancer 7, 64
  malignancies 7, 44
  neck dissection 64, *66*, *67*, *74*
  palpation 5, 7, *7*, *8*, *9*, 21
  sentinel node *see* sentinel node (SEN)
  swelling, case history 272, 273, 275
  ultrasound scan 62
lymphoedema 114, 236, 239, 240
lymphoma 7, 276–278

m

Macmillan nurses 76, 233, 273
magnetic resonance imaging (MRI) 62, *62*, *119*, 157
malignancy, second, after radiotherapy 114
malnutrition 78, 247
mandible
  grafts and implants 94, 95
  osteoradionecrosis in 63, 95
maxilla
  cancer defects, obturators for 231
  implants 95
maxillofacial surgeons 60
medical history 174, 177
melanoma 14, **15**, 16–17, *17*, 20
melanotic naevi ('moles') 17
mental health/well-being 3, 223
  after diagnosis/pretreatment 51–52
  after HNC treatment 95, 255–256
  during treatment 169–170
  emotional response to diagnosis 51, 52, 76, 95, 169, 219, 262, 273
  needs, in substance dependency 29
  supporting, restorative dentist 95–96
Merkel cell carcinoma **15**
metastatic disease 7, 44, 116, 118
methamphetamine 31, 32
'meth mouth' 31
Microsoft HoloLens 157, *158*
microvascular anastomosis 68, *71*
minimal access surgery 61, 129
mood, low (patient's) 169–170, 223, 255
morphine 250, 260, 265
motivational speaking *270*, 270–271
mouth cancer *see specific sites/types of cancer*
Mouth Cancer Foundation 13, *13*, 181
mouth care 218–230, 227
  before HNC treatment 219, 220–223
  during/after HNC treatment 223–227, 228
  essential, and part of holistic care 228
  obturator use and 233–234
  see also dental treatment; oral hygiene
mouth ulcers 144, **184**, 194, *195*, **258**
mouthwash 183
  alcohol-free fluoride 183, 222, 226
  before treatment 221–222
  chlorhexidine 183, 201, 221
  during/after treatment 226, 240, 264
  halitosis management 201
mucoadhesive disks 188
mucositis, oral *see* oral mucositis (OM)
mucous secretions **80**, 164, 216–217, 224
mucus, thickened 216, 223–224, 259
  management 216–217, 224
mucus glands 216
multidisciplinary team (MDT) 52, 57–59, 105, 141, 181
  composition/specialties 57, **58–59**, 60, 76, 78
    CNS as integral member **58**, 76, 77
    dental hygienists/therapists, role **58**, 141, 151
    restorative dentistry consultant's role **58**, 92–93
  meeting (MDTM) 46, 48, *53*, 59, 63, 262
  role and approach by 59, 93, 105
  as source of advice for patient 105, 170
  transoral robotic surgery sequelae 137
multidisciplinary team (MDT) coordinator **58**, 59
muscle
  loss/weakness 78, 81, 240, 246, 255, 261
  spasms 227, 239
myelosuppression 174

n

nasendoscopy *61*, 61–62
nasogastric tubes *81*, 81–82, 87, 136, 267, *267*
National Institute for Health and Care Excellence (NICE) 57, 76, 77, 92
nausea **80**, 105, 169, 211–212
  treatment 211, **212**
nebuliser 224
neck dissection 64, *66*, *67*, *74*
neutropenia 105, 174, 274
neutrophils, count 105, 174
NHS dental services 219
nicotine 24, 26, 27
nivolumab 117, 118
non-clinical dental team members 4, 5, *5*
nonmelanoma skin cancers (NMSCs) 14, **15**, 16
nonsteroidal anti-inflammatory drugs (NSAIDs) 250
nutrition 78, 81, 208, 247
  feeding routes *see* feeding routes
  pre-radiotherapy 111
  see also diet
nutritional supplements, in radiotherapy 114

o

obturators *94*, 231–235
  construction and material for 233, *233*, 234
  defects without, sequelae 231
  definition, and function 231
  definitive 94, 233
  dental implants attached 231, *232*
  for developmental defects 231, *232*
  in head and neck cancer 233, *233*
  immediate 93–94, *94*, 233
  interim 94, *94*, 233
  mouth care 233–234, 235
  quality of life 234
odynophagia **80**
oesophageal speech 88, 161
opiate dependence 29
opiates/opioids, pain management 250
oral and maxillofacial surgery (OMFS) 60–75
  multidisciplinary team **58**, 60–61
oral care plan 181, 219
oral health 218
  before HNC treatment 93, 179–180, 219, 220
  challenges for patients 219, 223
  complications of HNC treatment and 223–227, *225*, 259
  food and drink 183–184, 222
  nurse-led clinics *100*
  oral mucositis prevention 207
  poor, microbiota diversity reduction 30
  saliva role 177–179
  smoking and *see* smoking
  substance dependence *see* substance dependence
  in xerostomia 179–181
    home self-care 181–184, **184–186**
    professional care **184–186**
oral hygiene, in HNC 181–184, 218, 220
  advice and communicating it 261
  before HNC treatment 214, 218, 220, 268, 273
  during/after HNC treatment 224, 225–227, 256, 259, 261
    after radiotherapy 112, 214, 240
    after restorative dentistry 96
  halitosis treatment 201

oral mucositis prevention 207
poor, risk/prognostic factor in HNC 181
in xerostomia 181–184, **184–186**
see also mouth care
oral malodour *see* halitosis
oral moisturising jelly (OMJ) 188
oral mucositis (OM) 3, **80**, 205–210, *206*
assessment and diagnosis 206–207
case study/story 264
chemotherapy causing 104, 105, 144, 169, 205
description and features 205, *206*
grading scales 206–207, **207**
healing 208
initiation and duration 205
management **184**, 207–208, 224
pain management 207–208, 264–265
pathophysiology 144, 205
photobiomodulation therapy for 141, 144, 146, **147**, 208
evidence-based practice 146, **147**
mechanism of action 144, *145*, 146, 208
prevention 146, 207–208
radiotherapy causing 112, *113*, 144, 205
risk factors *145*, 205–206
severity, factors contributing to *145*
severity scale (WHO) *146*, 206, **207**
oral ulceration 144, **184**, 194, *195*, **258**
oropharyngeal cancers 61
oropharyngeal squamous cell carcinoma (OPSCC), HPV-positive 36–37, *39*, 116
biomarkers, prognostic 37
case history 262–268
incidence 36
outcome/prognosis 37, 38, 63, 116
pathogenesis, HPV infection 37, 38, *39*
persistence of infections 37, 38
risk factors 37–38, *39*
TNM classification 63
treatment 38
orthopantomogram (OPG) 62, *72*, *99*
osteoradionecrosis (ORN) 92, *92*, 114, 213–215, 240
after tooth extraction 92, 150, 213, 214
causes 63, 92, 95, 114, 150, 179, 240
definition 92, 114, 150
grading 213, **213**
in mandible 63, 95
prevention and management 114, 214
symptoms 114, 213
treatment 114, 214–215
photobiomodulation therapy **148**, 150
otolaryngologist 60, 61

p

p16 (tumour suppressor) 37, *47*
pain 3, 169, 249, **258**, 259
assessment 259, **260**
chronic 260–261
definition, and '3 dimensions' 249
dental, in substance users 32
impact (SOCRATES) 259, *260*
oral mucositis 169, 205, 207
radiotherapy toxicity 113
referred 227
pain management 249–252, 259
adjuvant medications 250–251
analgesic preparations 249–250, **250**, 260, 277
case study/story 264–265
nonmedical 251
in oral mucositis 207–208, 264–265
palliative care 260–261
topical analgesics 251
palate (hard/soft)
cleft 231, *232*
defect after surgery 93
examination 11, *12*
palifermin 208
palliative care 52, **58**, 258–261
chemotherapy 104, 116
dietitian's role in 79, 261
immunotherapy 116
radiotherapy 110
palpation of head and neck 5, *6*, 7, *7–9*, 21
paracetamol 249–250
parenteral nutrition 83
parotid gland(s)
palpation 7, *9*
radiotherapy effect on 113
tumours 157, 159
pathologists **58**
artificial intelligence/digital pathology aiding 48–49
care of HNC patients, stages 44
cancer resection specimen 48
initial diagnosis 44–48, *45*, *46*, *47*
postoperative care 48
pathology, digital 48–49, *49*
pathology report 48
patient-centred interviewing 33
patient education
motivational speaking by patient *270*, 270–271
oral health, in xerostomia 181, 188
patient journey *45*, *53*, 61–63, 64, 219
adjuvant treatment 69
see also chemotherapy (CT); radiotherapy (RT)
after HNC treatment 255, 256
case histories/stories
Anthony, Roy 262–268
Baker, Steve 272–274
Hemington, Debbie 275–278
Shah, Shrenik 269–271
clinical nurse specialist role 76
flowcharts *45*, *53*
MDT role 59, 63, 76
reconstruction of defect *see* restorative dentistry
recovery after surgery 69, *75*
speech and language therapy 85
see also diagnosis (of HNC); examination; follow-up; imaging; surgery
PD-1 protein 117, *117*
antibodies to/inhibitors 117, *118*, 120
PD-L1 37, *39*, 45, *47*, 117, *117*
antibodies to/inhibitors 117, 120
pedicled flaps 61, 68
pembrolizumab 117, 118
percutaneous endoscopic gastrostomy (PEG) **58**, 82, *82*, 111, 208
case studies/stories 263, 264, 265, *266*, 273–274
recommendations 268
periodontal disease **186**
before treatment 30, 31, 222
during/after treatment 227
halitosis in, treatment 201
photobiomodulation therapy for 149
substance dependence and 30, 31
PET/PET CT scans 63, 263, 273
pharynx, examination *12*
photobiomodulation (PBM) therapy 141–156
benefits on clinical outcomes 143, **144**
future directions 151–152
oral complication management 141, 144–150
parameters, units of measurement **143**
principle and mechanism of action 141–142, *142*
for oral mucositis 144, *145*, 146
for xerostomia 149
protocols (specific oral complications) **147–148**
safety and cautions 150
training/education on 151, 152
photons, interaction with biological tissue *142*, 142–143
physiotherapists **59**, 236, 237
role, advice for 236, 237
physiotherapy 236–237, *237*, *238*, 260
PICC lines 104, 105
pilocarpine hydrochloride **178**
plaque removal 182, 183

plastic and reconstructive surgeons 61
platelets, count 175
pleomorphic dermal sarcoma **15**
plucking, of intraoral hair *243*, 243–244
pneumonitis, immunotherapy causing **120**, *121*
position of patient, in dental chair 105, 224, *225*
positive margin 64
postoperative care 48, 69
potentially malignant disorders (PMDs)/lesions 44, 45–46, *46*
pregabalin 251
preoperative assessments 63–64
pre/post auricular lymph nodes, palpation 7, *8*
pretreatment (of HNC) phase
  dental treatment *see* dental treatment
  mental health and responses in 51–52
  oral hygiene 214, 218, 220, 268, 273
    see also oral health
primary care dental team 3–4, 220
professional mechanical plaque removal (PMPR) 182, 226
prognosis/survival 64, **110**
  OPSCC, HPV-positive 37, 38, 63, 116
  resection margin and ENE 64
prothesis care
  dentures 183, 222–223
  voice prosthesis 163, *164*
proton therapy (PT) 123–128
  challenges in UK 127, *127*, 128
  clinical trials 126
  costs, and optimal use estimates 123, 125, **125**
  evolution to 123–126
  indications for 126
  NHS plans *vs* European strategy 126, 127, 128
  normal tissue complication probability (NTCP) 126
  principle 124–125, *125*
psychoactive substances, effects 29
psychological well-being *see* mental health/well-being

q

quality of life 78, 95, 141, 218–230
  obturator use 234
  palliative care and 258

r

radial forearm flap 68, *69*, *70*, *71*, *74*
  intraoral hair growth after 241
radiation caries 91–92, *95*, 226
  photobiomodulation therapy for 149
radiation dermatitis **147**
radiation-induced fibrosis 239
radiologically inserted gastrostomy (RIG) 82, 83, 111
radiology, development 157
radiotherapy (RT) 69, 107–115, 123, 239–240
  aim and mechanism of action 107, 125
  case studies/stories *263*, 263–264, *264*, *265*, 269, 274, 276
  dental assessment/treatment before 110–111, 214
  dental treatment after 111
  follow-up after 114–115
  fractions, and duration of treatment 69, 110
  help for late effects 240
  for Hodgkin's lymphoma 276–277
  image-guided (IGRT) 108
  immobilisation device for 111, *111*
  indications 92
  information required before 109
  intensity-modulated *see* intensity-modulated radiotherapy (IMRT)
  organs at risk (OARs) 107, 108, 112, 125
  palliative 110
  planning 112, 214
    imaging for 62–63, 107, 112
  precision, evolution of 123–126, *124*
  preparation before 110–112, 269, 273, 276
  salivary gland vulnerability and protection 177
  target volume 112
  techniques 107
  three-dimensional conformal 107, 108
  toxicities/complications 98, 112, 144, 239–240
    acute effects 112–114, 169
    grading system 112
    late 112, 114, 239–240, 261, 277, 278
    for oral flora and implants 95, 96
    oral mucositis 112, *113*, 144, 205
    osteoradionecrosis *see* osteoradionecrosis (ORN)
    photobiomodulation therapy for 141, 149
    radiation caries 91–92, *95*, 266
    salivary gland damage 91–92, 113, 239
    skin damage/inflammation *see under* skin
    xerostomia 95, 113, 177, 191–193
reconstruction of defect *see* restorative dentistry
recovery, after treatment 255–256
recurrence of cancer 96, 106, 228, 256
recurrent aphthous stomatitis (RAS) 194, *195*
referral 13, *53*, 57, 259, 272
  case studies 262
  dental nurse role after 98
  to general medical practitioner 228
  NHS two-week pathway 61, 62, 259
reflux (gastroesophageal) **80**
rehabilitation 91, 260
  communication 85
  edentulous patients 95
  exercise programme 247
  problems related to 91–92
  respiratory 88
  speech and language therapy 85
  trismus 88
relaxation, sleep improvement 246
remineralising products 183
resection of cancer *see* surgery
resection specimen 48
respiratory diseases, e-cigarettes and 27
respiratory rehabilitation 88
restorative dentistry 91–97
  edentulous patients, rehabilitation 95
  flaps/grafts *see* flaps, types; free flaps
  function restoration 92
  importance/aims 91
  interventions 93–95, *94*, *95*
  long-term prevention/maintenance 96
  ongoing cancer surveillance 96
  reconstruction of defect 61, 68–69, *72*, 93–94
  rehabilitation problems 91–92
  restoring function 92
  supporting psychological well-being 95–96, 106
restorative dentists/dental consultants 91–97, 98
  interventions provided by 93–95
  at MDT meeting, role **58**, 92–93
risk factors, for HNC 4, 116
  carcinogens 31, 63, 96
  exercise to reduce risk 246–247
  lip cancer 20, 22
  mouth cancer 4, 20, 23
  OPSCC, HPV-positive 37–38, *39*
  poor diet 247
  sleep disturbances 245
  see also alcohol use; smoking
robotic surgery *see* transoral robotic surgery (TORS)
'rodent ulcer' *see* basal cell carcinoma (BCC)
root caries 226

s

saliva 91, 177–179
  composition 177, 179
  functions 177, 179, 184, 259
  normal volume and flow 177, **177**
  production increase 217, 223–224, 267
    by acupuncture 187, 191–193
    medication for **178**, **186–187**

role in oral health 177–179
substitutes 186, **186–187**
thick/sticky **184**, 216, 223–224, 259
management **184**, 216–217
volume/flow, compromised 177, 216, 222
after/during treatment 223–224
radiotherapy late effects 239–240
signs/symptoms and mitigation **184–186**
xerostomia 177, **177**, 179
see also hyposalivation
salivaMAX **178**
salivary glands 177
damage 176
by radiation 91–92, 113, 239
parotid gland palpation 7, *9*
swellings 7
tumours, high-definition MRI 157
Screening, Brief Intervention, and Referral to Treatment (SBIRT) 33
seborrhoeic keratosis 17
secretions, altered **80**, 164, 224
thickened mucus *see* mucus, thickened
weather affecting, stoma care 164
self-esteem 255, 257, 261
self-examination 13, *13*
sentinel node (SEN)
biopsies 67
SPECT CT scan 157, *158*
sexual behaviour, OPSCC risk factor 38
shoulder stiffness 224
sialadenitis 177, **184**
sialorrhea (hypersalivation) 217, 223–224, 267
sinus conditions 240
skin
anatomy and physiology 14, *15*
benign lesions 17, *17*
care 240, 279–280
health, promotion 18
inflammation, radiotherapy toxicity 112
radiotherapy toxicity 112, *113*, 114, 161, 240
case studies/stories 263, *263*, *264*, *265*, 274
rash, immunotherapy causing **120**, *121*
tightening/fibrosis, radiotherapy causing 114
UV radiation, penetration 14, *15*
skin cancer 14–19
diagnosis 17–18
early recognition, hygienist role 14
prevention *15*, 16, 18
suspected, management 18
types 14–17, **15**
skin graft 69
sleep
disturbed, oral cancer risk factor 245, 248
poor, reasons for 245
suggestions to improve 246
treatment impact on 169
sleep–wake cycle 245, 246
smoking 23–24, 26, *26*, 223
cessation 24, 26, 27
effects on oral health 23
as HNC risk factor *21*, 23, 38, 116, 245
social function/well-being
impact of diagnosis/pretreatment on 51–52
impact of treatment on 170, 224, 255, 274
restoring function and 92
SOCRATES 259, **260**
spasms 227, 239
'speaking valve' 161
SPECT CT 157, *158*
speech, impairment 85, 92, 224, 237, 261
after laryngectomy 88, 161, 269, 270
assessment and treatment 64, 85–86
impact on mental health 85, 92, 237, 255
radiotherapy causing 113
see also communication, by patient; voice disturbances
speech and language therapists (SLTs) **58**, *75*, 85–90
role **58**, 64, 85, 86, 88, 261
training 89
working with dietitians 85, 88, 261
working with physiotherapist 236
speech and language therapy 85–90
altered airways, managing 88
assessment for 64, *75*, 85
before radiotherapy 111
communication, role 85–86
see also communication, by patient; speech, impairment
exercises and advice 86, 87, 88, 111, 236
obturator use, coping with 94, 233
ongoing rehabilitation 85
swallowing, role 86–87, 261
trismus, role 87–88
squamous cell carcinoma (SCC) 44, 109, 116
diagnosis/specimen examination 45
lip 20, 21, *21*
oropharyngeal *see* oropharyngeal squamous cell carcinoma (OPSCC)
prevalence 109, 116
skin 14, **15**, 16, *16*, 98
treatment modalities 116
staging the cancer 48, 63
cancer distribution by stage **110**
sternocleidomastoid muscle (SCM), palpation 7, *7*, *8*
steroids 119, 208, 274
stoma 161
baseplate *162*, 163–164, *166*, *167*
care 161, *161*, 163, 166, 216
protection 166, *166–168*
shower aid for *167*
submandibular lymph nodes, palpation 7, *9*
submental island flap *242*
submental lymph nodes, palpation 7, *9*
substance dependence 29–35, *32*, 223
attitudes of dental professionals 32
definition, prevalence 29, 30
dental avoidance/access difficulties 32
oral health, impact on 30–31, *32*
support for patients, by dental professionals 31–33
treatment journeys 30, *30*
xerostomia due to/exacerbated 30, 177
sugar, consumption 81, 183, 184, 214, 246, 274
suicide, and suicidal intent 95–96, 223
sunscreens *15*, 16, 18
support network 223, 228
supraclavicular lymph nodes, palpation 7, *9*
surgeons **58**, *65*
surgery 63–75, 129
case studies 263, 269, 273
curative, plan and aims 64, 110
floor of mouth cancer 63, 64, *72*, *73*, *74*
impact on mental health 170
individualised, parotid gland tumours 157, 159
instruments 67–68
margins 64, 67
transoral robotic surgery 137–138
for osteoradionecrosis 214
planning programme *99*
reconstruction of defect 68–69, *72*, *74*, 91
recovery after 69, *75*
resection of cancer 63–64, *66*, 67–68, *74*, 91
tissue examination 48, 67
tongue cancer 64, *64*, *65–67*, 67
transoral robotic *see* transoral robotic surgery (TORS)
swallowing 86–87
assessment 86–87
difficulty *see* dysphagia
management by SLTs 87
tracheostomy impact 88
symptoms/signs of HNC 5, 13, **258–259**
systemic anticancer therapies (SACTs) 116
see also chemoradiotherapy (CRT)

t

taste changes *see* dysgeusia
telangiectasia 16, *16*, 114, *114*
therapeutic ratio 107
thrush 194, *195*
thyroid problems, radiotherapy late effect 169–170, 240, 275
tissue flaps *see* flaps, types
tissue processing 44–45
TNM classification system 48, 63, 64
tobacco products 24
tobacco smoking *see* smoking
tongue
  biofilm 201
  cleaning 182, 201
  examination 10, *10*
  reduced saliva flow affecting **184**
tongue cancer *62*, 63, *63*, *64*, *65*, *110*
  immunotherapy *119*
  laser excision 67, *68*
  Lugol iodine staining 64, *65*
  MRI *62*, *119*
  neck dissection 67, *67*
  reconstruction of defect 68
tonsillar crypt, HPV-positive tumours 37
tonsillar lymph nodes, palpation 7, *8*
tonsils, HPV-positive OPSCC 36–37
toothbrushes
  after use care of 183
  before HNC treatment *220*, 220–221, *221*
  suction 224, *225*
toothbrushing
  before HNC treatment 220–221, *221*
  during/after HNC treatment 224, 226
  nausea and vomiting, advice 212
  obturator use and 234
  oral mucositis prevention 207
  in xerostomia 182
tooth extraction 219
  before HNC treatment 219, 222, 226, 273
    before radiotherapy 93, 179, 214
  osteoradionecrosis after 92, 150, 213, 214
toothpaste 207, 268
  during/after HNC treatment 226, 228
  halitosis management 201
  obturator use and 234
  prescription, use before treatment 220, 268
  in xerostomia 182
tracheoesophageal tube 82, *82*
tracheostomy 88
training
  laser therapy and photobiomodulation 151, 152
  oral and maxillofacial surgery 60
  speech and language therapists 89
  on substance use 32
  for transoral robotic surgery 138–139
tramadol 250
transoesophageal echocardiogram (TOE) 278
transoral minimally invasive surgery 129
transoral robotic surgery (TORS) 129–140
  applications/sites for 129
  indications, contraindications 136, **136**, **137**
  outcomes 137–138
  postoperative care/complications 137, **138**
  procedure 136–137
  surgical setup/preparation 133, *134*, *135*
  training for, challenges 138–139
  see also da Vinci robotic surgical system
treatment of HNC
  aims 64, 91, 110
  complications after *see* complications of HNC treatment
  flowchart *45*, *53*
  see also specific treatment modalities
trismus 87–88, 92, 224, 261
  photobiomodulation therapy for **148**, 150
  radiotherapy causing 111, 114, 239, 261
  rehabilitation 88
'two-week wait' 61, 62, 259

u

ulceration, oral 144, **184**, 194, *195*, **258**
ultrasound scan (USS) 62
ultraviolet (UV) radiation 14, *15*
  lip cancer 20
  protection against *15*, 16, 18
  UVA and UVB *15*, 15–16, 18
unsafe swallow 83

v

vaccine, human papillomavirus (HPV) 36, 39
vaping 24–27
  types/options 24–25, *25*
videofluoroscopy 86, *87*
viral infections
  herpes simplex, recurrent 194, *195*
  HPV *see* human papillomavirus (HPV)
  stoma protection against 163
virgin olive oil, lycopene-enriched 188
virtual reality (VR) 157
vitamin D 18
vocal cord cancer 269
voice disturbances 4, 5, **185**, **258**
  hoarseness 5, 176, **185**, **258**, 269
  see also speech, impairment
voice prosthesis 88, 161, 163, *164*, 269
  care 163, *164*
  cleaning *164*
voice restoration 161
volatile sulphur compounds (VSCs) 199, 202
vomiting 211

w

water, drinking 222
waterjets and waterflossers 221, *221*, 224
weight loss 114, 223, 247, 277
work, cancer diagnosis impact 3, 52
World Health Organization (WHO), pain management 249–250, **250**

x

xerostomia 95, 169, 176–190, 223, 259
  before HNC treatment 176, 222
  cannabis and 31, 177
  case story 277
  causes 176, 177
    chemotherapy 105, 177
    radiotherapy 91, 113, 177, 191–193
  consequences 176, **184–186**, *223*, 224, *224*
  diagnosis and assessment 179, *180*, 192
  duration 177
  incidence 176
  management/relief 176, 184, **184–186**, 224
    alternative therapies 187–188
    prescribable products 186–187, **186–187**, 224
    see also acupuncture
  oral health care in 179–181, 259
    home self-care 181–184, **184–186**
  patient education 181, 188
  photobiomodulation therapy for **147**, 148–149
  prevention in HNC treatment 177, **178**
  treatment **178**, 179, **181**, 224
Xerostomia Bother Index 179, *180*
X-ray photons/beam 124, 125
xylitol 184, 226